God Is *Still* My Spinach

Robert Pickering Sr.

July is hot... Some quotes that sizzle.

Do you wonder what negative and scary dreams mean?
Are they punishment or weak faith? Or was it too darn much sugar in that desert eaten after dinner?
July 20th

In the case of Moses, he was not passive. He took on an Egyptian overseer, stood up to Pharaoh and hiked the desert for forty years. It is hard to see him as a wimp.
July 21

I do not believe that the Lord helps me with my golf game...
{ but I remember to}"Always be thankful when lining up my fourth putt."
July 27

What do the reverends say?

"Good reading Mr. Pickering."
Rev. Jim McChesney

"From the ground up, Bob helps us to see how God is at work in the stew of our daily lives."
Rev. Mike Miller

"...you will see how Bob can write about his faith. I want you to know that Bob lives his faith as well."
Rev Ed Dubose

Printed in the United States of America

First Printing 2022

ISBN 978-09883074-8-3

BSM Publishers
12000 Marion Lane West #1101
Minnetonka, Minnesota 55305

God is *Still* My Spinach

Robert Pickering Sr.

Acknowledgments

This book is an update and upgrade of God Is My Spinach, printed in September 2012. The marketing of Spinach led to a Christian support ministry through our blog and Facebook Group.

Several people encouraged and supported my efforts and deserve a note of thanks. Friend Tim Cerar who first suggested writing devotions rather than distributing other publications. My wife, June, has tolerated and contributed her love to the equation while putting up with my early morning ramblings.

The 100 or more people who received my weekly email devotion. Their feedback contributed immeasurably to this book.

Methodist Ministers, Rick Ireland (RIP), Lyle Christiansen (RIP), Mike Miller, Ed Dubose and Jim McChesney each contributed in spirit and have influenced this material

My editor and friend Steve Rossi helped me by posting the Good News messages on our church website and supported me, and designed Spinach in 2011. Without Steve, these books and ministry may not have ever developed.

The following have directly contributed to this ten year edition. Jordana Pickering, cover photographer. Claire Torrey and Gail A, Peach, proof readers, Stephanie Symmes, Simon Halsey, and Jackie Collins allowed their pictures to be used (credited) and Paulett Odenthal for allowing her image where appropriate.

Contents

January

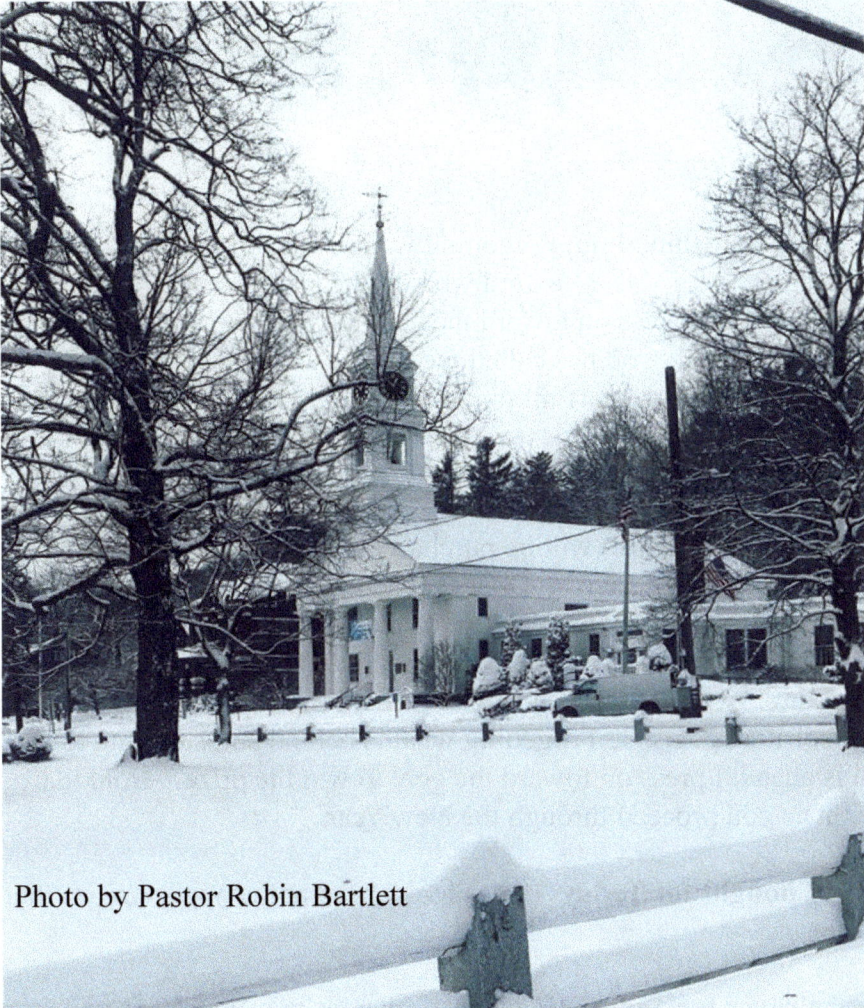

Photo by Pastor Robin Bartlett

The First Church
Sterling, Massachusetts
Gathered in the spirit of Jesus.
Committed to creating heaven on Earth.

Happy New Year

But one thing I do: Forgetting what is behind and straining
toward what is ahead,
I press on toward the goal to win the prize
for which God has called me heavenward in Christ Jesus.
(Philippians 3 vs 12-14)

Happy New Year. For the next few weeks, athletic clubs will be filled with "New Year's resolutionists." Diet programs will come and go, self-improvement books will be purchased, or at least the dust will be blown from last year's cover. Does that sound familiar? Have you had a few resolutions fall by the wayside? Paul would not have written the above on New Year's Eve, but it is appropriate. There are a lot of new goals today: weight, fitness, financial goals, etc. Paul is asking us to look at our spiritual goals. "...Forgetting what is behind and straining toward what is ahead, I press on toward the goal to win the prize." Hold that thought as you proceed through the New Year.

Thought for Today: Let us look ahead at the opportunities that exist for us.

Prayer for Today: Heavenly Father, as this New Year begins, hear our serenity prayer:
"God grant me the serenity
to accept the things I cannot change
the courage to change the things I can,
and the wisdom to know the difference."

January 1 Gray's Bay, Lake Minnetonka
Wayzata. Minnesota

Our Task for a New Yea

Let your light so shine before men, that they may see your good works and glorify your Father in heaven.
Matthew 5 vs 16

Happy New Year! We say and think that and have trouble living it because there are problems (illnesses, financial issues, family stress, etc.) that do not roll over at midnight on December 31st. "Happy New Year" is an excellent thought to have. If we are the light of the world, then we need to be happy and allow the light to shine.

When we hear or read the news, it can be depressing. There is our post-COVID world, racial violence seems on the uptike, and world economies seem lackluster. As Christians, we need to care and be concerned. However, we also need to pray and thank the Lord for the good news side of the coin. Our focus needs to be on the positive side; there is always more right than wrong, good than bad.

In a recent TV sermon, Joel Osteen asked, "The bible says we are the light of the world. Have you got your light shining out?" Focus on that with smiles and laughter, and show the light of the world.

Thought for Today: Today will be a great day. Yes, everyday things will occur like illness, stress, cranky kids, bad weather, and too much to do. There will also be great friends and family, fresh air, good food, and other positives. We need to keep our light shining so others may see it.

Prayer for Today: Dear God, we give thanks for the warmth and joy you give us in our hearts and our Christian love for others. We thank you for the happiness in our lives, the ability to share it. Amen

Bexhill On Sea,
East Sussex, UK   **January 2**   Page 3

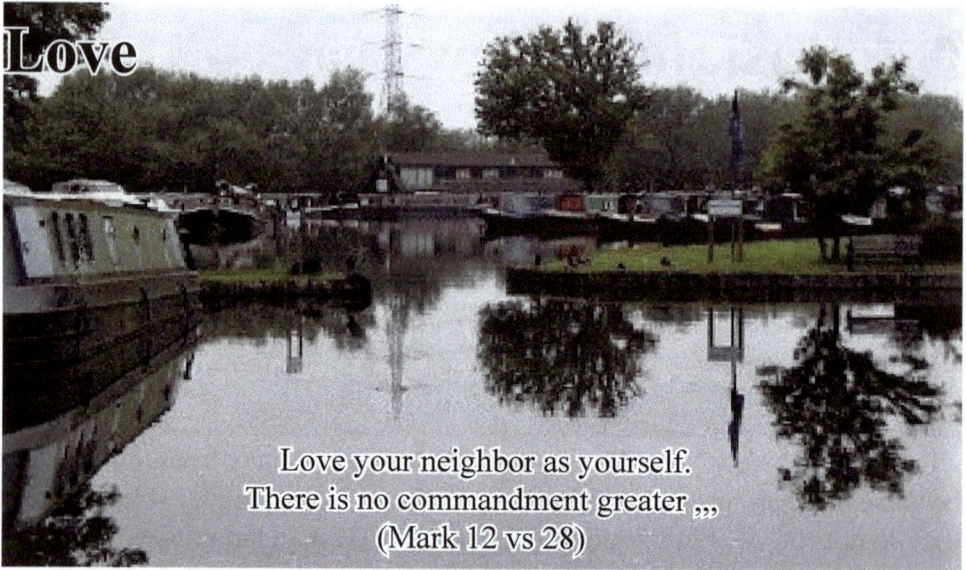

Love

Love your neighbor as yourself.
There is no commandment greater ,,,
(Mark 12 vs 28)

Do you remember the bracelets WWJD, "What would Jesus do?" There is no doubt about it; He would love you. Jesus was blessed with the ability to love completely, agape love. That term is used over 200 times in scripture. It may not be humanly possible to love as Jesus did.

There are times when our love is conditional; in a crowded place like a mall or airport, we do not feel comfortable with everybody. There are subconscious conditions on our love. Is it fear of the unknown, or common sense? Are we discriminatory? Somehow in public, the people surrounding us are not qualified as neighbors to be loved.

Real love is a complicated personal issue for your neighbor, enemies (wish I had a better word for this), bosses, etc. The secret is separating behavior from the individual self. The boss has to say no to implement a policy; the neighbor can come uncomfortably close. At the core, all people are lovable, and we need to love them.

Thought for Today: Today, let us make a special effort to search inside ourselves and feel affection and love for everyone we meet.

Prayer for Today: Dear Lord and Father, today we pray for the ability to care deeply for all of those around us. Please help us flush our conscious and unconscious prejudice and dislikes from our minds; help us be more like Jesus. Amen

January 3 Canal Harbor,
Pyrford, Surrey, UK

Persistence

Then Jesus told his disciples... that they
should always pray and not give up.
(Luke 18 vs 1)

Bob Dylan's lyrics said, "Times, they are a-changing…" and maybe not for the better. One of life's constants is change. It is like an endurance event or marathon. It takes persistence to get to the end. There will be ups and downs along the way that necessitates keeping our eyes on the prize. We need to "…always pray and not give up."

There is a long year ahead, and there will be changes and some stresses; careers, financial, health, to name a few.
The holiday season is a period of stressful joy due to all the activities. January is when reality comes to the forefront, the start of an annual endurance event called the year. Dr. Benjamin Mays wrote the poem "God's Minute."

I have only just a minute.　　I must suffer if I lose it,
Only sixty seconds in it.　　Give account if I abuse it,
Forced upon me, can't refuse it.　　Just a tiny little minute,
Didn't seek it, didn't choose it.　　But eternity is in it.
But it's up to me to use it,

Mays had it correct, but we need to think about a whole year.

Thought for Today: Let us take a minute to plan for the year ahead.

Prayer for Today: Heavenly Father, today we pray for smooth sailing through the rough seas of life as we will seek a way to do your will here on earth. Amen

Lake Harriet,
Minneapolis, Minnesota

The Serenity Prayer

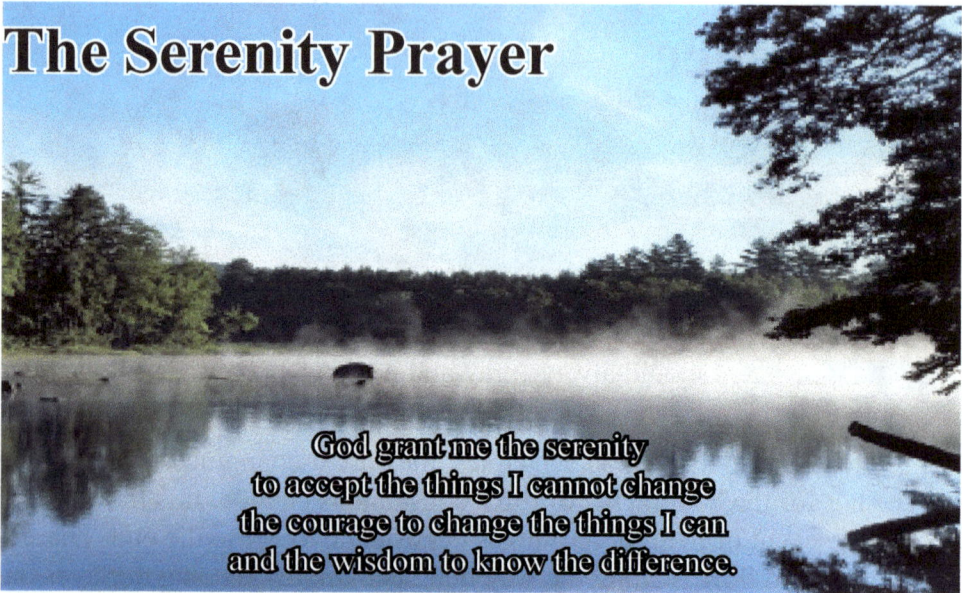

God grant me the serenity
to accept the things I cannot change
the courage to change the things I can
and the wisdom to know the difference.

At work and in our daily lives, we often fail to take the risk of allowing God to control and accept the spiritual help available. We will handle it all. Where is our humility when we try to do it all?

"... humbly accept the word planted in you,
which can save you."
(James 2 vs 1)

We are told to keep God at the forefront in our search for inner peace.

"And the peace of God, which transcends all understanding,
will guard your hearts and minds in Christ Jesus."
(Philippians 4 vs 7)

The serenity prayer is simple, and that is good. For the New Year, let's keep it simple.

Thought for Today: Let us focus on peace and tranquility in our lives; with our families, neighbors, and coworkers.

Prayer for Today: Let's use the serenity prayer this week and for the year, especially when overstressed.
Amen

Kindness

In his book "Bread for the Journey" Henri Nouwen acknowledged that "… All people, whatever their color, religion, or sex, belong to humankind and called to be kind to one another, treating one another as brothers and sisters. There is hardly a day in our lives when we are not called to do this."

It is a great feeling when someone treats us kindly, opens a door when we are carrying something, lets us into a traffic lane, or offers to help in any other way. We get an incredible feeling of gratitude and thankfulness. A few of these feelings each day contribute to a great day.

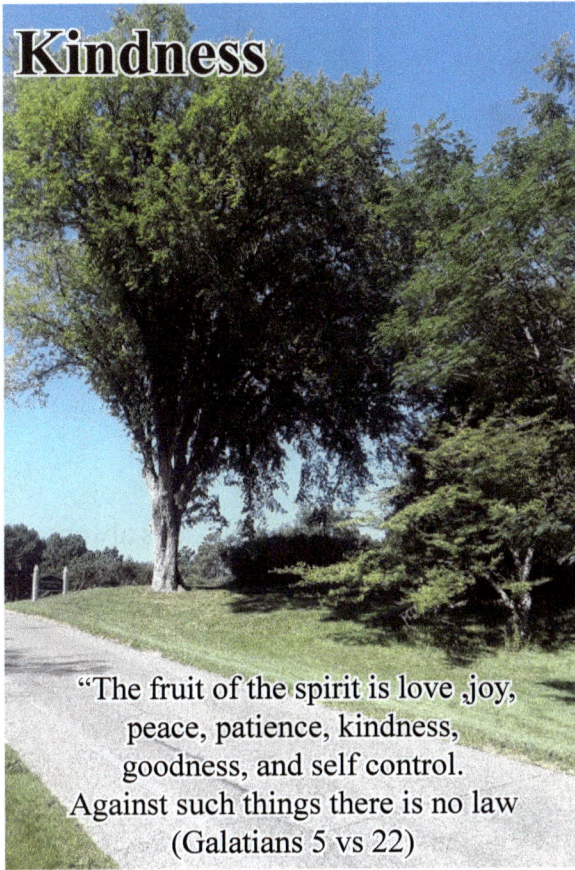

"The fruit of the spirit is love ,joy, peace, patience, kindness, goodness, and self control. Against such things there is no law (Galatians 5 vs 22)

A better feeling is when you are on the giving end, the door opener, courteous driver, etc. Contributing to others in such small ways seems to make the day smoother. The warmth of their smiles and the thank you make my day, and it will make yours also.

Thought for Today: Today, let us enjoy ourselves by smiling to show appreciation when others show kindness and acknowledge us.

Prayer for Today: Dear Lord, today we pray that we can contribute to others in a kind and considerate manner. We pray that when we interact with people, they will be glad and feel Jesus through our actions. Amen

23rd Psalm

The Lord is my shepherd. I shall not want.
He makes me lie down in green pastures,
he leads me beside still waters...
(Psalms 23 vs 1-2)

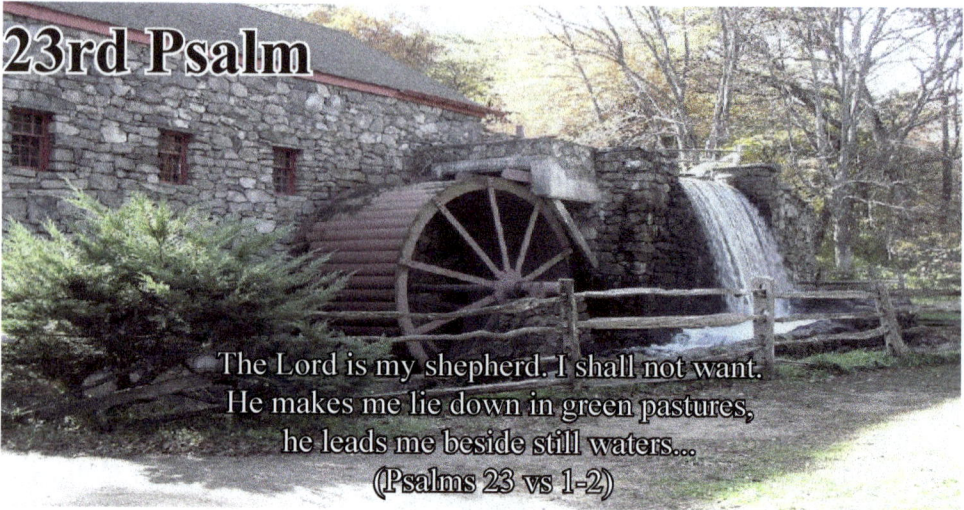

In the forties and fifties, public schools in Massachusetts always started with the 23rd Psalm, Lord's Prayer, and Pledge of Allegiance to the United States. Wow, by today's standards, that is powerful stuff. Look at this and see if we can apply it to our lives today.

The first two lines above lead us to tranquility. Faith will take care of your wants and guide you to that inner peace you desire and to the restful place beside still waters.

"He refreshes and restores my life;
He leads in the paths of righteousness for His namesake."
(Psalm 23 vs 3)

When things in your life need rebuilding, the way to get out of the dumps is to follow Him.

"Yes, though I walk through the valley of the shadow of death,
I will fear no evil; for You are with me;
Your rod and Your staff to comfort me."
(Psalm 23 vs 4)

Christians have beautiful tools to work with. The more we let God lead, the more we will be at peace.

Thought for Today: Let us reflect on this New Year and all of our goals and resolutions.

Prayer for Today: Heavenly Father, many times, stress builds up in our lives. We pray that when this occurs, we find a way to let you help and can accept the guidance, protection, and support promised through our Christian faith. Amen

January 7 The Mill at the Wayside Inn
Sudbury, Massachusetts

Trust

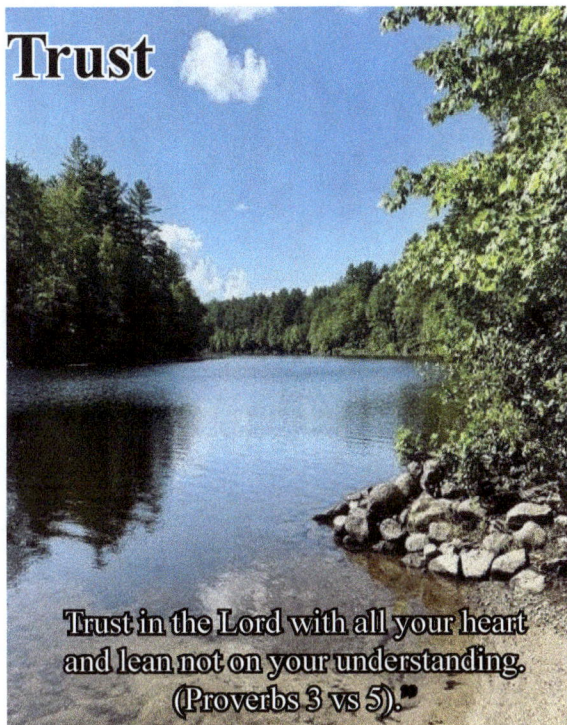

Trust is an exciting concept. There are camps and seminars focused on building trust in others. They take you on rope and cable courses in trees, sliding down zip lines at breakneck speeds, or standing straight up and falling backward, knowing that the team will catch you. Yes, that takes trust.

Your catcher, God, is always with you, but you need to trigger the catch. Often, we get caught once a week on Sunday morning.

Trust in the Lord with all your heart and lean not on your understanding. (Proverbs 3 vs 5).

reminded to let the Lord in for a bit, then out of the church for a busy week.

Indeed, all we do is necessary; it is on the calendar, made the commitments, etc. So here we are at midday, overstressed, the boss just dumped a big job on us, and there is no relief in sight. Now is the time to trust, count to ten, take a deep breath, and focus. It is time for prayer, even if only for a few minutes.

"…He will make your paths straight."

Thought for Today: Today, this week, or even this hour will not be stress-free. Suggestion by Bob: Try thanking the Lord for 30 seconds of peace the next time a traffic light stops you! When stress sets in, remember to stop and pray- Take a break.

Prayer for Today: Dear Lord, we will be dealing with our full and busy lives and may fail to acknowledge your presence. Today we thank you for being here with us and pray that we take the time to trust you to help us through the day.
Amen

Confidence

For you are my hope,
O Lord God, you are my trust...
And the source of my confidence.
(Psalm 71 vs 5)

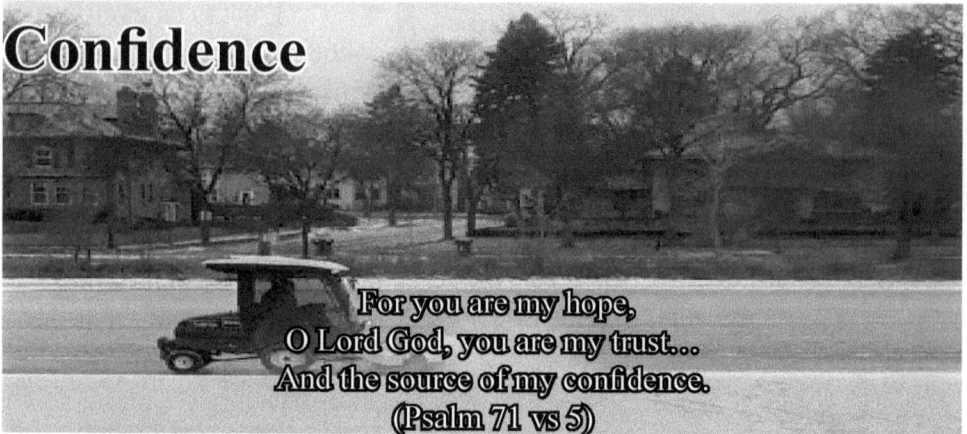

    The Psalmist above gives a strong message for a new year; we can develop confidence and trust through faith. Our news sources all seem to sell negativity to increase ratings. They think focusing on the negative is the way to sell their time. That is not an excellent service to the world. It is good to be aware of the news, even when negative. Reading the good news of Jesus to balance the books can and will overcome all the news media's negativity.

This Psalmist also said:

"But as for me, I will always have hope."
(Psalm 72 vs 14)
and
"You will increase my honor
And comfort me once again."
(Psalm 71 vs 21)

    Through the good news of Jesus Christ, we will all have a better life and live in a better world.

    Thought for Today: Grow in confidence and share our good news.

    Prayer for Today: Dear Lord and Father, we pray for the spiritual maturity and growth to be better at being a disciple and worker for You. We pray that we may find a clear vision of what we can do.
Amen

Park Department Rink,
Lake of the Isles
January 9 Minneapolis, Minnesota

Help Wanted

Do not think of yourself
more highly than you ought.
(Romans 12 vs 4)

"HELP WANTED"- When reading the newspaper, do you ever take a quick look at the help wanted section? Many of us do for a variety of reasons; searching for an improvement in a career position; a new career, salesmen sometimes spot new prospects; there are many reasons. The selection grows thinner than usual in hard times and slow economies.

When we attend church, we hear a message. Sometimes we listen and absorb and come away enthusiastic about the subject. We are pleasantly soothed and calmed at other times, and occasionally we are disinterested. It is OK to be in any one of those moods after hearing a message. We are all different, and even God can't send us a message on Sunday that affects all of us uniformly.

What does it mean when we are enthusiastic about a message? When it inspires us to think about action? Perhaps there is an opportunity to serve, help, increase our time or cash commitments. Whatever it may be, we have heard God's "HELP WANTED," and it is our choice to apply for the job. It is our opportunity to allow God's will to be done through us here on earth.

Thought for Today: Today, let us focus on our daily activities. Search our planners and calendars for Godly reasons to be busy. Allow some time to do God's will as we move through our busy schedules.

Prayer for Today: Heavenly Father, wars and conflict abound, hunger and poverty seem excessive in the world. This seem inconsistent with your will. We pray that we find a way to contribute, to serve society in your name, and respond to your "HELP WANTED." Amen

Perfection

> God is not unjust; he will not forget your work
> and the love you have shown him as you have
> helped his people and continue to help them.
> (Hebrews 6 vs 10)

In twelve-step programs, there is a reading called "How It Works." It recognizes that the program is about "spiritual growth," not perfection. We all tend to get into that perfect mode; perfect mom, perfect dad, perfect employee, and the list goes on. Each of us falls short of perfection.

In our daily lives, we make mistakes. We could count them weekly and judge ourselves as failures. The only one of us that does not make errors probably does nothing. Many people work their way into depression by counting their losses.

In our spiritual lives, it is not any different. We all have made mistakes and will continue to be less than perfect. We may feel inadequate or judge ourselves rather severely. However, "God is not unjust; he will not forget your work and the love you have shown...". We must remember that as we walk the walk.

Thought for Today: We will fail again at being perfect, so try to focus on the good we do, the encouragement we give others, and the love we have in our hearts. That will help us have a great day.

Prayer for Today: Dear Lord and Father, there is scary and awful news every day. Often we forget your love because of worry and concern. We pray that we may focus on your understanding and caring love. We pray for the opportunity to demonstrate and share your passion with others. Amen

January 11 Dartmoor
Devon, UK

Soar Like an Eagle

> They will soar on wings like eagles;
> they will run and not grow weary,
> they will walk and not be faint.
> (Isaiah 40 vs 31)

In the nineteen fifties, a bald eagle was a rare sight. Now 60 years later, they are soaring over shopping centers, eating fish out of the local lakes, and generally hanging out with us. Seeing them makes it easy to see why our founders selected them as a national symbol. They are big, majestic, and beautiful birds. Their revival as a species shows us how humans can contribute to God's creations and the world. We changed a few rules, respected the Lord's way, and the bald eagle is now a common sight.

We are always searching for ways to make a better world, a way to soar. There is a story about eagles rising above storms. They sense the storm coming and use the wind to rise above the dangerous currents and ride out the storm. In many instances in life, we need to keep our faith while staring at negativity, the storms of life. We count to ten, punch a pillow, and ask the Lord for support when we are wise. When we involve our faith while handling our storms, we minimize our stress and significantly improve our quality of life.

Thought for Today: Let us use our faith in the Lord to rise above the problems of everyday life.

Prayer for Today: Let us pray to find a way to serve "God's will" rather than "our will" as a country. Amen

Bring Love Home

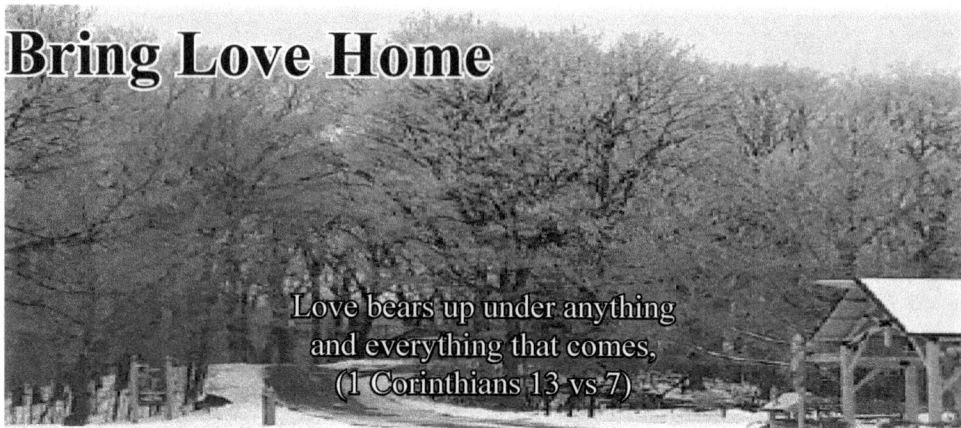

Love bears up under anything
and everything that comes,
(1 Corinthians 13 vs 7)

Are you having concerns regarding your financial future? Are institutions you trusted letting you down?
The world is changing how it operates and forcing us to live our lives differently.

Competing in a world market changed the rules. It is not the sixties or seventies anymore. In short form, our lives have become more stressful, and some frustrations have become anger. The benefits of spiritual growth through our faith are harder to see. Meditation can be a mood changer, problem solver, and relationship builder.

Mom and Dad head out for work every day in today's world, and the children head out for school. The family scatters for the day, and each member deals with their daily activity, which is often stress-related.

It is easy to bring our daily problems and frustrations home at night and into our family life. But why? Tonight, try sitting in the driveway, reading this message, and leaving the stress behind. Pray that you can go into the house in a loving and caring mood; contribute to a peaceful and loving environment called home.

Thought for Today: Let us all focus on preparing for the meeting with our families and with God, contributing to peace and tranquility.

Prayer for Today: Dear Lord and Father, today I pray for peace; peace in my family, my relationships, and throughout the world. Amen

Breaking Rules

*Then they would put their trust in God
and would not forget his deeds
but would keep his commands.
(Psalm 78 vs 7)*

Is the law the law? Do we always obey the law? Man's common law and the Ten Commandments get broken every day all around us. Drive the speed limit on a busy road, and someone will pass you. Around fifty-five percent of people surveyed answered that it was OK to cheat on their taxes. Have you broken a rule in the last 24 hours?

In the seventies, a radar detecting device designed to warn drivers a police radar was in the area; slangy called a fuzz buster. People purchased millions, and parents got a chance to demonstrate to their children that some rules could be ignored. Think about that. We teach by example.

The Psalmist talks about "...commanding our forefathers to teach their children." The facts are simple, we must teach our children, and the best way to do that is to live a Godly example for them to follow. That isn't easy.

Thought for Today: Let us focus on our habits regarding God's and common laws this week. Let's think about them regarding honesty and integrity. Let's observe where we may do a better job and patch up a few holes.

Prayer for Today: Heavenly Father, our children,are loved by you as much as by ourselves. We pray that we are doing them justice; that way learning your laws and ways from our teachings and examples. We pray for your guidance so that our children will follow and experience the peace that comes from loving you. Amen.

The Wayside Inn,
Sudbury, Massachusetts   **January 14**   **Page 15**

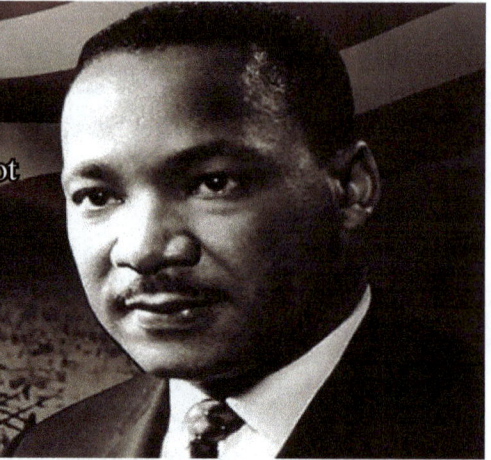

MLK Day

"It may be true that the law cannot make a man love me, But it can keep him from lynching me, And I think that's pretty important."
Martin Luther King

This quote is neither biblical nor spiritual but very genuine and honest. It does not make a tremendous philosophical statement, and there is no spiritual or social justice meaning; it is a simple truth. Living and having the right to pursue freedom always needs to be protected.

Other quotes by MLK have a deeper meaning spiritually. Below are the ones that seem to be popular in the media:

"Darkness cannot drive out darkness; only light can do that. Hate cannot drive out hate; only love can do that. Hate multiplies hate, violence multiplies violence, and toughness multiplies toughness in a descending spiral of destruction."
"Strength To Love," Martin Luther King, Jr.

A favorite is:
"Faith is taking the first step even when you don't see the whole staircase."
And as Christians, we need to demonstrate that we have the faith to take the first step.

Thought for Today: One word; acceptance.
Prayer for Today: Dear Lord, we do not pray for forgiveness of our forefathers' past discrimination and separatist social acts. We need to accept them and move forward. Today we pray for the guidance and will to contribute to peace and acceptance through Jesus's love. Amen

Win-Win

You made him lower than the heavenly beings
and crowned him with glory and honor.
(Psalm 8 vs 4,5)

There seems to be a win-lose philosophy running rampant throughout our society in America. There is a lot of hero worship devoted to overpaid athletes. We seem to have Henry Russell Saunder's (see note)* attitude, "Winning isn't everything, it's the only thing." That may be our world, but it is not God's world.

The Psalmist demonstrates that we were created a little lower than the angels and crowned with glory. There is plenty of God's love for each of us. When shared in God's way, there are worldwide resources that will do for all. We live in an incredible world with great people, and somehow, we taint it with our un-Godly behaviors.

As a young athlete in the 40's, I remember the great Grantland Rice quote, "It's not that you won or lost but how you played the game." That is an expression of a win-win philosophy—God's way.

Thought for Today: Focus on creating win-win situations in our lives. Open a door and allow for a few people. Sit forward in church and leave some room in the back for latecomers. We all can win.

Prayer for Today: Heavenly Father, somehow, we need you to guide us into a win-win world. We pray that we can find a way to spread your love to accomplish world cooperation. Amen

*Note: Attributed to UCLA Bruins football coach Henry Russell Sanders. In 1950, at a Cal Poly San Luis Obispo physical education workshop, Sanders told his group: "Men, I'll be honest, winning isn't everything; it's the only thing."

Lake Bde Maka Ska,
Minneapolis, , Minnesota

The Light

The eye is the lamp of the body...
If then the light within you is darkness,
how great is that darkness.
(Matthew 6 vs 22-23)

Have you ever had a person take unfair advantage of you? Lie about a deal? Sell you something that did not meet expectations? Perhaps a neighbor is encroaching on a property line?

Opportunistic behavior is alive and well. We live in a free-market society. Let the buyer beware. Competition for resources is a way of life. That is the American way. Or is the American way the golden rule?

Have you ever met someone in a church environment who was very aggressive in business? Maybe an all-out crook! (OK, so we should not judge, but that's another devotion.) The question is, "Can a person be an opportunistic shark in one part of his life, deal with a dark side, and be a Christian on Sunday?"

Well, the aggressive (dark) side exists, and it is God's place to do the judging and our place to be forgiving and welcoming on Sunday.

Thought for Today: Today, consider how much darkness exists inside our lives and make a conscious choice to let the light in and share it with others. Let us light up other people's lives in the name of Christ.

Prayer for Today: Heavenly Father, we offer prayers for peace. The world seems to be spinning out of control with diseases, riots, and political upheaval. It makes us ask, where is the world going? We pray that sharing the light brings common sense and tranquility to the world. Amen

January 17 Bexhill On Sea.
East Sussex, UK

Let The Glory Be God's

> The Lord is my strength and shield;
> My heart trusts in Him and I am helped.
> (Psalm 28 vs 7)

The "Super Bowl" takes place in January, and there are enormous numbers associated with it. Numbers like 150 million people watching on TV, six million dollars for a thirty-second ad, five hundred million added to the area economy- Oh yes, there are some competitors and coaches from both teams who will attend a prayer meeting and bible study Sunday before the game, members of the Fellowship of Christian Athletes.

My sports history goes back to age six as a YMCA swimmer, and my 60 plus years of associating with athletes have convinced me that they are not a group to be proud to know. Years of competition and "winning is everything" attitude have negatively influenced them.

On Super Sunday, there will be members of the "Fellowship" representing what a Christian needs to be: The best they can be with an appreciation of the Lord and Jesus Christ. Below is the last paragraph of their competitor's creed.

"I give my all every time.
I do not give up. I do not give in. I do not give out.
I am the Lord's warrior- a competitor by conviction and a disciple of determination.
I am confident beyond reason because my confidence lies in Christ.
The results of my efforts must result in His glory.
Let the competition begin and let the glory be God's."

Thought for Today: Let us enjoy today by being the best we can be while keeping the Lord in the forefront.
Prayer for Today: Father, today we pray that we will keep you in our lives, that we will be fair in our dealings and competitions. Amen

Storm Sky over
Minnetonka, Minnesota   **January 18**   Page 19

Friendships

Husbands, love your wives,
just as Christ loved the church
and gave himself to her."
(Ephesians 5 vs 25)

In his book Bread for the Table, Henri Nouwen stated, "Strange as it may sound, the table is the place where we want to become food for one another. Every breakfast, lunch, or dinner can become a time of growing communion with one another."

Intimacy is not only a marriage or "significant other" issue. In my business world, several of us have met the evening before sales meetings for a prayer dinner. Yes, we skipped the welcome happy hour and free buffet to be together. There is a closeness that exists within that group. Another business associate shared that his small company starts with a prayer breakfast each week. You can feel something special when dealing with those guys, even when you do not know precisely why.

Within a relationship, husband-wife, parent-child, good friends, or in other instances, intimacy makes a partnership. Closeness and intimacy create trust and confidence between friends and family.

Thought for Today: We all like to feel comfortable, and intimacy within a group creates a warmth that we all love. However, we are often guarded with our feelings when in groups. We are conservative and hold back. This week let us think more about letting others see our inner selves. Let us share our Christian love and create more intimacy with our friends and associates.

Prayer for Today: Heavenly Father, we seem to be living in a world with hate and revenge commonplace. Young mothers as human bombs, nations terrorizing other nations, and too many lose-lose negotiations in business. We of faith are searching for your will in all of this. Today we pray that we can understand and contribute to friendships and worldwide Godly solutions. Amen

Yellow Rose

Soar Like An Eagle

He has told us that you always have pleasant memories of us and that you long to see us, just as we also long to see you.
(1 Thessalonians 3 vs 6)

Good feelings are lovely, memorable moments that burn into our memories and last a lifetime. They vary in many ways. Often at a funeral, family and friends recall those feelings about a loved one who has passed. They make a grand celebration of life.

As an athlete, I have experienced a lot of self-induced memories. My favorites are a hole in one, championship swimming races, and a 1991 Triathlon with my daughter. The ones that set me on fire and bring tears to my eyes are from helping other people. The smile on the face of a nursing home patient when you visit them, for example.

Memories are warm feelings. In retirement, memories are a significant part of life. The did-do are more common than the can-do. The self-imposed memories are great, but people from the past often make your day. We have contributed along the way, something simple maybe; advice to a youngster at church, or perhaps something they observed.

Thought for Today: Today, let's take some time and do some serious thought about our past. Enjoy the memories.

Prayer for the Day: Heavenly Father, we thank you for the many gifts that you have given us, the feelings that we have when we use these gifts in our daily lives, and the opportunity to use them to serve humanity. We pray for the wisdom to discern what you want us to do and the will to do it faithfully and well. Amen

Great Bay,
Dover New Hampshire

A Place To Hide

The boundary lines have fallen for me in pleasant places;
You have made known to me) the path of life;
(Psalm 16 vs 6)

In the eighties, Ty Boyd, a speaker on the business circuit, was a Christian, businessman, and TV ad man who introduced me to the National Speakers Association. Ty taught that to be successful, and you had to be happy. Also, to be happy, you had to have a "life plan" that included all phases of life. It is early in the New Year, and we all have our resolutions and goals; that is a good thing. However, what is our plan to accomplish those goals?

Frankly, I do not care about the plan to lose weight or get fit, the resolution to be a better employee, etc. Let us recognize what has been given to us through Jesus to be successful and happy. This year we will need to use the Lord as a refuge, a place to seek peace.

The expression "When the going gets tough, the tough get going" is sporty and cute. My thoughts are that when the going gets tough spiritual people will recognize the pleasant boundaries given them by the Lord and be at peace. The closer we stay to the Lord and His plan, the happier and more successful we will become.

Thought Today Day: Today let us focus on staying close to God and let Him set us up for success and happiness.

Prayer for Today: Dear Lord, we are scared and concerned as we move forward through a changing world. We pray that we may hear your call and find refuge in your love. We pray that we may follow a plan to be close to you throughout life and do your will here on earth. Amen

God's Help Wanted

We have different gifts, according to the grace given us.
If a man's gift is prophesying, let him use it in proportion to his faith.
If it is serving, let him serve; if it is teaching, let him teach;
if it is encouraging, let him encourage;
if it is contributing to the needs of others, let him give generously;
if it is leadership, let him govern diligently;
if it is showing mercy, let him do it cheerfully.
(Romans 12 vs 6, 7)

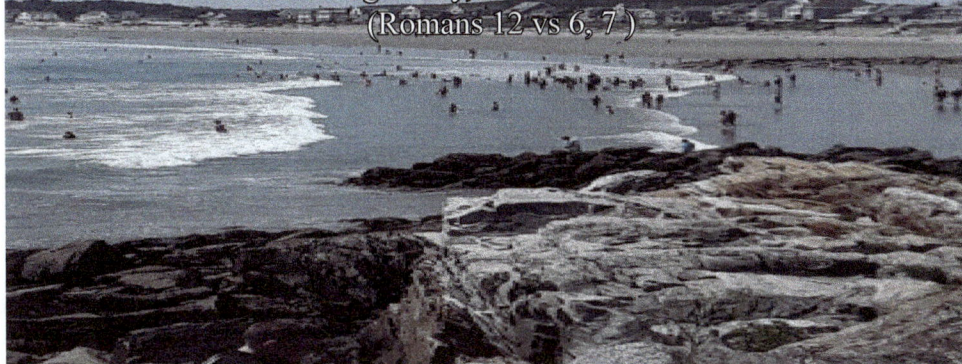

Paul's message to the Romans lists seven specific gifts. We have been blessed with some of them and can use them in our everyday lives. God's "HELP WANTED," asks us to use our gifts to do His work. We, therefore, have two challenges. One is to recognize the gifts given to us. The other is sharing these gifts in our daily lives.

The sharing of these gifts in a loving Christian way brings us peace.

Thought for Today: Today, let us focus on our gifts, understand them, and use them to help ourselves and others.

Prayer for Today: Dear Lord, we pray for an end to the pandemic, peace, and justice in a troubled world. We are trying to understand what everything means and our place in it all. We feel too small to help. We pray that we may recognize our gifts and use them to help the world. Amen

Rye State Park Beach,
Rye, New Hampshire

January 22

Service

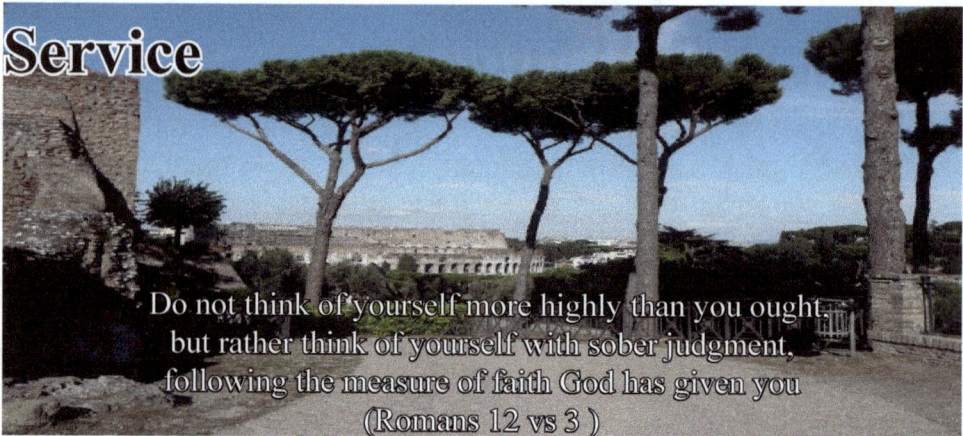

Do not think of yourself more highly than you ought, but rather think of yourself with sober judgment, following the measure of faith God has given you
(Romans 12 vs 3)

Consider the term "…measure of faith." in any context. It causes us to stop and wonder what scale we would measure it with, yards or meters? Euro vs. dollars? Pounds vs. kilograms? Faith, of course, cannot be measured in such easily quantified terms. The measure that probably matters is how well we use God's gifts.

"We have different gifts, according to the grace given us. If a person's gift is … serving, let him serve."
(Romans 12 vs 6 & 7)

When serving others is done as a passion, it is truly a gift from God. The warm feeling of having helped is always worth the effort. Many are famous because of this gift and raised to sainthood. The best part of the gift of service is we all have it and can feel it at some level. We all, at some time, will have the opportunity to be the "good Samaritan." We need to use this gift and enjoy the feeling that God gives us as His reward.

Thought for Today: Today, let us think about how we may help. Is there someone with an ill family member that could use a visit? Can we make time for coffee with a friend? If we can't plan an opportunity to serve, let us look during the week for a chance to use this gift.

Prayer for Today: Dear Lord, service to you is essential to us, but we are confused. Violence seems to invade our lives at all levels; There is violence and too many assaults in our cities. We pray for an opportunity to help others in a way that will benefit all. Amen

January 23

The Appian Way
Rome, Italy

Leadership

We have different gifts according to the grace given us.
If a man's gift is ...leadership, let him govern diligently;
(Romans 12 vs 6-8)

Leadership is one of God's greatest gifts. The world has experienced great leaders in many different forms. The ability to have a passion and develop followers that believe and follow the lead is truly a gift from God. In this regard, Jesus is, was, and will be the "King of Kings."

On a more human scale, we have leaders within our society. Many of us are leaders of our families; some of us are managers in business, youth sports, or at church. Often when in these leadership roles; decisions are made that are different than Christ would have made them.

Several years ago, the bracelet with "WWJD" engraved was popular. Those letters stood for "What would Jesus do?" The bracelet served as a reminder that it is always a good idea to consider our faith and leader when deciding. As normal humans, we will not achieve perfection. We can, however, strive toward it with every decision we make when asked to lead.

Thought for Today: Let's recognize and utilize our gifts from God. As Christians, we need to consider "What would Jesus do?"

Prayer for Today: Heavenly Father, we are all called to make decisions. Financial pressure, personal prejudices, and many other factors often cause us to drift from your will when making choices. Today we pray that we may all make decisions that fit your plan; that would be as Jesus would do. Amen

Parkers Lake
Plymouth, Minnesota

Teaching

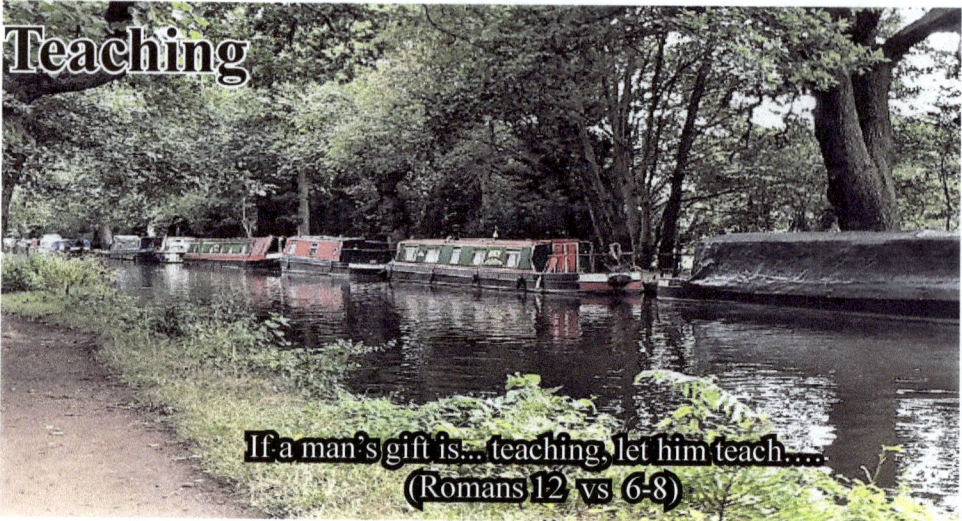

If a man's gift is... teaching, let him teach....
(Romans 12 vs 6-8)

Webster says that a teacher is someone who "... gives knowledge or insight to another." Yes, that is part of it all, and if that is the case, we are all part-time teachers. We can get through a day without sharing part of our knowledge base with someone. The scary piece is that we do not always know when we are teaching.

We are often teaching others through our public actions. One Sunday morning in church, I watched an older gentleman holding hands with his wife. Later he had his arm around her like a teenager on a Friday night date. Let me share that this guy and I had a very negative business relationship. However, he and his wife set an example for me and all around them that day. I grew to know them better and often used his "behavioral teaching" to improve my relationship.

June and I have observed many behaviors in our children that make us proud and some we wish they had not learned from us. Yes, we often teach our children the wrong stuff. Wouldn't it be great if they only saw us at our best? Within our families, parents are always teachers.

Thought for Today: Let us recognize our God-given roles as teachers. Each day let us share our behaviors, words, and actions, teachings that will make us proud. We did not ask for it, and we can not avoid it, so let us do it well.

Prayer for Today: Heavenly Father, today we ask that we feel your spirit so that we may act as a disciple of Christ. Let our behavior teach those around us that there is some good in the world. Amen

January 25

River Wey Navigation
Wisley, Surrey, UK

Contributing

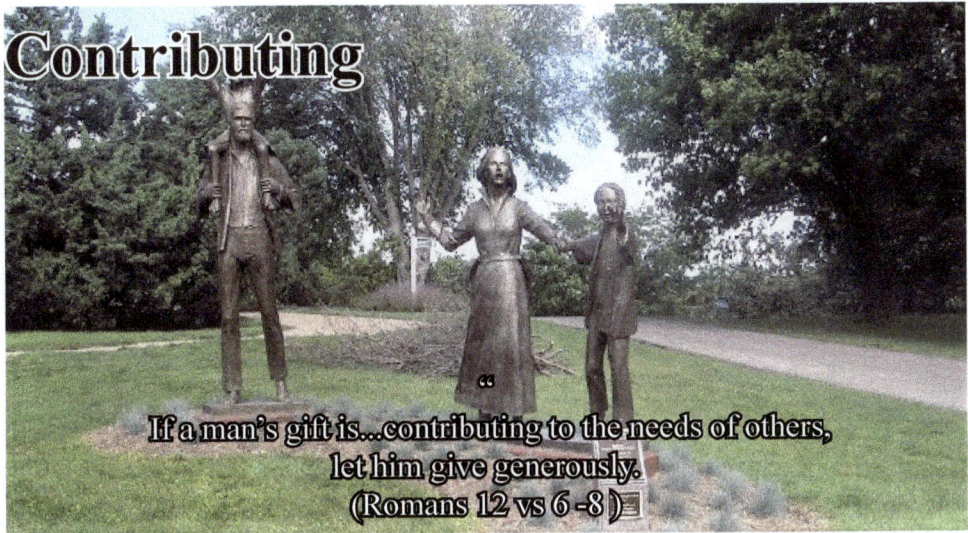

"If a man's gift is...contributing to the needs of others, let him give generously. (Romans 12 vs 6-8)"

When are we contributing to the needs of others? We rarely risk physical harm or sacrifice but contribute every day. Sometimes our contributions are intentional and planned. Often they are reactionary and just something that we do.

We often help serve at shelters through our Church, contribute to transients in the neighborhood, and many other ways. Many of us jump in when neighbors have projects or problems at home. Even the simple act of preparing food for someone who is ill is a contribution; a spiritual act. As Christians, we were all given this gift at some level, and we get a great feeling, a gift from God when we contribute.

Thought for Today: Let us contribute. Each day we walk past opportunities to contribute to someone in need, search them out and contribute to their tranquility. No, not some coins in the tip tray at a coffee shop or restaurant (but go ahead anyway.) Look for and find someone that needs help.

Prayer for Today: Heavenly Father, often the balance in our lives seems tipped toward being selfish. The immediate needs of our selves, family and occupy too much mind share. We tend to forget to reach out to others. Today we pray for improved focus on Your work. We pray for simpler lives to put "Your will" on our "to do" lists and calendars. Amen

Encouraging

If your gift is ...to encourage, then encourage...
(Romans 12 vs 6 - 8)

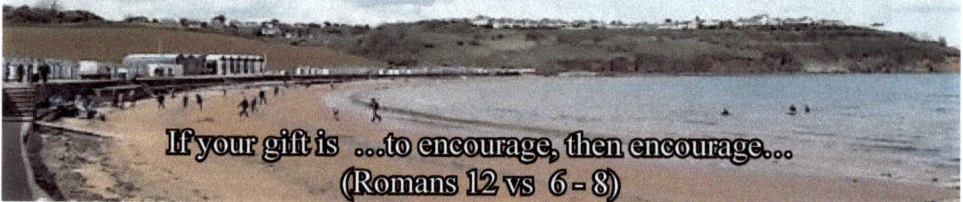

Another gift mentioned in Romans 12 is "encouraging." As leaders and teachers, we need to recognize that those around us often need encouragement. I grew up in the "Walk softly and carry a big stick" era. Parenting had yet to be enlightened.

Youth coaches face the challenge of teaching skills and attitudes. Former Chelsea striker, Didier Drogba, says it like this, "Coaches can teach you two things: confidence and technique." In an interview with Tiger Woods, after shooting eight over par and finishing near the bottom of a tournament, his comments were about all he did correctly. That is the attitude of positive thinking, that of a champion

One of my early mentors used to say, "Hurry up, make that mistake." Oops, that is counter-intuitive. He used every mistake as a learning experience in training and encouraged improvement. His reviews reviewed our progress and included an updated plan moving forward. He had the gift of encouragement.

Thought for Today: We will all have an opportunity to encourage someone this week. Let us recognize where we fit and utilize God's gifts in our lives to make God's world a better place.

Prayer for Today: Heavenly Father,the book says, "There are different kinds of working, but the same God works all of them in all men." We pray that the entire world comes to understand your many gifts. Amen

Mercy

"If it is showing mercy, let him do it cheerfully.
(Romans 12 vs 6-8)

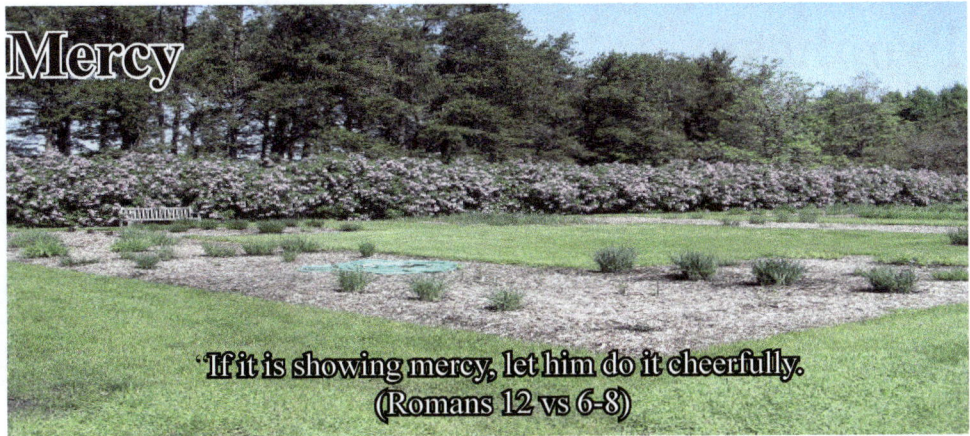

The gift of mercy is a hard one to define but an easy one to see. During the American civil war, Clara Barton organized a nurses' corps, and they risked their lives tending to soldiers in the field. That is a true gift of mercy.

We often listen to a speaker who presents his case with great emotion instead of logic. They demonstrate empathy, compassion, and sympathy rather than addressing things logically. Can that be mercy?

People with mercy pick up on the emotional response of others. They want harmony in their lives, at home, and work. Physical contact is highly valued, and they seem to understand the body language of others very well. As with other gifts, there are limitations.

Webster says mercy means to "console or succor one afflicted," and the Amplified Bible says, "He who does acts of mercy, with genuine, cheerful eagerness is blessed." Mercy is a gift from God to those who can keep on giving. Mercy leaps from the heart, and there is no resistance to care.

Thought for the Day: Let us think about who we are and what gifts God has given us. Let us learn to use these gifts in our lives and the lives of others better.

Prayer for the Day: Heavenly Father, today I give thanks to those that show mercy for others. They are a gift that the world needs. Amen

Prophesy

If a person's gift is prophesying,
let him use it in proportion to his faith.
(Romans 12 vs 6)

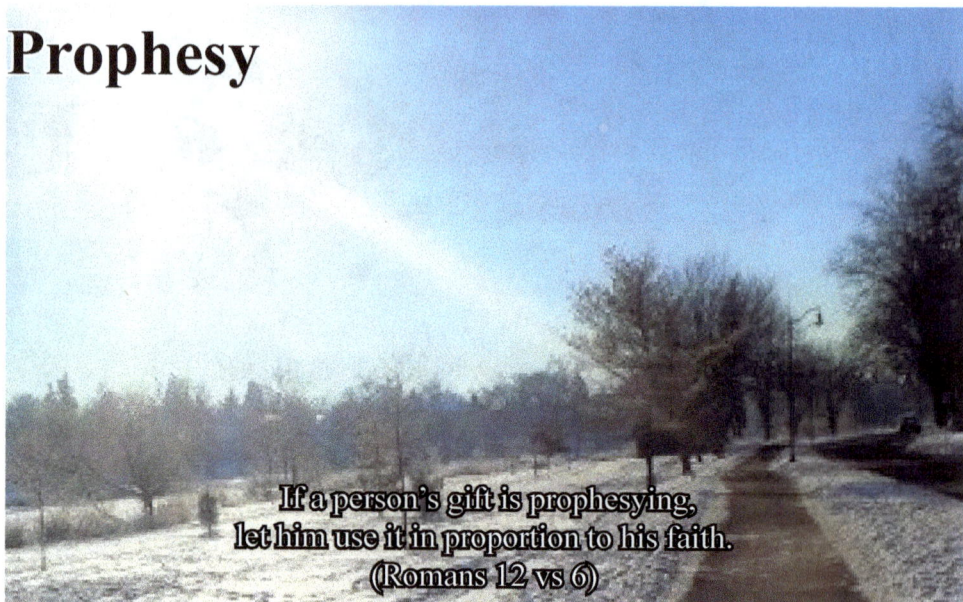

We look at prophets as old-time geniuses, people with wisdom who spoke their minds and often worked to correct societies' ills. They were different from most because they said their minds and were often controversial. They were rarely in doubt but not often considered correct.

Speaking out on controversial matters and society's ills is gutsy at the best of times. In our world today, our population seems to be split down the middle. Most votes are close to a 50/50 split. Today's prophets offend almost half the people when they speak out.

We are all given the gift of having prophetic ideas, but few have received the gift as Paul meant it in his message. Those few are the outspoken leaders and supporters of change in the world. They are still around and will be a blessing to future generations.

Thought for Today: Let us try to recognize our gifts and how we apply them in our personal lives within our community and our business lives.

Prayer for Today: Let us pray that the prophe0ts in our society continue doing the Lord's work. They have a natural gift that needs to be heard and not forgotten. Amen

January 29 Lake of the Isles
Minneapolis, MN

Soar Like An Eagle

"There are different kinds of working,
but the same God works all of them in all men."
(1 Corinthians 12 vs 4-6)

For a week, we have thought about our gifts from God. It is early in the year, and He wants us to use them. Paul talked about them in Rome and Corinth. None of us have received all the gifts, and we need to recognize which ones we have and apply them to doing God's work here on earth.

Here are some thought-provoking questions about the gifts God gave to each of us:

Have we developed an understanding of the gifts we each received?
Do we use them in our daily lives?
Do we have an obligation to use them to help others?

We need to think about our gifts and how we use them in our lives.

Thought for Today: Today, let us all recognize our gifts as we put them to use in everyday activities. Let us give thanks to the Lord for them.

Prayer for Today: Dear Lord, we live in a confusing world of negativity and frustration. Hate seems to dominate our news, terror and violence seem to dominate our local news. Today, we pray that we can recognize our gifts and skills while we pray for your guidance that we may contribute to expanding your love here on earth. Amen

February

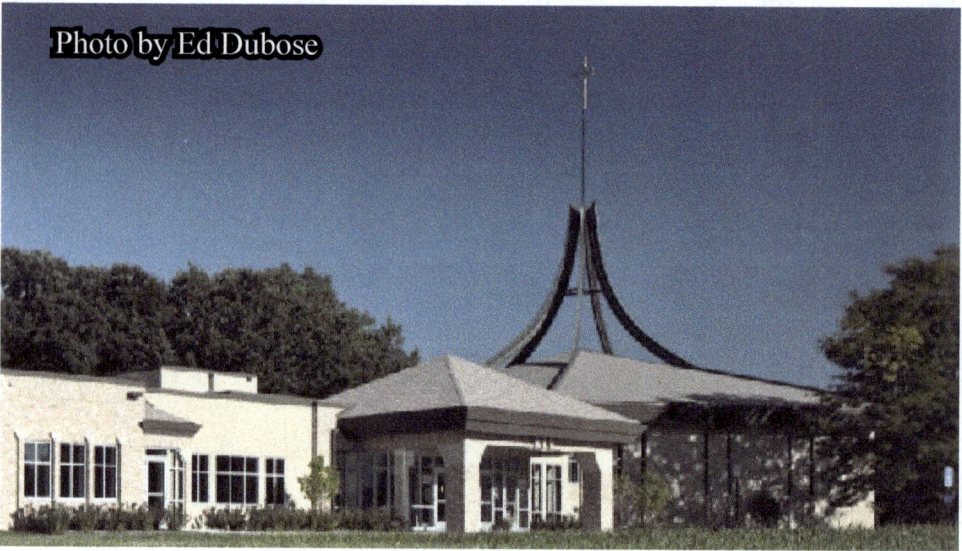

Photo by Ed Dubose

Spirit of Hope UMC

"We are called by God to be a radically inclusive, caring community of faith offering personal and social transformation though Jesus Christ."

Confidence Through Trust

One who trusts in the Lord is secure.
(Proverbs 29 vs 25)

A Pickeringism is a phrase or idea that is an absolute truth with no scientific basis. A favorite is "All days are not created equal." Truth in all areas of life. Marriages vary from day to day when one spouse has a gloomy day, or maybe both do. In the workplace, differences are problematic despite the rules and policies.

In Thomas Harris's book, I'm OK; You're OK," he reviews the four states of every two-person relationship. They are summarized as I'm" OK, you're not OK": when one person has some stress or discomfort with the moment. That position is reversed with the second condition, "I'm not OK, you're OK. A great place to be is home when all is well and comfortable; I'm OK, your OK; the state of marital bliss; The whole relationship may be a mess with the condition "I'm not OK, you're not OK."

Among all life's variables, there is a constant; power of one that can work on any day, in any condition: That power is our faith. Pickeringisms can be negated by confidence and the knowledge that God is with us. Joseph Kennedy, President Kennedy's father, is credited with saying, "When the going gets tough, the tough get going." We need to recognize that the going will often vary, and sometimes we need to pray for guidance and help.

Thought for Today: Today, let's be secure in knowing that the Lord is with us and will help us through.

Prayer for Today: Dear Lord, today we give thanks for your support in our everyday lives. We are grateful for your blessings. We are thankful that no matter how the world changes, you will be there when we need you. Amen

Lake of the Isles
Minneapolis, Minnesota

Punxsutawney Phil

We know that an idol is nothing at all in the world, and that there is no God but one.
(1 Corinthians 8 vs 4 & 5)

On Groundhog Day every year in Pennsylvania, they forecast the end of winter. Today, Phil's shadow was not seen, and they declared that winter would end early! Well, you see, Phil is never wrong because somewhere there will be an early spring, probably not here in Minnesota.

Phil is a character, not even a legend. He is no Paul Bunyan, Johnny Appleseed, or Ichabod Crane, and he is just a groundhog being disturbed for a group of people in Pennsylvania to have fun. Frankly, he is not a good idol.

Would it be fun if they opened Phil's den next year and Jesus stepped out? Picture him in a white robe, the sun beating down on him with a heavenly glow leaving the crowd speechless. Imagine Jesus saying something like, "Sorry folks but even I refuse to do a long-range weather forecast. There will be more bad weather here in the north country but do not fear, for the Lord will be with you." He would then give his blessing and arise toward the heavens.

Bless you, all, and may we have an early Spring.

Thought for Today: The Lord blesses us and keeps us 365 days a year.

Prayer for Today: Dear Lord and father, we pray for those who deal with fire and ice in the north. May they take the time to appreciate the seasons and the beauty of it all. Amen

February 2

Hwy 394 View
Minnetonka, Minnesota

Peacemakers

**Blessed are the peacemakers,
for they will be called children of God.
(Mathew 5 vs. 9)**

A peacemaker is not a person who avoids issues but resolves issues, one that will go where others avoid. Some do it because it is their job, some because it is their passion. I view a peacemaker as one who stirs the pot. That is generally a negative saying, but it also is the way to solve problems and bring good (peace) by generating a deeper discussion.

The puzzle of our times is that we have become a polarized sound bite society, leading to polarization. There is not enough understanding of the issues. Peacemakers try to stir the pot to bring awareness and a reasonable solution. Peacemakers strive for win-win and have a tough job today.

We often have difficult discussions in our church because both sides believe God is on their side. Jesus wants us to contribute, to stir the pot for acceptable solutions. Paul advised the Romans:

"Let us, therefore, make every effort to do what leads
to peace and mutual edification."
(Romans 14 vs. 19)

Thought for the Day: Today, we will hear sound bites and snippets of reality, and let us ask what Jesus would do with that snippet.

Prayer for the Day: Dear Lord and Father, today, we pray for the ability to think and ponder what is between the sound bites of our society. We pray for the ability to follow Jesus and understand your will. Amen

Sky over the River Nene,
Cambridgeshire, UK

February 3

Page 35

Self Respect

Then God said, "Let us make man in our image, in our likeness."
So God created man in his image.
(Geneses 1 vs 26 & 27)

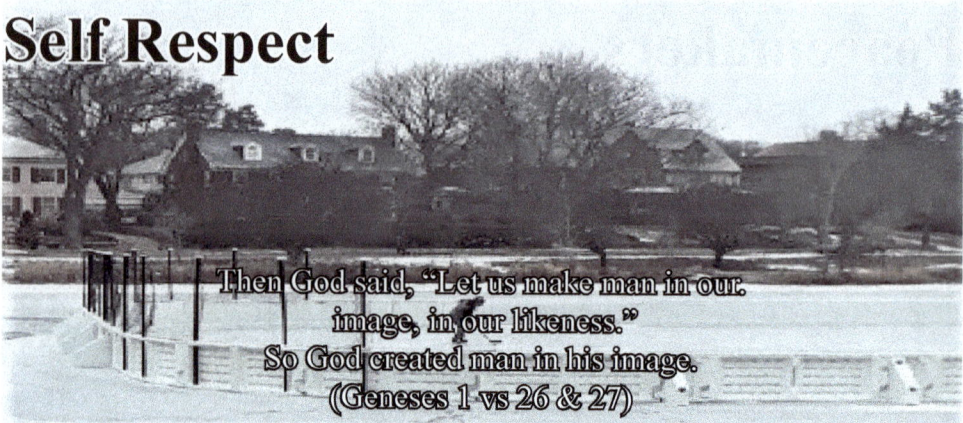

God made us in His image. But one of humanity's significant problems is people suffering from low self-esteem and a lack of self-respect, including substance abuse and depression.

Twelve-step programs have been very good at dealing with these two issues. They work because people admit there is a power greater than themselves (God), and their goal is spiritual growth. Spirituality, self-respect, and confidence go hand in hand. Understanding that the Lord is with us every day makes for a satisfactory lifestyle.

If you are reading this, you probably have life under control. Meditation is one way of recharging our spiritual batteries. We need to do that for ourselves, our families, and others around us. When we have self-esteem, others will want what we have. That is when we can help.

Thought for Today: Today, when we look in the mirror, let's look past the visual image of ourselves. Let's look into our own eyes and try to see inside where our heart and soul reside. Take that thought out for the week and display our pride, self-respect, and faith in the Lord to others.

Prayer for Today: Dear Lord and Father, we live in a beautiful place surrounded by beautiful people. Some let differences separate us and come between us. We pray that we can contribute to dissolving and understanding those differences. We pray that with our strength through you, we find a way to do your will and accept spiritual differences by respecting others. Amen

February 4 Minneapolis Parks Rink
Lake of The Isles, Minneapolis, MN

It's Only Money

Photo by Stephanie Symmes

Who of you by worrying,
can add a single hour to his life?
(Matthew 6: vs 25 & 27)

Several years ago, my pastor and I had coffee at his request. His concern was some business stresses affecting June's and my lives. We talked about money, lawsuits, and tough decisions in my life. Often these decisions are financial and made without remembering today's passage.

My comments made Pastor Rick laugh harder than I had heard him laugh in our seven-year relationship. They were that "June and I felt that God had a plan that we had not yet seen and that somehow we were serving His needs." He challenged my decisions based on standard financial logic as we talked about my life strategy. Then I made a slight error and slipped into some studio language, " After all, it is only f@^%#g money." Pastor Rick almost fell out of his chair in laughter.

There is a message there somewhere. Matthew 6:27 above asks what "worry" will do for us. But we still worry. What will worry accomplish? Higher blood pressure? Broken relationships? Jealousies? Maybe we should pray more than we worry. After all, our faith says that God is with us at all times.

Thought for Today: Today, let us think about Matthew 6:25-27 and try harder to enjoy the week. Think about how great it would be to get through the week without "worry." Let's "Let go and let God."

Prayer for Today: Heavenly Father, there are wars and conflicts globally; many of us are unemployed or concerned about our future, and of course, COVID... It seems that there are endless reasons to worry. We pray for the faith and sound judgment to let you help us. We pray rather than worry. Amen

Excellence

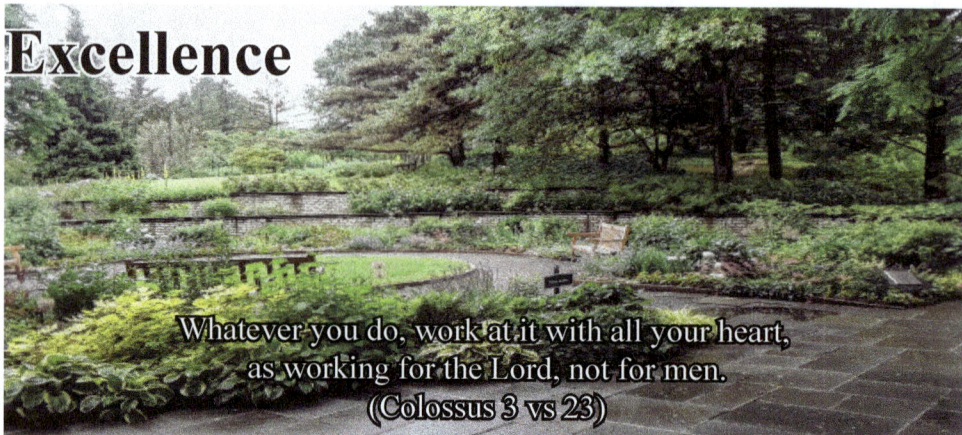

Whatever you do, work at it with all your heart,
as working for the Lord, not for men.
(Colossus 3 vs 23)

Earlier I wrote about my "Pickeringism" that all days are not created equal. Here is another example. There are days that we are full of boundless energy and others when we are as flat as pancakes. However, these feelings are mental, physical, and emotional states, and they do not affect our hearts, just our performance or output.

As a long-term weekend athlete, there have been too many days when only the heart showed up for the workout; the arms, legs, and head wanted to go back to bed. There were many days when that's how the day started, but the performance was in the excellent range when it ended.

One of my best friends and four-time Olympic athlete relates to this. Pat has trained every day of his life, and he can relate to the fact that the heart and head often lead the body, " … work at it with all your heart, as working for the Lord," and you will be rewarded with excellence. Excellence starts with believing in yourself and the Lord, and the rest will follow.

Thought for Today: Today, let us remember that "All days are not created equal." On the day we want to go back to bed, let us trust our hearts and move out, take and the leap of faith and give ourselves the chance to exhibit the excellence that God wants us to share.

Prayer for Today: Dear Lord, we give you thanks for your ongoing presence in our lives. When we are physically worn, you help us recover, and when emotionally drained, you recharge our spirits. We give thanks that you are always with us. Amen

Rule Number One

> It is the Lord Christ you are serving.
> (Colossians 3 vs 24)

Early in my engineering career, I had a boss who had the following sign on his wall:

"Rule number One-The boss is always right.
Rule number 2- When the boss is wrong, see rule number one."

Exactly who did he think he was? He was a real controller and taskmaster. The sign was right on when we consider our God the boss to apply his words to our lives.

Many of our readers have young families, two careers, and a busy family schedule. My daughter has two jobs in our family, her husband one, and two middle school students. Life seemed easier when June and I had our four, or maybe we were younger and could juggle more balls in the air. Either way, we lost track of the actual boss more than once. There were coaches, sales managers, the tax man, and the list seemed endless. Somehow it all fell into place.

In our history and future, especially today, the BOSS is always right. It is our choice daily to decide who is boss; "…as working for the Lord."

Thought for Today: Today, there will be challenge, stress, and we will run out of time. We will meet the challenge and remember who we are and what we are working for through Jesus

Prayer for Today: Today, we give thanks for our blessings. We pray for a simple day of peace and joy with a minimum of stress. Amen

Roman Collusium
Rome, Italy

February 7

Page 39

Trust And Faith

> When I am afraid, I will trust in you.
> In God whose word I praise,
> in God I trust.
> (Psalm 56 vs 3)

We will all experience times in our lives when our trust level is low. These are usually times when we must let a situation be under someone else's control. A teenager spending a weekend away with friends, at camp, or going off to school. We fear what they may find to do. A family member is not home at an expected time. We fear an accident or other harm.
It would be easy to think that today's subject was fear rather than trust.

There is a direct link between a weak faith and trust in the Lord and high anxiety and stress levels. Yes, there are days when we are strong and have no fear, then there are days when we are weak need to meditate. Leave the news turned off, put down the newspaper and get closer to God.

Call upon me in the day of trouble; I will deliver you,
and you will honor me.
(Psalm 50 vs 15)

Thought for Today: When we have doubts, stop, take a deep breath, and try to place our faith in God. When we do, our reactions to doubtful situations will be less stressful.

Prayer for Today: Heavenly Father, it is easy to forget you as we go through our busy schedules. We seem not to trust you. We try to control, manipulate, and alter our lives to fit "our will" and lose sight of "your will." We pray that we can slow down, consider your will for us, and increase our trust in you. Amen

Intimacy

Then the Lord said
It is not good for the man to be alone.
(Gennesis 2 vs 18)

I want to update the passage to "It is not good for a person to be alone" because loneliness is a problem for everyone, and faith and godly interaction is a great help. We all appreciate intimacy and being close.

But what does it mean to be close, and how do we get there? What is our responsibility in the equation? First comes openness, followed closely by honesty. We need to be open with the other person and straight-up honest. When two people can be that way with one another, intimacy has a fighting chance.

My observations are that when we are very young, we are often too impetuous to allow intimacy. Relationships seem to stay on the surface, and interaction is activity-based which is rarely heartfelt. Middle age, say, 30 to 60, seems when people have the most confidence and are willing to be close. Unfortunately, I see a retraction as people age.

In summary, I do not think we can help the youth become intimate; that is a growing thing greatly helped by wisdom and spirituality. I have significant concerns and prayers for us as we grow older. We lose capabilities and want to hide the losses. We often lose intimacy and become more distant from our loved ones as we age. That is sad and worth our prayers.

Thought for Today: For today, let us focus on our open and intimate relationships. Let's be sure that they are intact and growing. Let us involve the holy spirit in our lives.

Prayer for Today: Today, we pray for the lonely, those that cannot open up their hearts to others; share their fears and wishes. We pray that they find the spirit of intimacy through our Lord Jesus. Amen

Intimacy

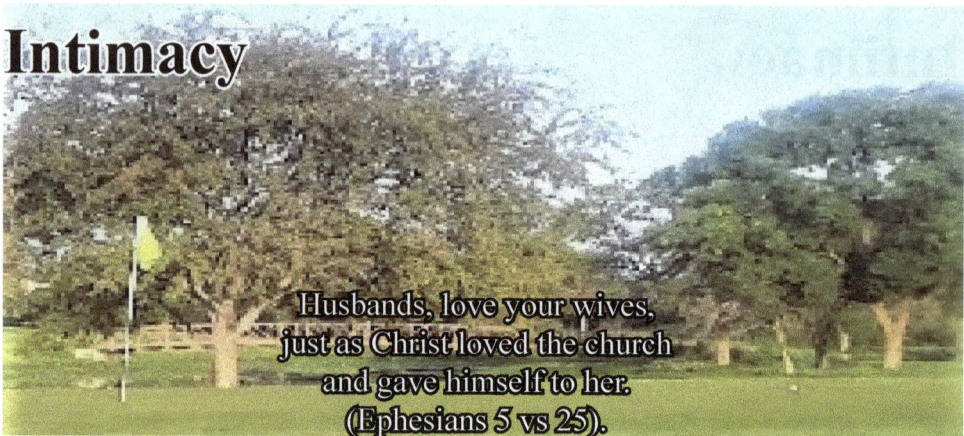

Husbands, love your wives,
just as Christ loved the church
and gave himself to her.
(Ephesians 5 vs 25).

I want to alter Paul's message here to "Love your spouse just as Christ loved the church and gave himself" because a relationship is a two-way street, and it is vital to love and pray for each other in a relationship.

In the early years, what I call my dark period, June's and my relationship was one-sided. There was deep love on both sides but not intimacy. She was the glue that supported me and my schedule, and I was busy building a business, endurance training, and being self-focused.

During my dark period, June was my light at the end of the tunnel, and through the grace of God, I saw that it was not a train coming from the other end. Today, our relationship is balanced and giving, perhaps too much, if possible.

The Lord gives us an unlimited supply of love when we are born, and it is never-ending, always available to offer, and we have a chance to share it with our spouses every minute of the day. As my favorite philosopher, NIKE, says, "Just Do It!"

Thought for Today: Let us each tell someone close, friend, or family how much their relationship means to us.

Prayer for Today: Dear Lord, today we give thanks to those close people in my life. We share our love for them as Christ did for the church. Amen

Februsry 10 Brookview Golf Course, Golden Valley, Minnesota

Strengthening

For the eyes of the LORD range throughout the earth to strengthen those whose hearts are fully committed to him. (2 Chronicles 16 vs. 9)

We, males, are strange; we don't ask for directions, fail to speak up, and hide our feelings. Our egos seem to hurt our lives, so we unnecessarily challenge ourselves. Unlike us, women will ask for help, give directions, admit when they don't know something, and learn.

We can conceal weaknesses and inequities from each other but we cannot hide them from God. He will support us even when we do not know, ask, or want Him to. A good life goal is acknowledge our weaknesses and pray they go away.

Recently we headed out to a visit at a hospital we had not been to in the past. As the driver, I checked Google maps, my old map book, and wrote all the contact information down on paper; Sure enough, we got to the freeway exit and followed the signs into the parking lot and then into the lobby. I wasn't going to have to ask for directions.

Sometimes I wandered around a bit lost but eventually figured out where to get help. Fortunately, I have been willing to ask for and take spiritual direction throughout my life. It seems that the eyes of the Lord have always been on me as they are on you. He sees and strengthens us all.

Thought for the Day: Today, there will be times when we need more strength, and let us find it through Him, prayer, and meditation.

Prayer for the Day: Dear Lord and Father, today I give thanks for the beautiful day, the people around me, and the strength to deal with whatever happens. Amen

Lincoln

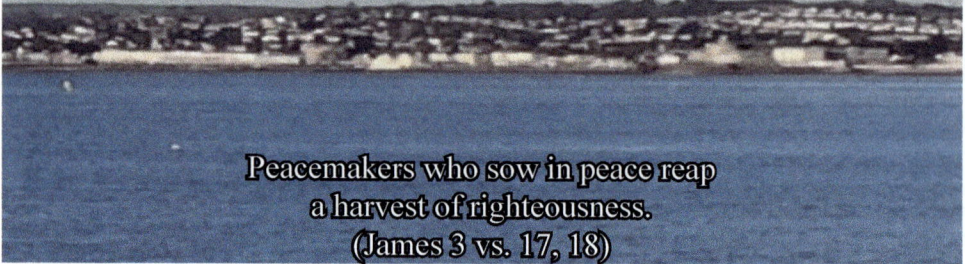

Peacemakers who sow in peace reap
a harvest of righteousness.
(James 3 vs. 17, 18)

President Lincoln presided over a war that was one of the bloodiest in the history of our country. He could not have done what he did without his strong faith. His bible was often at his side in meetings and had dog-eared pages from continual use. It reinforced his belief that he and the union were doing the right thing.

It brings to my mind the old joke about disagreements in church congregations. The arguments are often fierce because both sides feel God on their team. We are not making decisions that cause battles where 10,000 plus soldiers die in church politics or people getting assassinated, brothers fight brothers, and a race's freedom is at stake. Still, somehow we do the Lord's will.

Often Lincoln felt badly after a traumatic field report and would lean on the Biblical hope offered to him (and all of us. Today's verse was one he often used when he needed reassurance. He would say to his cabinet and all who would listen, "Let us renew our trust in God and go forward without fear and with manly hearts." (Note from Walking With Lincoln)

Happy Birthday, Abe.

Thought for Today: Our summons is to be happy Christians, be the light of the world, and share and contribute through our faith. Today let us shine our light brightly.

Prayer for Today: Dear Lord and Father, we thank those great men who had gone before us. We pray that we contribute in some way to accomplishing your will and create a world of peace and love. Amen

February 12   View of Duxbury from
Plymouth, Massachusetts

Respect

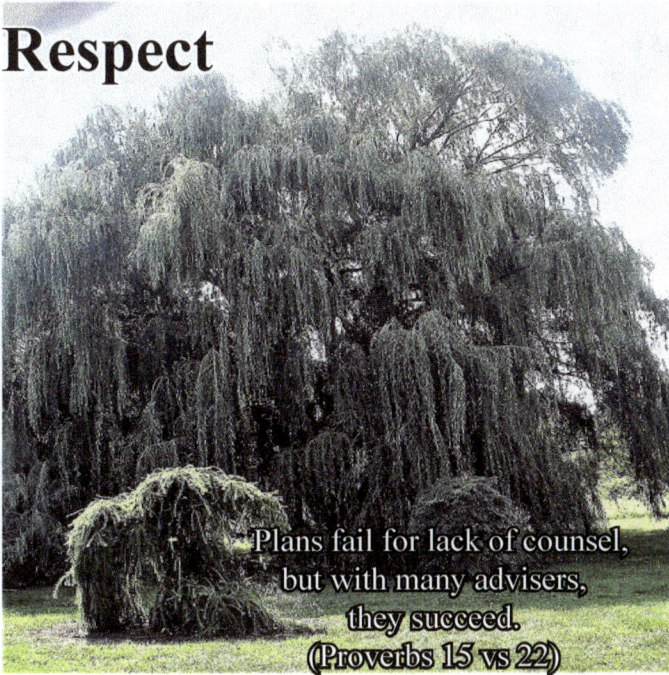

Plans fail for lack of counsel,
but with many advisers,
they succeed.
(Proverbs 15 vs 22)

Earning respect is an ongoing challenge throughout our lives. According to the book of Proverbs, communication will make other people want to connect with us. Proverbs 15vs22 talks about the benefits of good counseling, sound advice.

To earn respect, be a willing advisor. Share your experiences, your knowledge, and goodwill with those in need. Share that precious intellectual property that God has allowed you to accumulate. Earn respect through sharing.

Thought for Today: Let us think about helping others through our experienced advice. Listen and share as Proverbs advises us and observe how much better we feel when we practice sharing. Try hard to let others help us.

Prayer for Today: Dear Lord, we pray for peace and tranquility for those around us and throughout the world. We pray that somehow our life's experiences shared and used as an example of your will. Amen

Be My Valentine

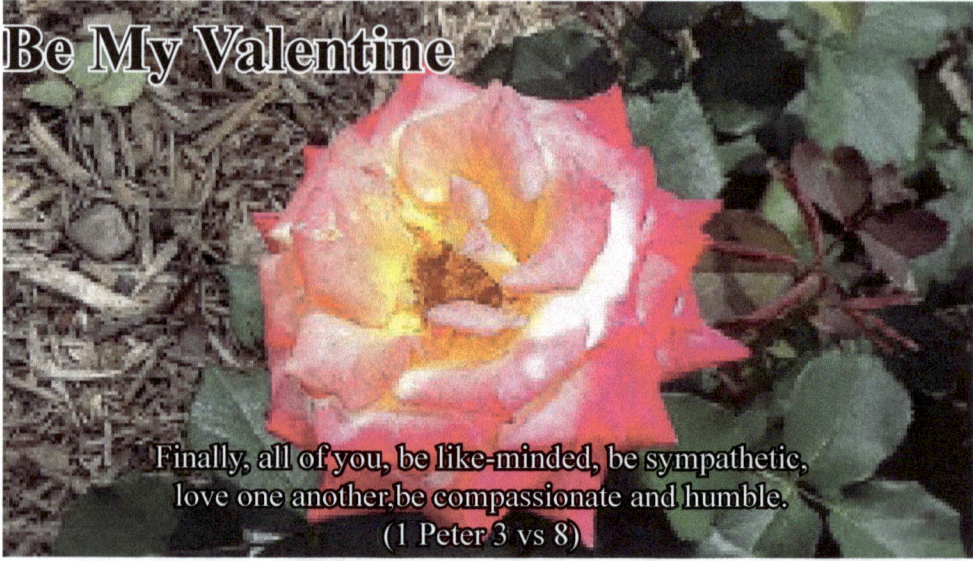

Finally, all of you, be like-minded, be sympathetic, love one another, be compassionate and humble.
(1 Peter 3 vs 8)

"Love one another" is a great idea, and it does not include any qualifiers or reasons to separate people from the group; it means all, every day and moment. That is our Christian charge, and it means everyone, every day.

Valentine's day in America has become a symbol of romantic love where symbols seem to replace reality. It is good to have a day when we symbolize our love, caring, and dedication. It is good to focus on those around and dear to us, and it is kind of fun.

Happy Valentine's day. As Christians, we believe that we were made in God's image. To love everyone, we need to have God's heart and capacity to care, and we are reminded of that today.

Thought for Today: Today, we will focus our love on those closest to us; our families, significant others, moms and dads, etc. That is great but let's also try to care for everyone!

Prayer for Today: Dear Lord, today we give thanks for our ever-expanding hearts that seem to have enough love in them for everyone. We give thanks for the ability to understand and care for all. Amen

Also Ran

> Then the LORD said to Joshua, "Do not
> be afraid; do not be discouraged.
> (Joshua 8 vs 1)

Being an also-ran is a way of life. We rarely finish first. Russell Sanders uttered the famous quote, "Winning isn't everything. It is the only thing." It is not valid, and here are some: My friend Pat McNamara qualified in four different Olympics and did not win a medal. Ted Williams and Carl Yastrzemski played years for the Red Sox and never received a World Series ring. None of the above is a loser, and all were proud of their accomplishments.

In my instance, I have three triathlon trophies out of 21 races; a second, a third, and an only. There was always someone faster until the Summer of 2011 when no one else my age competed. Did I lose? Never. In each Triathlon that I did, I would well up with tears of joy from the sheer pride in my accomplishment in the last mile of the run. The pain experienced during the run would go away, the legs would seem fresh again, and the finishing sprint would feel and look great. Second, Third, or twentieth did not matter; I was winning inside.

We rarely are number one, but we are always winners since God is always with us.

Thought for Today: Today, we will have battles we do not expect. Let us be winners with God's help, no matter which way the battle turns out.

Prayer for Today: Dear Lord and Father, today we thank you for being with us at all times in every place. We thank you because when you are along, we will be winners. Amen

Rose Garden Sign
Minnesota Landscape Arboretum

Marriage

*A wife of noble character who can find?
She is worth far more than rubies.
(Proverbs 31 vs 10, 11)*

Many of you have heard me discuss the benefits of a good marriage: great mutual support, care when illness arrives, joint celebrations of the many events that occur. Yes, marriage is truly a remarkable institution when things are well and blessed by God.

Many times it has been stated that marriage is the world's most challenging job. Let me quote from The Mystery of Marriage by Mike Mason.

"Marriage, even under the best of circumstances, is a crisis; one of the major crises of life. It is a dangerous thing not to be aware of this. Whether it turns out to be a healthy, challenging, and constructive crisis or a disastrous nightmare depends largely upon how willing the partners are to be changed, how malleable they are."

"Crises" seems a bit extreme. Still, marriage is a great opportunity for life fulfillment, and it certainly is not without its "opportunities" for success or failure. A marriage blessed by God, one in which the partners have allowed God's love to grow in their relationship, is one of the world's most incredible experiences.

Thought for Today: We face many distractions in our daily lives; work, busy schedules, terrorism, war, deficits, and many more. Let us look at our primary relationships. When things are okay in our relationships, the outside problems seem less intense.

Prayer for Today: Heavenly Father, we are in a world of hurting people, a world of fear. Today we pray for love within our lives. We pray that somehow we can feel your presence and overcome our doubts. Amen

February 16 Lake Harriet, Minneapolis, Minnesota

Let's Talk

"You must go to everyone I send you to
and say whatever I command you."
(Jeremiah 1vs7)

The city of Boston has a public area called Boston Commons, and it is a central park set up as a common grazing ground for city-owned live-stock. Even today, all Boston residents have the legal right to graze their cow on "the common."

"The Common" is now and always was a meeting place where people meet to discuss the day's issues, and it still serves that function today. There are people on every corner, some standing on soapboxes, discussing whatever they choose. You can generally find a "talker" that represents your ideas no matter what you feel.

The most common subjects the "talkers" address are issues of faith. There will be conservatives on one corner and liberals on the next using the same Bible passages to reinforce their beliefs. Often, they engage their audience in debates that may be very intense. "The Boston Common Talkers" represent America's free speech at its finest.

Most of us shy away from publicly sharing our faith with others. Jesus wants us to share, but we generally do not have the confidence to speak out in public. We need to realize that we need to share and "…say whatever I command you."

Thought for Today: Today, let us all look for a chance to tell someone about our faith, invite someone to share, someone we may help, and possibly even ask them to join us at a service.

Prayer for Today: Heavenly Father, I pray for the strength to do your will here on earth. I pray that I may share the story of my life with You with someone. Amen

Gray's Bay,Lake Minnetonka
Wayzata, MN   **February 17**   Page 49

Love Each Other

"Accept one another, then,
just as Christ accepted you,
in order to bring praise to God."
(Romans 15:7)

God is adding ingredients to America's melting pot, so a change in the brew constantly challenges us. Growing populations of various nationalities and religions seem foreign to us. Yes, some of these make us uncomfortable. Must we accept and love them all?

Picture yourself leaving a movie tonight and walking through a parking lot. You see a group of youths of your race coming toward you. They could be a street gang, a church youth group, or your friends going to the next show. At first, there is some doubt, then recognition, and then, hopefully, comfort.

Sometimes we are uncomfortable with who is approaching, and we get nervous as a safety precaution that may be justifiable. Often it can be a sign of subconscious or even conscious prejudice. Yes, often, our biases show up in this way. As Christians, we need to recognize this when it happens.

Growing up in a white suburb of post-WWII Boston, we were taught to "stay with your own kind." In 1948, author Stetson Kennedy stated that WASPs (White Anglo Saxon Protestants) gang up and take their frustrations out on whatever group is handy- Negro, Catholic, Jewish, Japanese, or whatnot.

Boston was the city where companies posted, "Irish need not apply." It was a terrible environment. With that said, the Catholic girls would not date a Methodist. I often heard from mom, "We don't need those kinds of problems." Whatever that meant.

Several of us discussed that subject at our fiftieth-class reunion in 2007. Friend Marie and I never dated because of it, even though her brothers and I were best friends. Their folks did not want a Methodist in their home, and I was discouraged from bringing Irish or Italian friends home. I did not ever understand why. It was shocking to hear that they were advised the same.

Today, in our 80s, looking back, it seems ridiculous. Today June and I walk through our complex and pass black, brown, red and white, Muslim, Hindu, and Christian; and we live together. My mom would not live here. Unfortunately, our world still has not changed enough, but as Christians, we must never stop trying,

To get back to the question, "Must we accept and love them all?" the answer is clear. John quotes Jesus in chapter 15:17, "This is my command: Love each other," and Jesus left no one off the list.

Thought for Today: Today, look at our fears, prejudices, and the way we view the diverse elements of our society. Let us ask if we can learn to exhibit Christian love toward these elements. We will understand that we can when we try.

Prayer for Today: Dear Lord, help me reach out to people. Could you help me understand the undesirable? There is still terror and the threat of war throughout the world. We are confused and have difficulty loving our enemies, and we pray for the ability to understand and follow Jesus' command for love.

Forgiven

You set aside all your wrath
and turned from your fierce anger.
(Psalm 85 vs. 3)

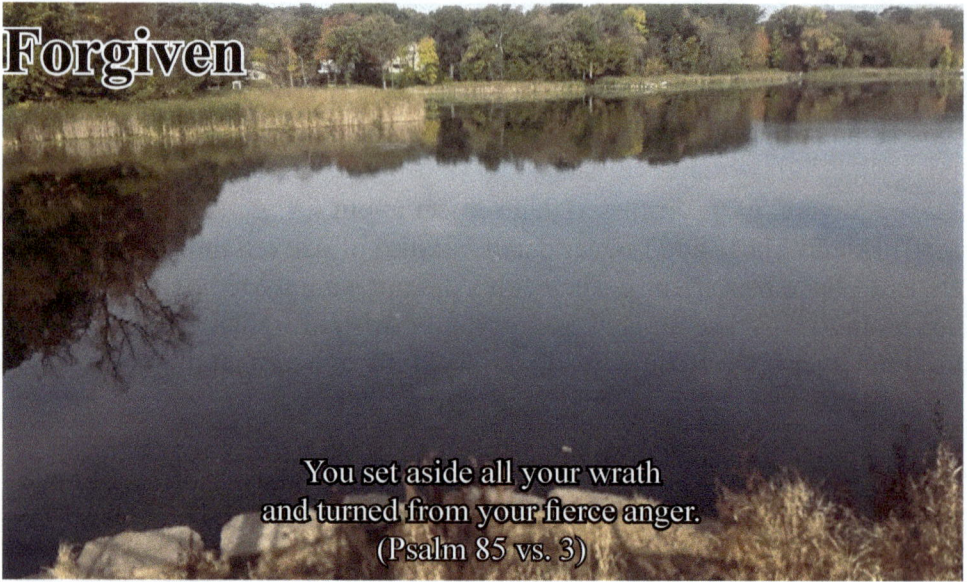

In twelve-step programs, the eighth and ninth steps are about making amends to people. Often these amends are greeted with a curious look because the offended person had forgotten the incident. We are our worst enemies when it comes to forgiveness, and we will forgive others and hold on to our feelings of remorse for years.

It is the sixth week of the New Year, and statistically, 90 percent of New Year's resolutions have fallen by the wayside. Most of the resolutionists are disappointed and sometimes remorseful because they did not make it. Why?

We all need to think about that. It is honorable to try to improve and make resolutions, and it is not dishonorable to not succeed. We need to accept forgiveness and grant it to ourselves; Jesus would.

Thought for Today: For today, let us forgive ourselves for our perceived shortcomings and look forward to our future successes.

Prayer for Today: Heavenly Father, today we pray for our future success. We do your work and do not seem to succeed but know you are with us. We thank you for your patience and forgiveness. Amen

February 19

Gleason Lake
Wayzata, MN

Don't Give Up

**Then Jesus told his disciples...
that they should always pray
and not give up.
(Luke 18 vs 1)**

The entertainment business has a lot of examples of persistence and success, living dreams of fame. To some, it comes fast, and they go from teenager to star. But many others need time to grow into their goal.

Remember Barney Miller, the cop played by Hal Linden? Very few people watching knew that this hilarious cop was a Broadway star. After high school in the 1950s, he spent time as a band singer and chorus member in shows, and his persistence paid off with TV and Broadway shows.

Barbra Streisand did not attend college. After high school, she went to Manhattan and worked from cabaret singer to star.

Barry Manilow differed in that he studied at the New York College of music. However, he still started his career in the bars of New York and wrote jingles for advertising agencies. Developing his skills and using his God-given talents prevailed, and he never gave up.

All of our lives need to start someplace. We often do not control our destiny and need to keep on plugging. Joel Osteen uses the term "…keeps on keeping on." I like, "Today is the first day of the rest of my life." Jesus said, "…always pray and not give up".

Thought for Today: Today, let us focus on what we want to be when we grow up. Our lives are constantly changing; we need to have our faith in hand.

Prayer for Today: Heavenly Father, we learn that life is an endurance event, not a sprint. Today I pray for stamina, guidance, and the patience to keep at it until you deliver me to your place. Amen

Green Heron Pond
Minnesota Landscape Arboretum

Thanks For The Memories

In The name of our Lord Jesus
always give thanks to God the Father.
(Ephesians 5 vs 20)

The following is a personal story that may relate to that.

We recently had the opportunity to have lunch at a seaside restaurant in my hometown of Saugus. We had our first date there in July of1967. This place had a family history. My aunt Virginia was a waitress there in the 40s, and my uncle Ken played guitar in a group there. It was an after-the-ball game hang out for my old gang in the 60s. It was a place with memories for us.

In the '60s, my friend Ralph and I carried too many drunks home. There was Larry, Dave, Pierre, and others. Oh yes, Ralph and I are programmed reformers today. Those are some of the growing pains of the past.

The place was also the start of a great experience; my life with June. I do not think she was very impressed at first. The place smelled of fish. It had uncovered Formica tables, and the crowd did not even come close to that of an English pub. However, the baked stuffed lobster for $ 3.75 and the 25-cent beers were impressive. It was not a place where one would typically go in search of the Lord. Unknowingly, we started our journey with Him that evening. You see, we were not looking, we were not in search of God, but we were open, willing suspects. Paul's message to the Ephesians says, "…Always give thanks for everything to God the father." We do.

Thought for Today: Let us pause when we are stressed out. Take a break from the bad weather, the office stress, the youth sports playoffs, and think back to our blessings. Take a time out each day to thank the Lord for who we are.

Prayer for the Day: Today, Lord, I thank your presence in my life and the many gifts you have given me. Amen

February 21   The Promenade
Torquay, Devon, UK

Washington

"As Mankind becomes more liberal, they will be more apt to allow that all those who conduct themselves as worthy members of the community are equally entitled to the protection of the civil government. I hope ever to see America among the foremost nations of justice and liberality."
George Washington

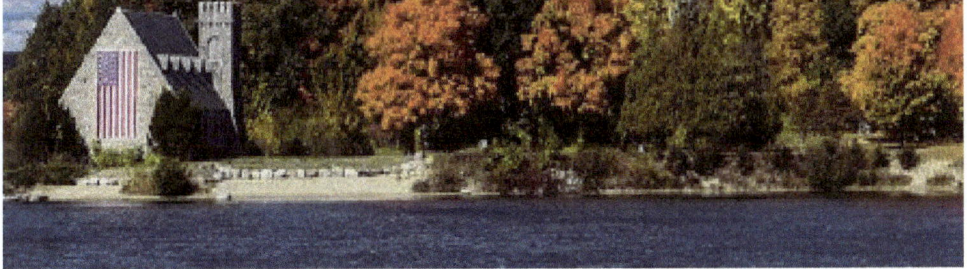

Today is George Washington's Birthday. There are many stories and fables about his life. He allegedly chopped down a Cherry tree and threw a silver dollar across the Potomac. These are unproven myths but great folklore.

It takes a great man to recognize a weak position and make the proper corrections. He was a man of great vision and envisioned that his ragtag army could defeat the British. He realized when he was wrong and intelligent enough to involve the French as allies.

The quote above expresses his dreams for America, and it is also a stated Christian dream delivered through Jesus. Today, our challenge is to accomplish the justice and equality these two men desired. We all need to do a little every day.

Thought for Today: Take a step toward bringing equality and justice to our world.

Prayer for Today: Today, dear Lord, we pray for equality and the opportunity to contribute to creating a just and equal society. Amen

Giving

Each of you should give what you have decided in your heart to give, not reluctantly or under compulsion, For God loves a cheerful giver.
(2 Corinthians 9 vs 8)

There is a feature of retirement that I call "The all I am ever going to have syndrome." I see it all the time in retirees and am fighting it every day in my own life. Dr. Joyce Meyer says that you cannot be selfish and happy.

In our hearts, we would like to give everything away, help people but in practice, we have a bit of the syndrome. As a former financial chair at our church, I need to share two stories. The first was a lady who came forward with a three-year gift that made her our largest giver. It was a significant blessing to the church but an even more incredible blessing for her. Another year a widow called me in December as we were trying to balance the budget and wanted to talk. I was concerned because although she was a lovely lady, we were not close, and she was not the easiest person to approach. We had coffee, and she offered to balance the budget with a five-figure check.

Both of these ladies insisted on absolute confidentiality, and we honored that even down to masking the donations in the accounting system so nobody could trace them. However, we could never hide these generous people's feelings, their smiles, and their enthusiasm. You see, they gave from their hearts and did not hold back.

Today's message is that money is essential, and we need our cash. However, listening to our hearts is also crucial if we are going to be happy and satisfied with our lives

Thought for Today: Today, let us focus on giving to someone.

Prayer for Today: Heavenly Father, today we pray for those in need. We pray that we may recognize that need and contribute to them in some meaningful way. Amen

February 23 The River Nene, Peterborough, Cambridgeshire, UK

Let God Lead

**Commit everything you do to the Lord.
Trust him, and he will help you.
(Psalm 37 vs 5)**

God works in many ways when we allow Him to help us. Yes, he is always there, but not always present in our minds. We have a way of being self-centered, focusing on business issues, personal problems, etc. We want to be in control, and we can deal with it ourselves.

Twelve-step programs focus on spiritual growth and simplify the process with slogans. When we try to control a difficult situation, they advise us to "Let go and let God." Our house had this on a four-inch refrigerator magnet. We tend to be control freaks. Worrying or controlling things outside our sphere of influence will make us "tired, …weak…and worn". (Take My Hand, Nina Simone)

It is easy to become frustrated when things are beyond our control, and it is customary to try to control. It is better to recognize our place and let God take our hand, lead us home.

Thought for Today: Today is the first day of the rest of our lives, and we do not have to function the same way as we did yesterday. Take a look at God's influence on our decisions and allow Him to help us.

Prayer for Today: Heavenly Father, we are concerned about others in our society that have less, some without food, housing, or a job. We are worried about the many people who are afraid they will lose their jobs and security. We pray for our society in general, that somehow everyone can be at peace, that all children have food and that our riches are shared as You would have us share them. Amen

Evening Sky
Minneapolis, Minnesota   **February 24**   Page 57

Let Go

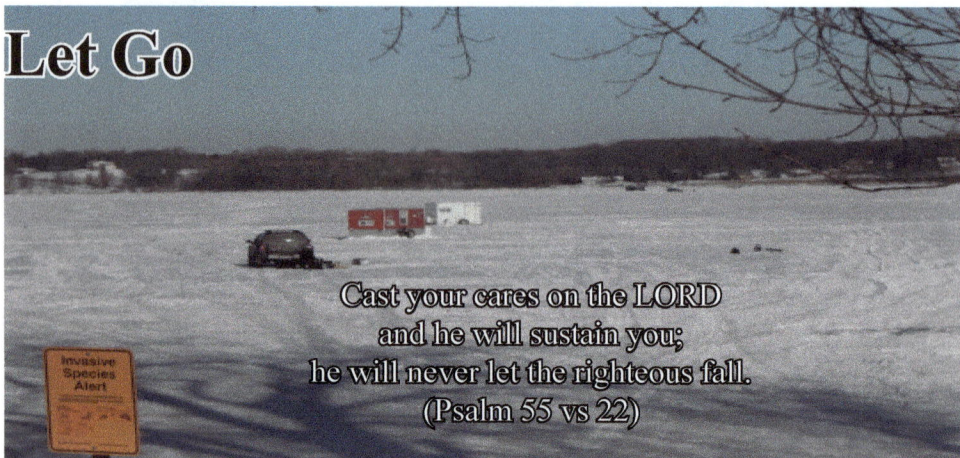

*Cast your cares on the LORD
and he will sustain you;
he will never let the righteous fall.
(Psalm 55 vs 22)*

This week a good friend talked to me about some resentment bothering him. This individual has extreme integrity and was an officer of a corporation. He was let go for taking a stand on the side of ethical and legal corporate behavior. He has a problem forgiving his former associates and is wondering where God is in this equation.

We all need to practice letting go and letting God deal with offenders. For our own sake and the sake of our families, we need to have God deal with our resentments while we look ahead to our future. Keeping grievances inside, holding ill will within us, causes a cumulative effect that hurts those around us. Resentments manifest themselves into anger, sometimes paranoia, and a lack of trust.

As Christians, the Lord will open doors of opportunity when a negative situation occurs in most cases. We need to pray and remember that things happen for reasons we do not often understand. Remember that "…he will never let the righteous fall."

Thought for Today: Today, let us all look toward the future and leave our worries behind. Leave resentments and hurts in the hands of the Lord and focus on taking our lives to a higher level through faith.

Prayer for Today: Today, Lord, we pray for all who are pressured by people of influence to perform in a non-Christian manner. May they find a way to keep their Christian ethics and their career. Amen

February 25 Medicine Lake, Plymouth, Minnesota.

God's Love and Grace

Know therefore that the LORD your God is God;
He is the faithful God,
(Deuteronomy 7 vs 9)

June and I are close to people of varied faiths. We believe that all worship the same God in different ways, and experience God's grace.

Several years ago, we became good friends with the family of an executive from Pakistan, and it was our first real close relationship with a Muslim family. We were close to them in 2001 and observed the frustration that a true Muslim felt regarding September 11.

Recently, a Jewish friend whom I have known and liked for years shared that he does bible studies to learn about the Christian perspective. His strong family values, general upbeat personality, and strong ethical standards make him someone I am glad to know.

To avoid making this a 10,000-word essay, let me summarize some of our other relationships: A son in law who is a Southern Baptist, a brother in law who is a Catholic priest in the UK, a Buddhist sister-in- law, a Mormon best friend who lost touch with his faith, a Native Amercan friend who has involved us in some spiritual activities.

In each instance mentioned, June and I have experienced good friendships and observed solid, godly values in our friends. We have observed God working in our friends' lives in most instances and see God's grace at work in many ways. Most importantly, we have experienced God's grace through our friends.

Thought for the Day: Recognize those around us that are different and try to befriend someone new. Seek out someone that looks at God differently. The Lord blesses them also.

Prayer for the Day: Dear faithful Lord and Father, the world is an incredible and wonderful creation. There are many peoples of all colors and beliefs. We pray the ability to bring unity to the world. Amen

Tamaracs
Minnesota Landscape Arboretum   **February 26**   Page 59

Commitment

Whatever your lips utter,
you must be sure to do.
(Deuteronomy 23 vs 23)

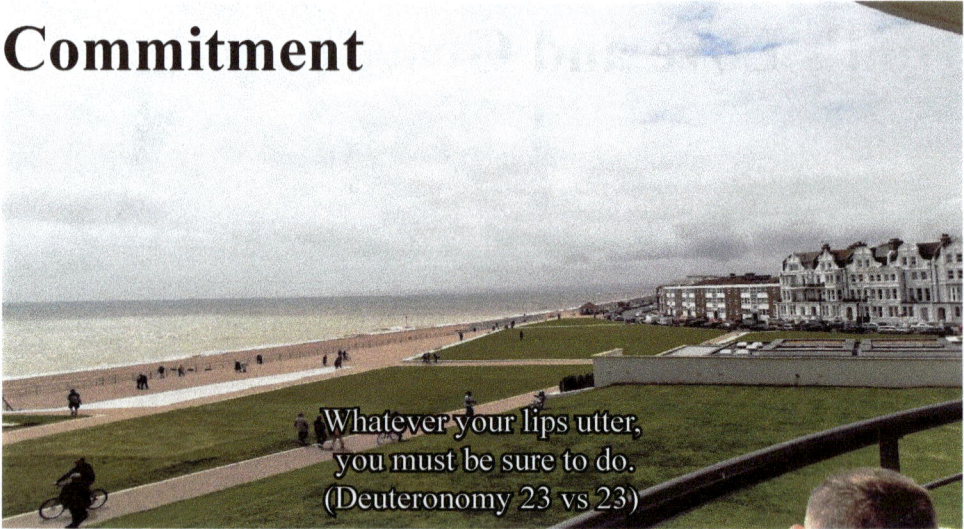

One of the ways to be successful in life is to keep all of your commitments. If you say it, make sure you do it, even after having second thoughts. Become known as one hundred percent reliable. It is probably impossible, but the closer you are, the more you will benefit.

Do you have friends who cancel at the last minute? …show up late? …or not at all? Are you one that lives that way? We all have missed a few deadlines, and some make it a lifestyle. At work or in business commitment is even more critical. On the job, it can determine your future success or failure. In sales, it generally means to win or lose. Abraham Lincoln said it this way, "Commitment is what transforms a promise into reality."

At some time in your life, you committed to God. Today we have the opportunity to review that commitment and recharge our batteries, stay engaged, and on track in a world of distractions.

Thought for Today: Today, be committed. First to God and then to ourselves by being the best we can be.

Prayer for Today: Dear Lord and Father, today we thank you for our many blessings. We give thanks for being Godly people that will be accepted and liked by others. Our families, friends, and people that we do not know yet. Amen

February 27 Sky over Bexhill on Sea
East Sussex, UK

He Comes Through

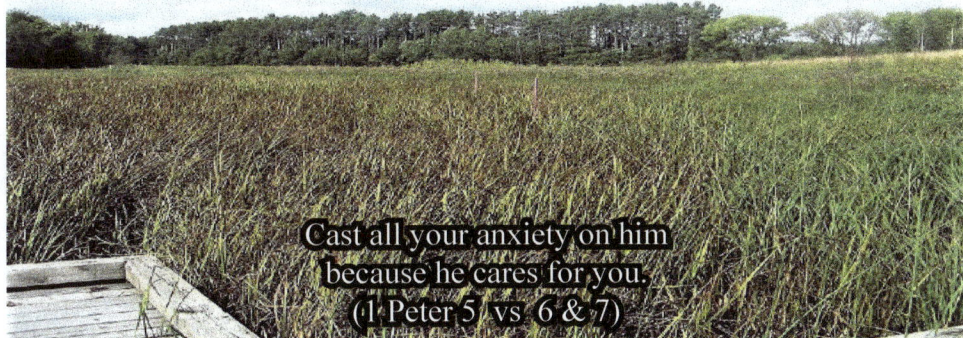

Cast all your anxiety on him
because he cares for you.
(1 Peter 5 vs 6 & 7)

Grand events are lovely. We just took three family matriarchs, octogenarians, out to lunch, my mom for her 89th birthday, and two aunts from her generation. It is always great to hear them reminisce about old times.

All three have gone through good times and bad. They were all widows, and there were new knees and hips at the table and a lot of arthritis. But wow, that was not the conversation. There was an attitude of joy and pleasure, smiles all around. The good times were the focus.

It was February in New England, the roads were terrible, and it was snowing. There were opportunities for sadness. Each was nearing an end of life experience, and the lunch was in a nursing home, and one had a son with terminal cancer. It was a festive lunch reminiscing about their lives and families.Great moments of joy are a gift from God. Seek them out, and enjoy them.

Thought for Today: Today, let us focus on casting away our angst and turning our lives over to the Lord. Let us mainly focus on the older generation, and let us reach out to them with love and share the good times.

Prayer for Today: Heavenly Father, we pray for ourselves, our friends, and our loved ones. Many are ill and experiencing fear, uncertainty, loneliness, or hurt. Many need You in their lives and have not found You. We pray that we may be the conduit that strengthens their faith and eases anxieties. We pray for a way to do your will in this way. Amen

Paul's Sales Training

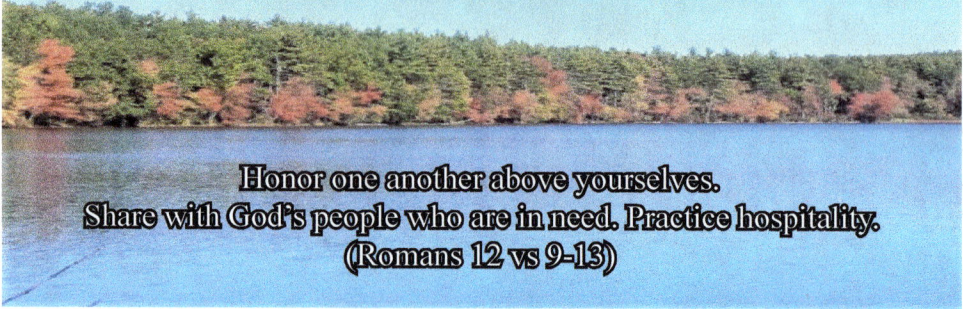

**Honor one another above yourselves.
Share with God's people who are in need. Practice hospitality.
(Romans 12 vs 9-13)**

Paul's message to the Romans has a lot to it, and it is an excellent way to live your life. Today, I share a personal story about my sales mentor and trainer, George. In the years he spent training me, he sounded just like Paul in his message to the Romans. He would not tolerate sales bluster- he always was sincere and expected the same from me.

George did not like evil, like late deliveries, a bad product, or cheating on pricing- he liked what was good; fair deals, integrity, and ethics. He taught me to respect and honor both the manufacturer and the customer and that they had to come before me- that was not always easy.

Verses eleven and twelve have to do with keeping a positive attitude, a difficult thing in life, especially in sales. No salesman has more than half of the market share, so they lose more than they win by definition. We had about a ten percent share in my business, so we lost nine out of ten. With that said, George taught me always to be upbeat, "Never be lacking in zeal… Be joyful in hope, patient in affliction."

George was not a church person; just a great guy sent to me by God to be my mentor. We now have a different relationship, friends of each other, of the Lord and Jesus. I will hear from him when he reads this.

Thought for Today: Focus on Paul's important message in verses 11 and 12. Keep our attitude upbeat so that we may positively affect those around us.

Prayer for Today: Dear Lord and Father, we thank our mentors, those who have influenced our lives, including Jesus, Paul, and all you sent to guide us. Amen

February 29 West Waushacum Pond
Sterling, Massachusetts

March

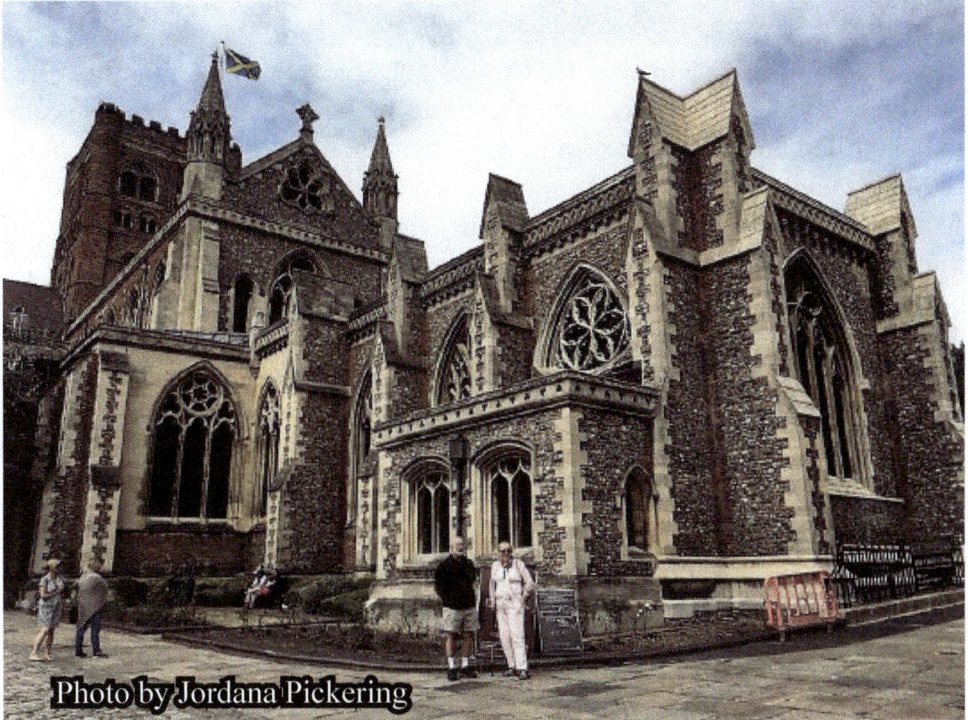

Photo by Jordana Pickering

St. Albans Cathedral
St. Albans Cathedral exists to glorify God and proclaim Christ's message of love.

A Still Place

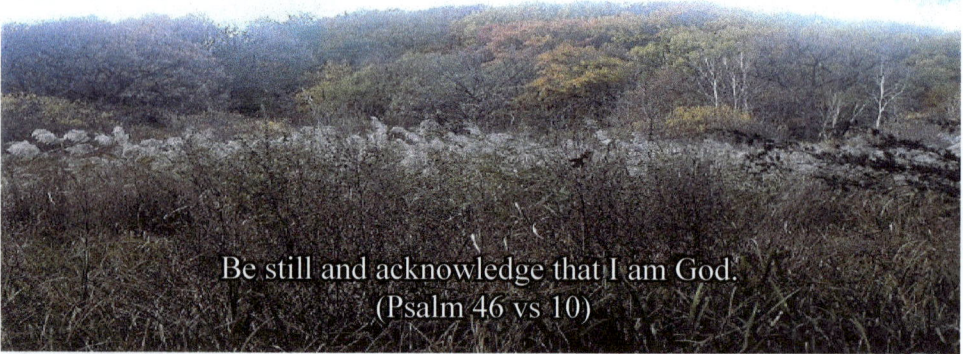

Be still and acknowledge that I am God.
(Psalm 46 vs 10)

The world is a busy place. Americans are overbooked; families are tied up every day with career and children's activities; empty-nesters seem to have filled the time with commitments; often, retirees do not know how they ever had time to work! That leads to a lot of stress, tension, and often family failures. That's correct; the family that plays too much together may not have enough quality time to survive. They do not have time to call for help.

In his book Bread for the Table, Henry Nouwen says it this way, "These are words to take with us in our busy lives. We may think about stillness in contrast to our noisy world. But perhaps we can go further and keep an inner stillness even while we carry on … It is important to keep a still place in the "marketplace." This still place is where God can dwell and speak to us. …with that stillness, God can be our gentle guide in everything we think and do."

Do you have a still place? How do you keep your sanity?

Thought for Today: War, sickness and other varied conditions in our world are causing many of our friends and neighbors to go through unplanned changes in their lives. Let us pray that God will be a presence in their lives as they pursue the opportunities presented to them.

Prayer for Today: Heavenly Father, the world around us is confusing, sometimes cruel, and always challenging to understand. Please allow us time to step aside and dwell upon "your will" rather than "our wants and needs." Let us find the peace or stillness to allow "thy will to be done on earth as it is in heaven." Amen

Raising Expectations

> "...set your hearts on things above, where Christ is seated at the right hand of God. Set your minds on things above, not on earthly things. (Colossians 3 vs 1,2)

We have talked about how the head and heart lead our bodies. How often our thoughts may be negative, leading us to depression. Let's face it, when we read or listen to the news, they talk primarily about adverse events. However, most of what goes on in the world is positive. We need to focus on that!

Billy Rose wrote the words to the old song, Great Day, "When you're down and out, lift your head and shout. It's going to be a great day." Sometimes we meet up with the local curmudgeon, the person who finds fault with everything. Let's face it, they are correct. It is always too hot or too cold. Too rainy, or their lawn needs watering. Things are too expensive, and coffee is too weak or strong. Pray for them; they need us.

We will have negative influences in our lives, but we have the tools to deal with them in our lives. I read this on a sign in front of a local church recently, "The Lord does not guarantee us smooth passage, just a safe landing." It is up to us to use our Christian tools to stay positive and be happy.

Thought for Today: Today, we will have to deal with negative issues. Let us turn them into a positive experience by acting promptly.

Prayer for Today: Today is the day you have made for us. Unfortunately, the roads have bumps, and there are unknown troubles out there awaiting us. Today we pray that your presence will guide us through the challenging moments. Amen

Life of Victory

Blessed is the man who remains steadfast under trial, for when he has stood the test, he will receive the crown of life, which God has promised to those who love him.
(James 1vs 12-14)

The elderly can often be curmudgeons, maybe angry. They are focusing on the past rather than the joys they have now. A good goal in life is to have your grandchildren remember you as happy, content, and proud.

Life comes at us in waves or phases; the rapid learning years of childhood and youth; the wealth-building, family, or working years; the secure phase or empty-nesting; the retirement years winding down to an end of life experience! Each stage is unique, different, and memorable, filled with both joy and sorrow, and that is life.

We make choices with our focus. We could always use more money, more company, less pain in our joints, etc. Every day of our lives, the sun will rise and set; we will wake and sleep. The Lord will be with us, and we will have great memories of our past. Focus on them! Television evangelists, Joel Osteen, likes to say, "Keep on keeping on!"

Thought for Today: Negative influences will occur, and we can either dwell on them or deal with them. Today, let us focus on moving on with our lives and faith.

Prayer for Today: Dear Lord and Father, the world is full hate. There is trouble in the mid-east, deranged people shooting up our sacred institutions and some awful winter weather. We pray for the ability to understand it all and put it into the context of your plan. We offer special prayers for the older generation as they move onward. We pray for peace, understanding our place in your world. Amen

March 3 Lake of the Isles
Minneapolis, Minnesota

Spring

Let my teaching fall like rain, and my words descend like dew, like showers on new grass, like abundant rain on tender plants. (Deuteronomy 32 vs 2)

Spring is an excellent time of the year. In the north, we enjoy the transition from winter wonderland to green, and in the desert, we transition from the rainy season to a desert bloom. Longer days bring brightness to our lives. In its simplest form, children can play outside after dinner in the daylight. (So can mom and dad.)

In spring, we become affected by positive energy. We see more smiles on people's faces and interact with neighbors. We can visibly see the work of the Lord at work, appreciate his blessings, and renew our faith.

Thought for Today: Today, let us all observe and enjoy the wonders of spring, appreciate the many things being reborn, and feed off of the Lord's energy and beauty of spring.

Prayer for Today: Dear Lord and Father, today we give thanks for the rebirth of spring flowers, green grasses, and the blessings of warmer weather. Thank you for these reminders of your love and power. We thank you for always being with us.
Amen

Lake of the Isles
Minneapolis, Minnesota

March 4

Grow Rich

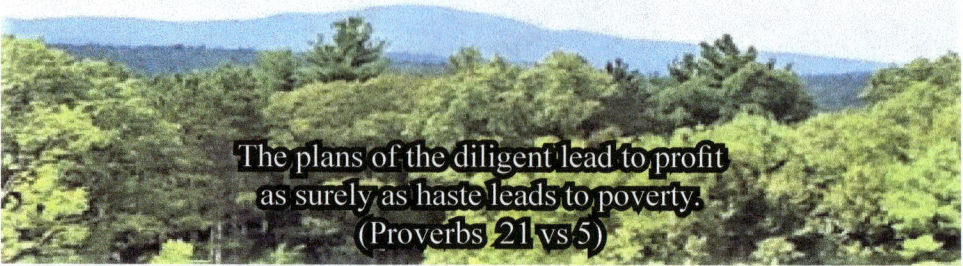

> The plans of the diligent lead to profit
> as surely as haste leads to poverty.
> (Proverbs 21 vs 5)

In his book, Think and Grow Rich, Napoleon Hill stated, "A quitter never wins, and a winner never quits." Today we live in a fast paced society that seems to demand instant gratification. In the business world, everyone is looking for the"low hanging fruit"; the diet fads are advertising fast weight reduction. We want what we want when we want it and often fail to be diligent, persistent, and patient.

In the eighties, sales trainer Ty Boyd did a presentation called "The Life Plan" about making a plan for life as we do for business. He preached that we needed to set goals for life and focus on attaining those goals.

A vital factor in keeping a life plan in order is spirituality. It gives us the ability to focus on the good rather than reacting to negative issues. Having the ability to forgive and pray helps us get through tough times and focus on the plan. In verse twelve, Paul advises, "Never be lacking in zeal, but keep your spiritual fervor, serving the Lord. Be joyful in hope, patient in affliction, faithful in prayer." That needs to be a part of every life plan.

Thought for Today: Remember where we want to go. There will be both positive and negative distractions. Give thanks when things go as planned and pray when they do not.

Prayer for Today: Dear Lord, we are busy working on our plan every day. We pray for success, positive memories, and that our plan fits your plan. Amen

March 5   Mount Wachusett from Tower Hill
West Boylston, Massachusetts

Friend, Spouse ?

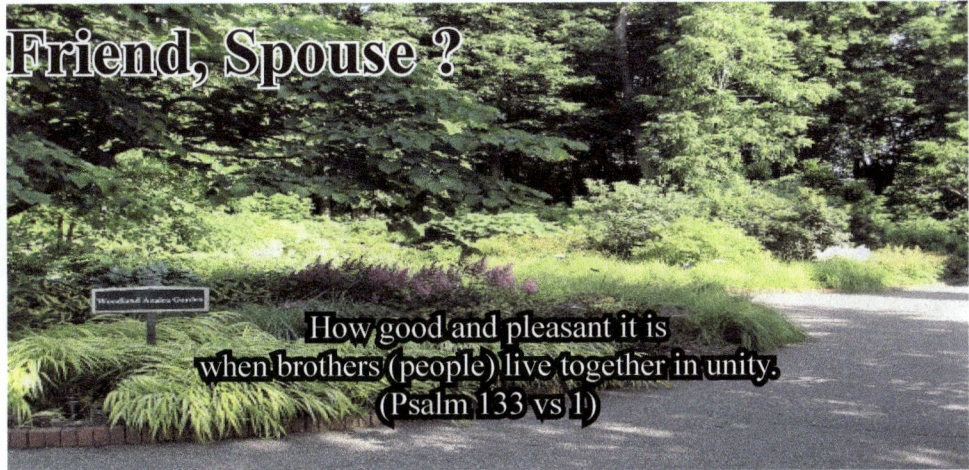

How good and pleasant it is
when brothers (people) live together in unity.
(Psalm 133 vs 1)

Did you marry your best friend? Can you still phone your best friend from high school? Or does the psalmist above mean those we interact with now? The ideal answer is yes to all the above.

In his book The Seven Stages of Marriage, Keith Brown lists them as; Passion, Realization, Rebellion, Cooperation, Reunion, Explosion, Completion. We will not address these today but list them to reinforce that marriage is hard work and will not always feel like unity.

Love is the most important commandment in life, family, and marriage. Sometimes couples do not agree, and need to find a way to be "…together in unity".

The psalmist may not have talked about marriage, and his words are valid in relationships, work, church, neighborhoods, etc. We need to live in harmony and focus on being good friends to make that happen.

Thought for Today: Focus on working on being a good friend; in the workplace, the neighborhood, at church, and home; focus on sharing our space with others in unity.

Prayer for Today: Dear Lord, we pray that you help us become better friends to those around us. You are with us, and we pray that your light shines through us and on our friends. Amen

Hope Through Prayer

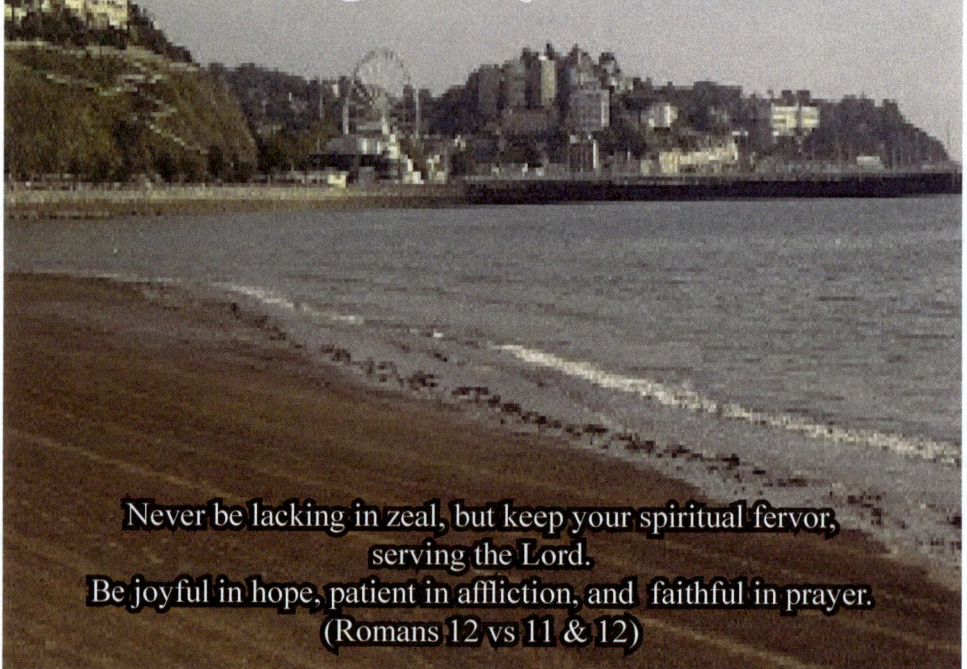

Never be lacking in zeal, but keep your spiritual fervor,
serving the Lord.
Be joyful in hope, patient in affliction, and faithful in prayer.
(Romans 12 vs 11 & 12)

Hold on to your faith; keep holding on. When the going gets tough, when choices are hard, when the stress builds, pray about it; turn it over to God. Paul's letters repeat that time after time, and often we do not hear it. Our faith is not always strong, and we can be confused.

He talks about a great way to get through a day, week, or month in his message above. He is preaching a way of life through faith to confidence and peace.

Memorize this one, try it, and you will like it.

Thought for Today: Let's attack today with "fervor," being "joyful," and by all means prayerfully.

Prayer for Today: Dear Lord, we give thanks for the day you have made for us to have. We thank you for the opportunity to do your will and contribute to each other's peace. Amen

March 7 Torre Abby Sands
Torquay, Devon, UK

Motivation

I saw that there is nothing better than that all should enjoy their work, for that is their lot;
who can bring them to see what will be after them?
(Ecclesiastes 3 vs 22)

Books on business often point out that no long-term, overachieving salesperson does it for money. The stresses of sales, the treatment received from the public, dealing with suppliers' failure to meet the customer's expectations are not worth the money. Long-term overachieving salespeople somehow believe they are helping others. Many believe that God blesses them for the opportunity to contribute.

With all that stated, greed can slide into the equation, and when it does, the situation gets ugly When money tilts our lives out of balance, we spin out of control. We will thump along out of sync with our faith like a bad tire on a car. We will wear out quickly if we don't re-align and balance our lives.

Democracy and free enterprise encourage competition and overwork. Motivation is good. Working hard is the American way, but we also need balance. Jesus' words in Luke 12:15 state, "Take care. Be on guard against all kinds of greed…." Motivation is good when it is pure; balance always needs to be at the forefront.

Thought for Today: Focus on our balance, communicate with our loved ones, and be sure that our lives are running without unnecessary bumps. Keep our spirit, mind, and body in harmony with Jesus' teachings

Prayer for Today: Dear Lord and Father, today we give thanks for all we have received and have. We pray that you will guide us through the maze of life to contribute to doing your will here on earth. Amen

Gleason Lake
Minnetonka, Minnesota
March 8
Page 71

Endurance and Life

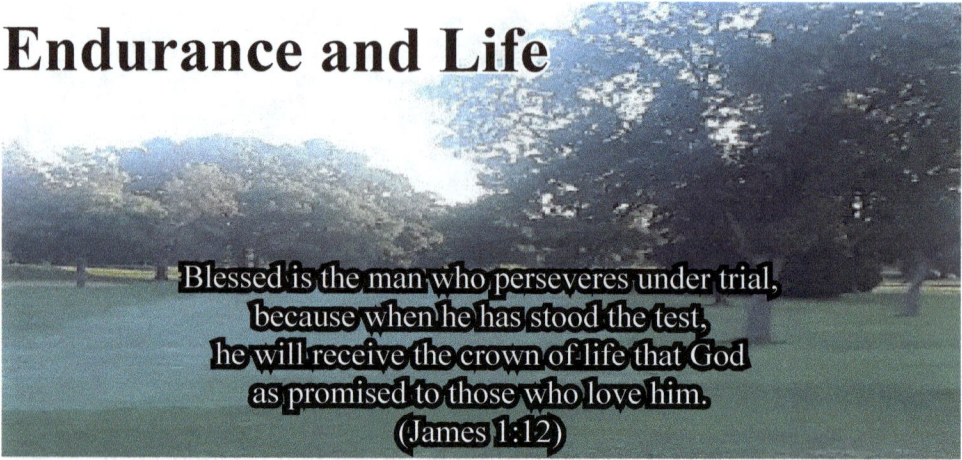

Blessed is the man who perseveres under trial,
because when he has stood the test,
he will receive the crown of life that God
as promised to those who love him.
(James 1:12)

In our seemingly endless search for tranquility, we tend to "want what we want, when want it." We want our victories to come via the easy route, rarely a reality. Life is not a sprint; it is an endurance event, a marathon.

As an amateur triathlete, getting to the starting line took hours of practice, alone; sometimes in pain; in all weather. What for? Why do that? In a typical triathlon one experiences anticipation and excitement during the national anthem. A feeling of spirituality during the blessing. There was a period of fear during the swim in all my races. Boredom, pain, doubt, and an entire array of other feelings occur during the bike ride and run. Then comes the good time, the approach to the finish line.

The finish line generally has a crowd of 5,000 to 20,000 spectators. Positive energy radiates out to be absorbed by the competitors. My fellow racers agree that the feeling of finishing, accomplishment, and of course, just being done, is special. Many finish with tears of joy in their eyes. I hope that you can see the parallel between racing and life. Be patient, meet challenges, and look forward to receiving your "crown of life."

Thought for Today: There is too much to do, too much work, not enough playtime. Today, look toward the future, knowing that patience and perseverance will bring us tranquility and happiness.

Prayer for Today: Heavenly Father, we pray for patience to discover your will, the courage to implement it, and the knowledge to recognize your presence in our lives. Amen

March 9 Brookview Golf Course
Golden Valley, Minnesota

Draw Near To God

..let us draw near to God
with a sincere heart in full assurance of faith...
(Hebrews 10 vs 19)

We often slip into moods that weaken our spirituality and faith. Fear, anger, and lack of trust (doubt) often get more attention than they deserve in life. It is normal to let negativity dominate our thoughts, but it is not a healthy way to live.

"Each morning we are born again.
What we do today is what matters most."
Buddha

There is a high percentage of unhappy people within the elder community, even angry. As they get closer to their end-of-life experience, they are anxious, while others seem loving and at peace. The difference appears to be acceptance through spirituality. Acceptance of the mystery of life, the words of Jesus seem to make the difference.

We need to live somehow closer to Jesus' example, forgive, and believe that peace will come out of this life. Draw nearer to God. Spirituality and faith are works in progress. Let God take our hand to find peace and tranquility and continue spiritual growth.

Thought for Today: Let's selfishly believe about ourselves and our faith. There will be opportunities to be angry and frustrated. When that occurs, act more like Jesus and "draw near to God with a sincere heart in full assurance of faith... ".

Prayer for Today: We pray for our world leaders; that the world draws near to you and that peace will prevail. Amen

Judgements

Do not judge, or you too will be judged.
For in the same way you judge others,
you will be judged, and with the measure you use,
it will be measured to you.
(Matthew 7 vs 1-3)

We often judge others based on an impression that did not fit our personal model. As Christians, our model is trusting and we expect others to be honorable.

Often, we observe an impression of others that generates doubt in our minds. It may be their dress, a display of anger or aggression, or something they said. We make judgments without drilling into and knowing the person's inner self. Sometimes that is referred to as a snap judgment. It is an error when we judge others this way.

What we know as Christians is that it is not our place to judge, and it is our place to accept, forgive, and love. When someone or something in our lives is unacceptable and needs to be changed, we need to change it Christianly. That means with love, compassion, and often prayer.

Thought for Today: We will need to make many choices as we go through the day. As we interact with others, we try to accept rather than judge. Work with them, help them when we can, and take them for who they are.

Prayer for Today: Dear Lord, we are concerned about world health and terror. Governments make judgments that we do not understand. We pray that we, the people, may find a way to support your ways rather than the ways of governments and worldly forces. We search for solutions through prayer and meditation. Amen

Fitness 1

You made all the delicate, inner parts of my body and knitted them together in my mother's womb.
(Psalm 139 vs 13)

Today I want to address the body rather than the mind. We are an incredible machine/animal, born with feelings, the intellect to apply logic to our lives, and without sin. For most, it is all downhill from there. Society allows us to pursue pleasure through wealth, eating great foods, and entertaining ourselves while sitting down. The pure hearts we were born with become hidden by our pursuit of worldly materials, and the "…the delicate, inner parts…" become hidden with excess weight.

TV personality Johnny Carson summarized reviewing his old family photo albums as watching himself gain and lose a thousand pounds. He meant to be funny, but there is a truth to his humor. Being physically fit, flexible and pain-free is a dream and a worthwhile goal that most do not attain.

My warning today is not about exercise but weight and eating. It is something like this: In your 50s, you can only eat two-thirds as much as you did in your 20s. Also, in your 80s, if you get that far, you will only be able to consume two-thirds of that. Ouch! Yes, a Pickeringism on eating.

Thought for Today: Today, let us focus on our physical selves. Let us be as good as we can be. Let's park a bit further from the door, say no thanks to the dessert tray, walk the stairs as we are able.

Prayer for Today: Father, we give thanks for who and what we are and the many helpers you have sent us along the way. Amen

Flowering Crabapple
Minnesota Landscape Arboretum

March 12

Page 75

Fitness II

"Thank you for making me so wonderfully complex...
Your workmanship is marvelous."
(Psalm 139 vs 14)

Today I write about two of my spirit, mind, and body mentors.

Bob D is a friend in Christ I met in my years of excessive training for triathlons and running. He once had a business career, but that went away, and he became a personal trainer. There was a challenging transition from commercial cash flow to a club trainer. His strength and faith have kept him a positive role model, and he has contributed to people as both a social and physical example. People emulating his example will be better for it in spirit, mind, and body in challenging times.

George was a church elder who impressed me when we started attending church here in Minnesota. He was a leader to emulate and a blessing in Friday bible studies. and a positive example of fitness and spirituality. Early on, I can remember sitting in an annual meeting hoping that someday I could contribute as much to the church.

In summary, the Lord gave us marvelous equipment and opportunity, and he supplies ongoing help. We need to take care of our spirit, mind, and bodies in His name.

Thought for Today: Today, let us focus on our physical selves. Let us be as good as we can be. Let's park a bit further from the door, say no thanks to the dessert tray, walk the stairs as we are able.

Prayer for Today: Father, we give thanks for who and what we are and the many helpers you have sent us along the way. Amen

March 13 The Green Heron Pond in Winter
Minnesota Landscape Arboretum

Be Positive

Therefore encourage one another and build each other up, just as you are doing. (1 Thessalonians 5 vs 11)

Our coach was a negative motivator in my high school years of football. It seemed everything we did was wrong. The compliments we received were a "good job, but...". The criticism after 'the but" was all that most of us ever remembered. None of us believed that we were very good and we were not having any fun. In 1956, three of us quit the team to go to private schools for various reasons. There was an extensive article in the local paper about how significant a loss was to the local high school team because they lost some great players. We were all surprised at the compliments given to us by the coach.

I found my way to a swim coach named Al Houston at my new school. Al was a caring man, a positive motivator, and would have two or three swimmers at each Olympic games. The team all felt good and worked hard. We liked Al and each other. We were also the best team in the northeast. We learned to care about excellence, not letting each other down, and generally care about each other.

We need to follow the lead of Christ, stay positive, and demonstrate our love and caring during these challenging times.

Thought for Today: Today, we will have the opportunity to be negative. When that happens, stop and meditate, *"Therefore encourage one another and build each other up."* Let's have great day.

Prayer for Today: Heavenly Father, we pray for those with unhealthy ideas and aggression toward humans and their victims. We pray for them and the opportunity to influence them positively. Amen

Thankfulness

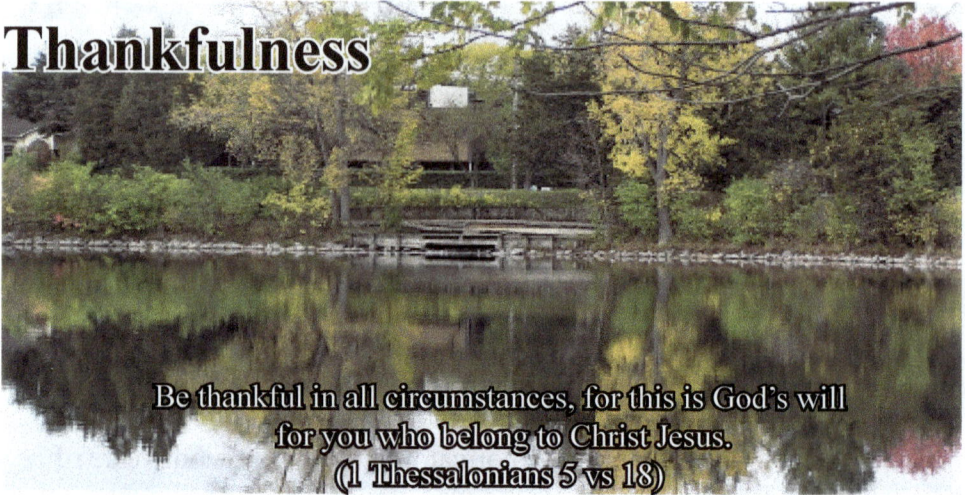

**Be thankful in all circumstances, for this is God's will for you who belong to Christ Jesus.
(1 Thessalonians 5 vs 18)**

It is sometimes hard to be thankful and gracious. Often, we have a problem seeing reasons to be grateful. The human-animal has a beautiful way of focusing on the negative and not remembering the Lord's gifts.

June and I visited my brother Wayne when cancer had metastasized into his bones and he was nearing his end of life experience. We reviewed our lives through the memories of our swimming careers, recalling the people and competitions we shared. The Tufts University staff had made a gift honoring him as his era's top swimmer, and we delivered it to him, which triggered an upbeat afternoon of fond memories.

When things are bleak, we need to focus on our blessings. God is with us and wants us happy under all conditions. "Let us then approach the throne of grace with confidence, so that we may receive mercy and find grace to help us in pour time of need" (Hebrews 4v16) and "Give thanks… because of what the Lord has done for us."

Thought for Today: Today let us acknowledge and recognize our blessings. Things will not go perfect, and something will surely go wrong. Let us choose to turn the negativity over to God and thank the Lord for the good times.

Prayer for Today: Dear Lord, we ask for special prayers for those with severe illnesses. We pray for their peace and tranquility and the ability to support them with your help. Amen

March 15 Cedar Lake
Minneapolis, Minnesota

Live in Peace

Live in peace with each other. ...be patient with everyone.
Be joyful always; pray continually;
...give thanks in all circumstances.
(1 Thessalonians 5 vs 16- Be joyful always; pray continual-

Each week our pastor starts with similar words. Something like, "We gather together to celebrate what we know is true; Our God is a loving and caring God who loves all humanity." We were made in his image so hold that thought.

If we accept those statements as truths, why are we sometimes resentful, angry, depressed, and concerned? Indeed, none of us are perfect, and we have these emotions and thoughts. If we could "...Live in peace with each other. ...be patient with everyone..." we would be meeting God's expectations and free ourselves of many of the anxieties of life. Paul, in his letter, tells us how "...Be joyful always; pray continually; give thanks in all circumstances..."

Thought for Today: Today, things will not always go in our favor, and we will have opportunities to be resentful or angry. We must choose to be thankful, caring, and joyful. In the words of Nike, "Just do it."

Prayer for Today: Dear Lord, our world seems to have slipped into a hate-driven society. Around the world, there are wars, terrorism, and discrimination based on too many issues. We are confused by it all. Today we pray for some understanding, knowledge of your role in this, and insight into how we should react. We pray that each of us may find a way to contribute to a joyful and peaceful society. Amen

St. Patrick's Day

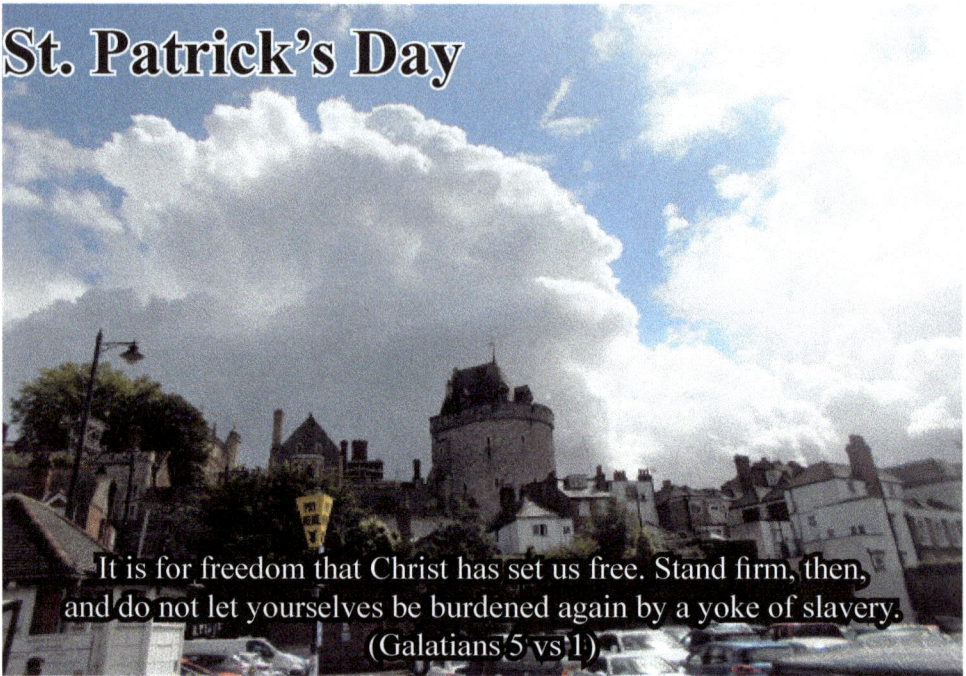

It is for freedom that Christ has set us free. Stand firm, then, and do not let yourselves be burdened again by a yoke of slavery.
(Galatians 5 vs 1)

There was always a large St Patrick's Day parade and celebration when growing up in Boston. It was great fun, mythical fun without a grain of truth to it. There were stories about a saint who drove the snakes out of Ireland, green beer, and buttons that said everyone was Irish today.

Wikipedia does not mention green beer or parades but tells of a great man who converted a country. St Patrick was an Irish saint who lived from 387 to 461. He is credited with bringing Christianity to Ireland. He allowed the Irish to become free of their demons (maybe snakes?) and experience the grace of Christ. We need to honor him for that today.

Thought for Today: Today, let us honor a person who spread our faith and the grace of Jesus to the heathen population. Maybe by drinking a toast with green beer.

Prayer for Today: Dear Lord and Father, we thank Saint Patrick and the many saints of the first millennium. They brought the grace of Christ to the world and made our lives special. We pray that, in some way, we carry on their work. Amen

March 17

Castle in the Storm
Windsor, Berkshire, UK

Old Salt

You are the salt of the earth. But if the salt loses its saltiness, how can it be made salty again? It is no longer good for anything except to be thrown out and trampled underfoot.
(Matthew 5 vs 13)

We know that the Romans used salt as money. It was life-giving, necessary for survival, and needed by everyone. So when Matthew called us the salt of the earth, it is a high compliment; praise in its highest form. It was one of my grandfather's favorite expressions, but he used it sparingly, and you had to do something well to hear it.

I considered leaving out the "no longer good" lines but changed my mind. There is in my thoughts no person who should be "thrown out and trampled." Somehow, we all have hope, and as Christians, part of our task on earth is helping people, preventing them from being "trampled." Our mission is first to be strong in our spirituality and faith and offer it to others through invitation. Demonstrate that we are at peace and invite people to join us.

Unlike commercial and sea salt, a person can be made salty again by becoming infected with the spirit.

Thought for Today: Today, we will meet someone who is down spiritually, and we will have a choice to talk and invite or turn the other cheek and do our own thing. For today and every day, let's try to help through invitation.

Prayer for Today: Heavenly Father, today is a great day, you made it for us, and we will use it for you. Today we give thanks for the opportunity to help others to recharge their saltiness. Amen

Magnolia In Bloom
Minnesota Landscape Arboretum

Hope

God, fill them with all hope, joy, and peace that they may abound in hope by the power of the Holy Spirit...
(Romans 15 vs 13)

There must be some lucky guy out there married to a woman named Hope. Isn't that a great thought; awakening every morning with hope, drinking morning coffee with hope; never being too far from thinking about hope? The reality is that we can be all those things because the Lord is always with us, and hope abounds through Him.

Losing hope in today's world is easier than having a hopeful mindset. Focusing on the positive gives us hope and feeds positive thoughts. Norman Vincent Peale, in his book, "The power of Positive Thinking," said it like this, "Change your thoughts, and you change your world."

One of the most incredible things about being a Christian is having hope. When we look toward the future, we must remember Proverb 23 verse 18. "There is surely a future hope for you, and your hope will not be cut off."

Thought for Today: Let today be a day of hope and light.
Prayer for Today: Dear Lord and Father, we give thanks for our everlasting hope and joy available to us through Jesus. We look forward to a day that we can contribute by showing others the way by example through our hope and light. Amen

Pope Francis Said:
Hope is bold. It can look beyond convenience
And open us up to grand ideals that make life beautiful and
Worthwhile. Advance along the paths of hope.

March 19

Tower Hill Garden
West Boylston, Massachusetts

Good Things Happen

And we know that in all things God works for the good of those who love him.
(Romans 8 vs 28)

Each day is an excellent opportunity for us. Paul said, "God works for the good of those who love him." Yes, each morning, we chose from our many options. Classic options are the TV news, the newspapers, daily meditation or prayer, and exercise. Each of us needs to choose every day or go back to bed.

The sun will rise tomorrow and every other day, and how we greet it is our choice. Not all days will go our way. If they did, Rabbi Harold Kushner's book "Bad Things Happen to Good People" never would have been written. Maybe each day when we wake up, before the newspaper and TV, before the exercise, perhaps we need to remind the Lord we love Him.

Cat Steven's song "Morning has Broken" finishes with "Praise with elation, praise every morning, God's re-creation of a new day." Yes, tomorrow shows promise through God's love, and we need to accept it and move ahead.

Thought for Today: Today, let us look forward to the sunrise and the opportunity of each new day. Let's bring the Lord with us, let him support us, and let us give thanks for His presence in our lives.

Prayer for Today: Dear Lord and Father, today we are blessed with another day. We pray that we may use it to spread your word and blessings.Amen

Tower Hill Garden
West Boylston, Massachusetts

March 20

New Beginnings

I press on toward the goal to win the prize for which God has called me heavenward in Christ Jesus. (Philippians 3 vs 14)

Those of you that have known me long enough understand that on March 21, 1978, my family and I started a true "New Beginning." I started treatment for alcohol abuse and adopted the slogan, "This is the first day of the rest of your life." They supported me, as did my friends and business associates. Each year, we can have a good life through faith and friendship. I thank all of you that have been my friends and associates since then.

Recovery stories are repeated in our society every day with the grace of God ever-present in the process. Often as Christians, we see a need and get a chance to help. One of the beauties of being Christian is the act of helping.

Thought for Today: Today, we will be out in the world interacting with friends and business associates. We may see a need to help, and many people will back away. Let us recognize needs in others and step forward with God's support and offer the Christian assistance that is needed.

Prayer for Today: This week is the Serenity Prayer:
"God grant me the serenity
to accept the things I can not change,
the courage to change the things I can,
and the wisdom to know the difference."

My blessings to all of you.
Bob

March 21

Granite Pier from Back Beach
Rockport, Massachusetts

Worst Enemy

*Wash away all my iniquity and cleanse me from my sin.
For I know my transgressions, and my sin is always before me.
(Psalm 51 vs 2, 3)*

Self-forgiveness is always a challenge. My worst characteristic is holding on to my transgressions and errors, feeling bad about things that happened 50 years ago! I believe that most people are that way, but I pray that they are not.

In twelve-step recovery programs making amends to people you may have harmed is part of the process. Working with people over the years has shown me that at least half of those contacted do not remember the offense! That has always intrigued me. If my first statement is a fact, at least half of our internal remorse is unnecessary. We hang on to things that do not matter; we are our own worst enemy.

That is not the case written by the Psalmist above. David talks about his affair with Bathsheba, and his conscience is bothering him deeply. He is praying for cleansing and forgiveness and will receive it. The question is can he accept it? We are very hard on ourselves in our human world and need to develop more robust spiritual growth to find acceptance.

Thought for Today: Today, let's move on with our activities unencumbered by our internal memories. Let's leave remorse behind and generate some positive memories!

Prayer for Today: Dear Lord and Father, like David, we have been holding on to past transgressions. Today we pray that we may let them go and escape so that they do not affect the work we can do for you in the future. We know you will forgive us, and that is not our issue. Amen

Bearskin Neck
Rockport, Massachusetts

March 22

Harvest

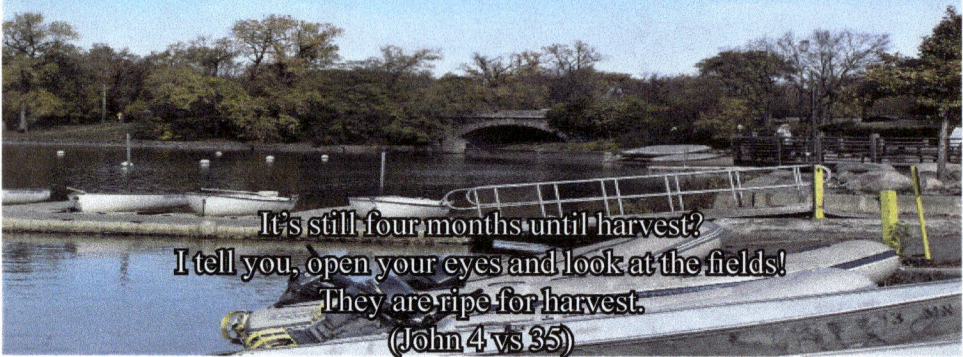

It's still four months until harvest?
I tell you, open your eyes and look at the fields!
They are ripe for harvest.
(John 4 vs 35)

It is spring, and our fields are softening. It is approaching planting time, and harvest will be in the fall. That is how the world works in my upper Midwest mentality. We till, plant, weed, water, prune, and harvest when we are lucky. Along the way, there is wind, rain, hail, heat, and all the forces of nature that we cannot control.

Jesus is not talking about a food harvest, and his disciples are. Jesus talks about making converts, telling the story, inviting people to worship. There are no seasons for that, there are harvest times in our churches when we are more invitational than others. Times when we are open to inviting people to worship: Easter, Christmas, Rally Sunday, and special events throughout the year. It is relatively easy, and most of us feel comfortable inviting people to join us at those special times. Throughout the year, Christians tend to hold back on invitations to worship.

We are all proud of our faith, congregations, and church and are willing to share on special occasions. Jesus asked to "…open your eyes and look at the fields." Let's invite a friend to join us soon.

Thought for Today: Christian church attendance is declining. Let's think about why.

Prayer for Today: Dear Lord and Father, our troubled world often seems to take control of our lives. Today we give we pray that we can choose to contribute to doing your will here on earth by following Jesus' teachings. Amen

March 23 Lake Bde Maka Ska,
Minneapolis, Minnesota

Tradition

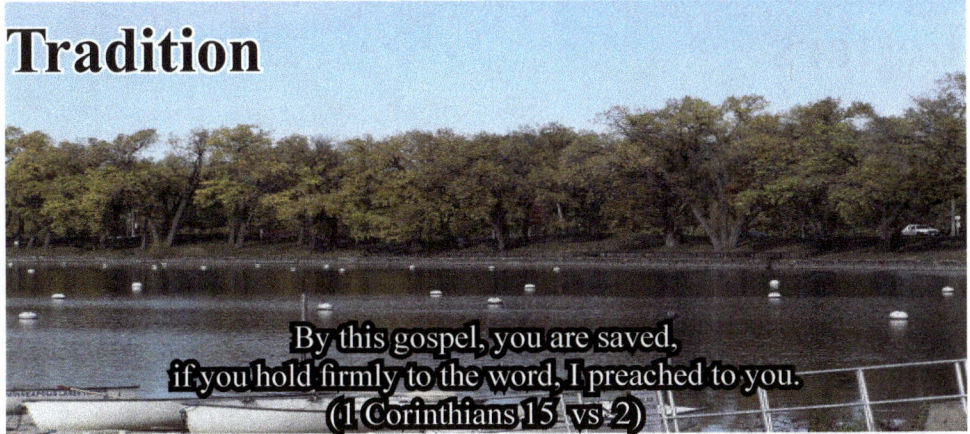

By this gospel, you are saved,
if you hold firmly to the word, I preached to you.
(1 Corinthians 15 vs 2)

In thirty years as a sales engineer, I saw a lot of changes. In the seventies, selling was called "show and sell." We drove thousands of miles with our sample cases bringing solutions to the customer. Often, we had new technology and served as an educational force and consultant.

Technologically, the products and sales process evolved as the advent of email and the internet minimized personal visits. In today's world, the customer reviews the product options online, and the sales challenge is to assist in his selection process. In the 2000s, sales engineers are online with the customer reviewing products and applying them. The style is different, but our message is the same. We can meet your needs.

Our church is trying to adjust to 2000 years of a changing market. We need to TWEET, POST, Email, and use the latest technology to send a 2000-year-old message to an ever-changing population. Our services are overhauled, so we refer to them as traditional, blended, and contemporary. It is a challenge to service present-day needs.

Our communication has changed, the message has not and cannot. Present generations will find the help they need in an ancient message. Over these new mediums and through the different styles, we must hold firmly to the word.

Thought for Today: For today, let's marvel at the message; never changing, always true. The Lord is with us.

Prayer for Today: Heavenly Father, our calendars are full, and technology gives us very little time to meditate. Wwe pray for your guidance through it all. We pray for grace and solitude through Jesus. Amen

Lake Bde Maka Ska
Minneapolis, Minnesota

Letters

> You show that you are a letter from Christ,
> the result of our ministry,
> written not with ink but with the Spirit of the living God.
> (2 Corinthians 3 vs 2, 3)

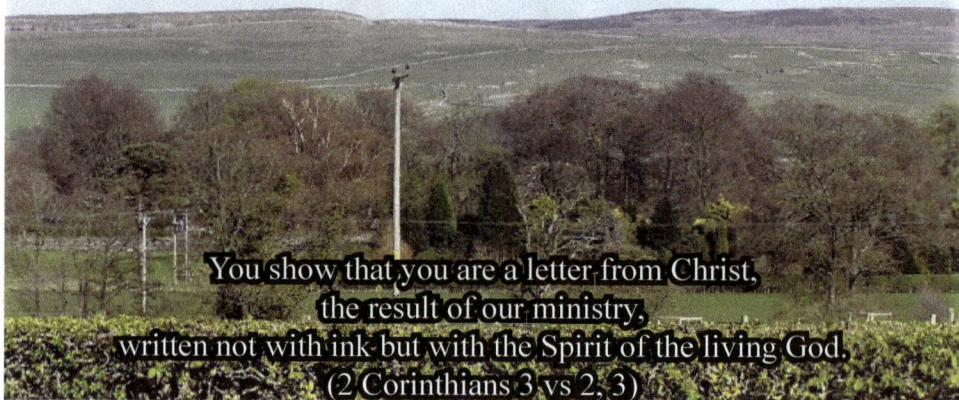

Wow, it sure is scary to think that we are a letter from Christ. Are we qualified to represent Jesus in our everyday lives? That is undoubtedly a challenging thought, and Paul was indeed challenging the people of Corinth. Was he challenging us, or can we discount his word here as too ancient?

I want to talk today about the difference between qualified and certified- two words that are not interchangeable but used in the same context. There is a big difference in the spirit world regarding representatives of the Lord. Ordained pastors are certified to give communion and baptism, many other things I do not even know. However, we are all ministers of the gospel, and through our spirituality, we are the light, the message, and the Spirit, and we are qualified through our covenant to shine that light.

Thought for Today: Today, I recognize my qualifications given to me by my covenant to my faith. I will share them and use them through the Spirit given to me.

Prayer for Today: Heavenly Father, for today help me live as an example of you, as a window into the Spirit. For today let others see you through my eyes. Amen

March 25

Pennine Range
Kirkby Stephen, Cumbria, UK

Righteousness

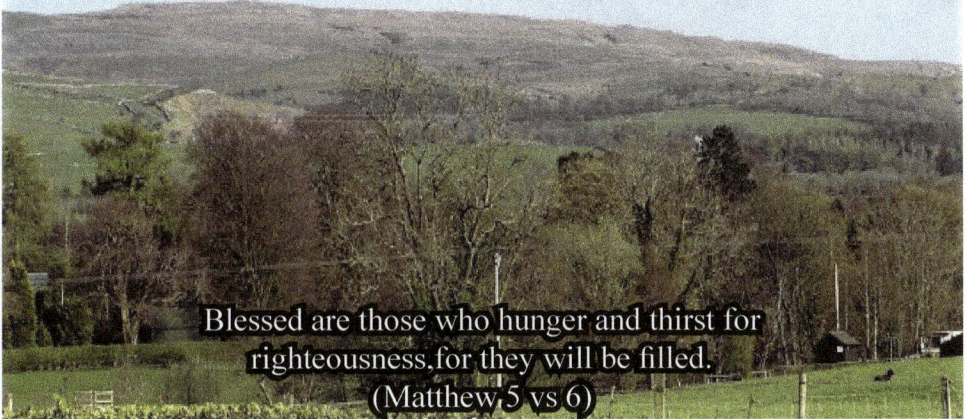

Blessed are those who hunger and thirst for
righteousness,for they will be filled.
(Matthew 5 vs 6)

You aim for righteousness when you strive to align your lives with the Lord's commandments. Trying to be the best we can be is a daily battle. Twelve-step programs teach small steps "one day at a time." Often it is an hour or even a minute at a time. There needs to be a persistent hunger and passion. That is an excellent thought.

Every day is a new day made by the Lord. Every day we will make choices that are both good and bad. By having a hunger and passion for being good and righteous, we will make mostly the right decisions. However, we will mess up; that's human! Our faith is about forgiveness when we do, but our humanity wants to hold on to the guilt. That's what Sundays are for; to recharge our spiritual batteries and be at peace.

Thought for Today: Let us go out and feel our hunger and passion and finish the day fulfilled.

Prayer for Today: Dear Lord, we give thanks for being part of your team. We go forth with thoughts of righteousness and doing your will here on earth. We pray for your guidance in our daily efforts. Amen

Pennine Range
Kirkby Stephen, Cumbria, UK

Character

*... keep his commandments,
for this is the duty of all humankind.
(Ecclesiastes 12 vs 13)*

What a wonderful world it would be. We are all aware of the rules and will have a chance to break them daily, weekly, etc. The temptation is always around, and none of us is perfect. Each morning we need to pray, "Dear Lord, for today I pray to be perfect." There is no coveting, jealousy, anger, or aggressiveness toward others (that must mean complete stops at the stop signs!). Ok, when done reading this, try again.

There are only ten rules to obey for a great life and a wonderful world. Most of us try, many of us fail. That's why we go to church on Sunday and pray daily. Somehow we end the day wishing we were better; we were perfect.

Each day we strive for perfection; we try to build character. We attend church and pray, and that generates spiritual growth. Building character is slightly different but parallels it. The closer we are to the pirit, the easier it is to have that perfect character we all desire.

Persistence is the word, and perfection is the goal. Never give up being the best you can be. Pray daily, obey the commandments daily, and life will be good.

Thoughts for Today: Today, let us be aware of the commandments in all of our activities.

Prayer for Today: Dear Lord, today we give thanks for our beautiful lives and the hope we have for the future through our belief in Jesus. We pray for the strength and judgment to be obedient and of the highest character. Amen

Relationships

Do nothing out of selfish ambition or vain conceit.
Rather, in humility, value others above yourselves,
(Philippians 3 vs 3-5)

Paul's message above sure says it all, and it would lead us to a perfect society. Unfortunately, we have not quite arrived at the point of grace. Our society and our world are competitive by design. We are in what they call a world economy, and nations compete for resources. Can it be that Paul was wrong? Should Paul have said something like, "Grab the brass ring before the other guy gets it?" Or maybe "Do unto others" and leave off the finish of the golden rule. I do not think so.

Our competitive world works best when people team up and work together. People working together can do more good than working as individuals. Indeed, the same is true of nations working together.

Paul's message may describe utopia or the world at peace, an excellent thought that we can never forget. Perhaps it will start with us as individuals, spread through congregations and nations.
That has to be the dream, if not the goal.

Thought for Today: For today, let's be unselfish and humble in our activities.

Prayer for Today: Dear heavenly Father, we give thanks for the many blessings we have. We pray that somehow, through our actions, we may bring our surroundings and the world closer to peace. Amen

Becoming Like Him

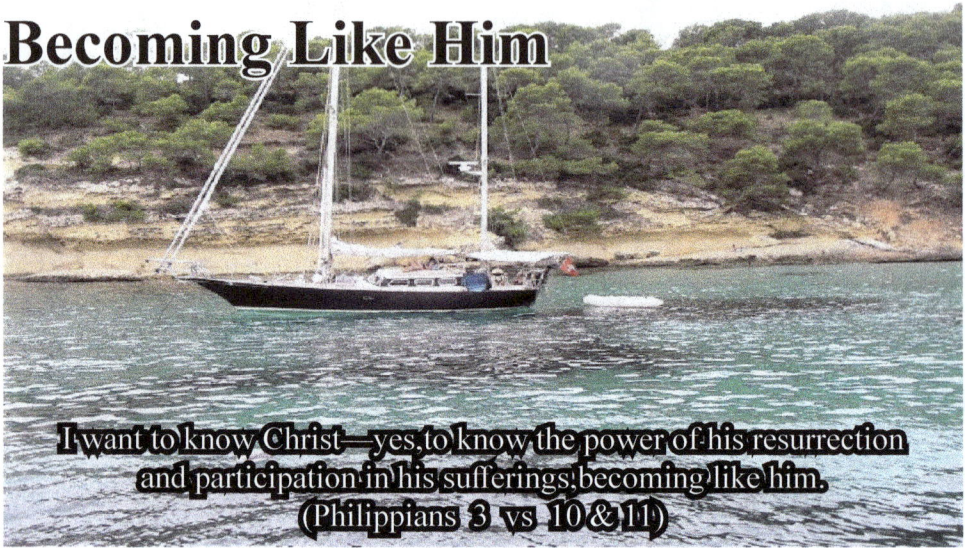

I want to know Christ—yes, to know the power of his resurrection and participation in his sufferings, becoming like him.
(Philippians 3 vs 10 & 11)

"Becoming like Him" is a great goal, and it speaks of faith, hope, and charity, three beautiful assets. Fortunately, we all have and experience them, just not all of the time. Sometimes, we are not faithful and occasionally let our minds drift away. There are times when disappointment or depression lead us to lose sight of the hope we need. And charity often takes a back seat to perceived necessity.

Ok, this is not Sunday, and I do not do sermons. None of us are perfect, and we will probably never attain anything like perfection. However, if you are reading this, you are doing the right thing at this moment; meditating, enjoying a quiet moment, hopefully drinking your favorite beverage, and thinking about "What Would Jesus Do today?"

As Christians, our lot in life is to strive for perfection, work daily on our spiritual growth, and be comfortable in our lives through Jesus.

Thought for Today: Let's look at our calendars for the next 24 hours and ask ourselves the question; What would Jesus do today?

Prayer for Today: Dear Lord, we want to thank you for resurrection today. It is spring, and the message is all around us; holy week speaks about the roots of our faith, and the coming of spring reminds us of the wonder of your powers. We are blessed and give thanks. Amen

March 29

Mediterranean Sea
Mallorca, Spain

One for All

I have other sheep that are not of this sheep pen.
I must bring them also.
(John 10 vs 16)

My former pastor used to say that we invite a guest to church every twelve years or so. He blamed our lack of invitation for not having congregational growth. A second pastor came along and tried to motivate us with a sermon about our style and referred to us as "the frozen chosen." Neither pastor grew the congregation during their tenure.

Several years ago, a new pastor showed up and talked about having an invitational ministry. That was a new term, and he invited us to join him in that task. So we did, and the church grew—what a concept.

You see, when Jesus was talking to his disciples, even he said that he needed to get out and talk to others. We are supposed to have open doors, hearts, and minds but need to remember that there may not be anyone coming through the opening without an invitation!

Thought for Today: Today, let's go about our business with our hearts and minds open and receptive to the needs of others.

Prayer for Today: Heavenly Father, thank you for the many friends and the fellowship we have together. This week we pray for the opportunity to help others with their spiritual needs and growth in your name. Amen

Mediterranean Sea
Mallorca, Spain

March 30

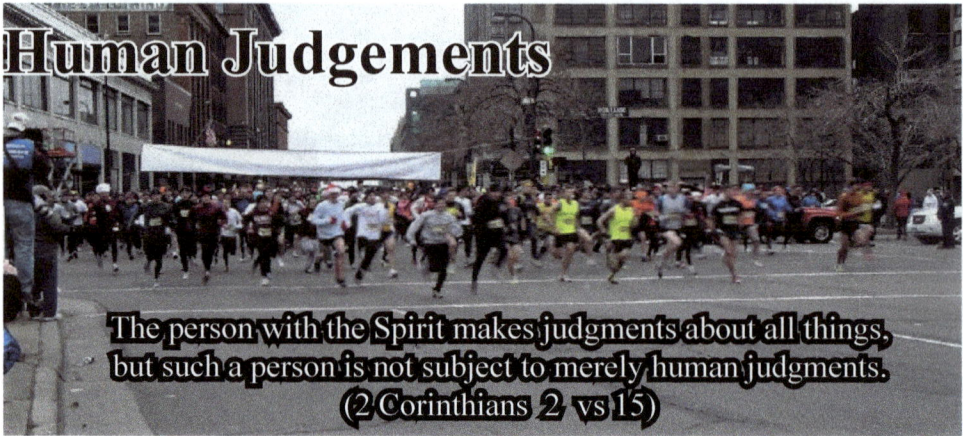

Human Judgements

The person with the Spirit makes judgments about all things, but such a person is not subject to merely human judgments.
(2 Corinthians 2 vs 15)

When our faith is strong, we are comfortable in our beliefs, and our lives are good. That is when we make decisions quickly without stress and doubt. We make hundreds of decisions and judgments every day to get through life. Most are easy and automatic. Some are not

We learned that it takes six weeks to change a habit and establish a new one in counseling training. That's why we have difficulty with self-improvement. Captain Marvel used to shout "Shazam" in the old comic books, and everything around him would fall into place. Our lives are not like that, not comic book simple.

Twelve-step programs are a way to find contentment through spiritual growth, starting with a belief system. Judgments become spiritual, based on God, which improves a person's life.

It is always great to see someone grow spiritually.

Thought for Today: Today, let's continue to be on autopilot and do the simple things we always do. When we get to the tough ones, let us turn them over to the Lord and be sure He is our actual pilot.

Prayer for the Today: Dear God, we give thanks for our routines, the things we do stress-free and on auto-pilot. We pray that your presence in our lives leads us to Godly decisions and positively impacts those around us. Amen

Starting the Arena 5K
Minneapolis, Minnesota

April

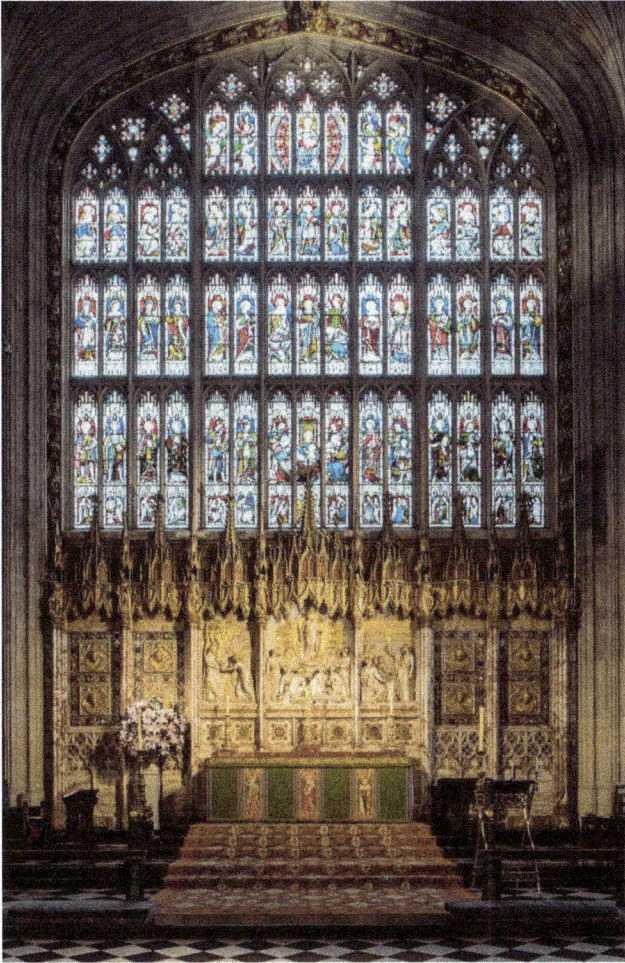

St George's Chapel

provides a haven of peace and quiet for prayer and reflection, or simply a pause on the journey.

The Alter of St. George's Chapel
Windsor, Berkshier, UK

Boldness

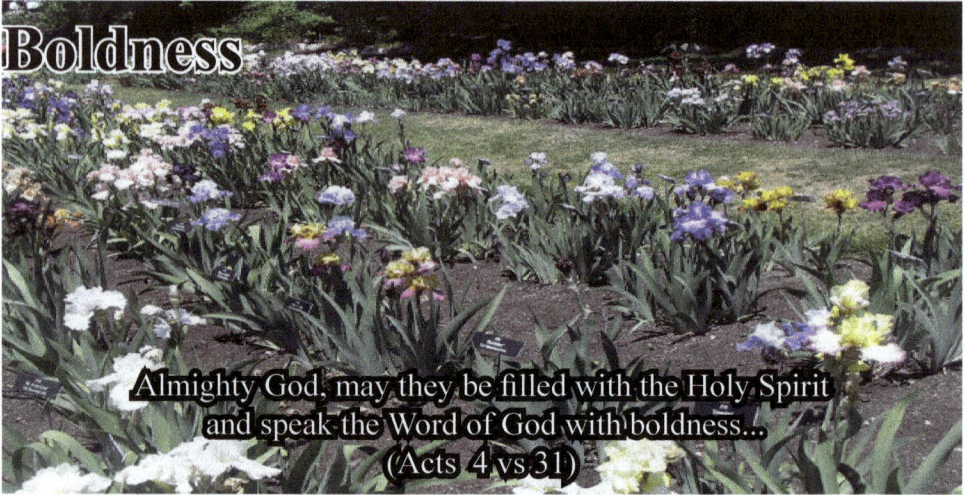

Almighty God, may they be filled with the Holy Spirit and speak the Word of God with boldness...
(Acts 4 vs 31)

April fool's day is a day of practical jokes, misleading emails, and general tomfoolery. That will not work because we cannot hide from God, who loves us. So, let's skip reading our devotional and forget the Holy Spirit and our Lord so that we may participate.

Today the comics in the newspaper will have Fool's Day jokes, the news and sports programs will be full of them, and there will be a few bogus press releases to get your attention. If I were to write a press release for today, it would be "Bob shoots par at St. Andrews!" or "... wins the Ironman." People would immediately recognize these were jokes, and some would know they were my fantasies.

Like all days, I hope this devotional puts you on track to recognize the Holy Spirit in your life and its role in you. While others are playing jokes, we need to be sure that we are bold in our faith.
Blessings to you all, and enjoy the start of April.

Thought for Today: Today, we will be bold in our faith and remember that it is ok to be a joker.

Prayer for Today: Father, we give thanks for all that we are and have. We thank you for having the freedom to enjoy a good joke, a great laugh, and the faith to know the absolute truth. We pray for good health, world peace, and prosperity for all. Amen

Fortress

The Lord Almighty is with us;
the God of Jacob is our fortress.
(Psalm 46 vs 7)

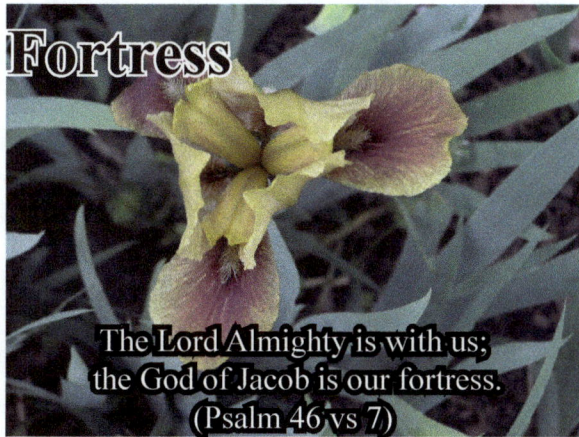

While writing this, a news flash can across my computer screen that a shootout on a local highway had recently shut down the road. The police were searching the parking lot, and the area was on lockdown.

So what? I am here, safe in my home. Well, the scene was in clear view from my deck. I did not feel very secure at all

We are always wary when we travel but not so careful when at home. When a crime occurs in "our neighborhood," we ask, "How could this happen here?" The truth is that tragedy and violence can happen anywhere. None of us is immune, and anything can happen at any time.

The author of the 23rd Psalm wrote these familiar words, "Even though I walk through the valley of the shadow of death, I will fear no evil, for you are with me." The psalmist does not say that we will not have to walk through the darkest valley or that evil does not exist. Instead, the psalmist reminds us that we need not fear or be overwhelmed because God is with us at all times. God will see us through. The ground and content of our hope is the promise that nothing in all creation can separate us from God's love.

Absolute security cannot come from walls and fences; real security comes from having a relationship with God.

Thought for Today: Let us feel secure in our faith, neighborhood, and relationships.

Prayer for Today: Heavenly Father, hold us close to you and remind us that you will never leave or forsake us. You alone are our hope and security. Amen.

Don't Forget To Call

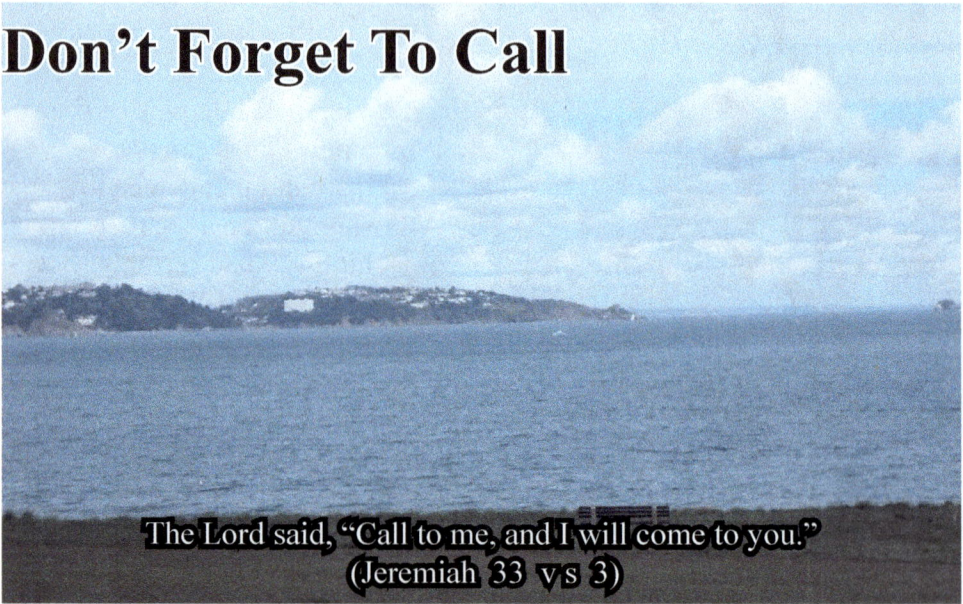

The Lord said, "Call to me, and I will come to you."
(Jeremiah 33 vs 3)

It is easy to go through a busy day without acknowledging the presence of God in our lives. Sometimes when we get to the end of a day and look back, the day seems un-Godly. We have not done the best job of caring for ourselves when that happens. That is our fault.

Confusion and stress seem to find their way into our lives. We will have busy and stressful days, and bad things will happen to us. It is advisable to put ourselves first for a part of each day, which requires a bit of selfishness. Alone time shared with God will make us better workers, parents, and people. There is nothing selfish about that.

Henri Nouwen called it a still place "…This still place is where God can dwell and speak to us. It also is the place from which we can speak in a healing way to all the people we meet in our busy days." We all need to think about that.

Thought for Today: Let us remember to be selfish, take a break, and allow God to support us.

Prayer for Today: Let us pray that God will be present in our lives as we pursue the opportunities before us. Amen

April 3

Torbay from Broadsands
Paignton, Devon, UK

Nervous Breakdown

And the peace of God will guard your hearts and your minds in Christ Jesus.
(Philippians 4 vs 7)

J.L. Glass has written a humorous article titled "Five Ways to Have a Nervous Breakdown." Below are four of them.

1. Try to figure out the answer before the problem arises. "Most of the bridges we cross are never built because they are unnecessary." Matthew 6:34 says: "Do not worry about tomorrow, for tomorrow will worry about itself."

2. Try to relive the past. Paul's letter in Romans 8 verse 28 states, "And we know that in all things God works for the good of those who love him, who have been called according to his purpose." As we trust Him for the future, we must trust him with the past, and He can use the most checkered past imaginable for His good.

3. Try to avoid making decisions. Doing this is like deciding whether to let weeds grow in our garden: while we choose, they are growing. Decisions are made while we procrastinate. Choice is a man's most godlike characteristic.

4. Demand more of yourself than you can produce. Unrealistic demands result in beating our heads against walls, and we damage ourselves. Romans 12:3 says, "Do not think of yourself more highly than you ought, but rather think of yourself with sober judgment."

Thought for Today: Let us feel the Lord's presence in our daily lives to keep our stress levels low.

Prayer for Today: Heavenly Father, we are masters at leaving you out of our lives and building obstacles in our paths. We pray that you will guide us through the day and minimize our troubles. Amen

The Promenade
Torquay, Devon, Uk

Power

You are awesome, O God, in your sanctuary;
the God of Israel, whose power is in the skies.
(Psalms 68 vs 34, 35)

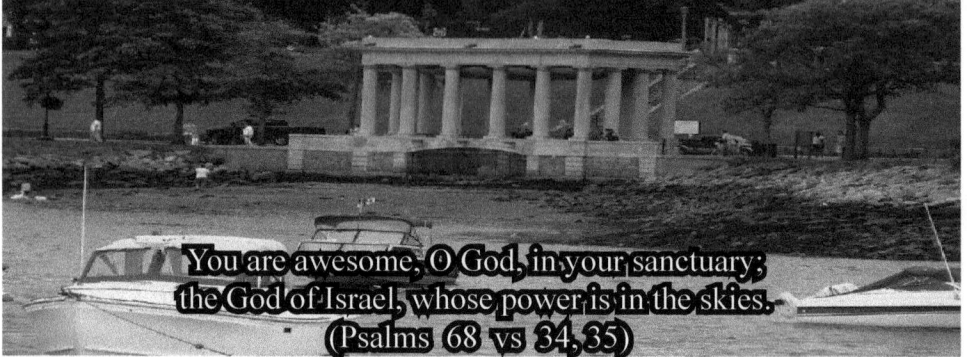

Power- what a word. What a feeling. We come into the world looking for power and equate power with security and control. We hear about power brokers. Books on leadership tell you how to gain, use and retain power. The feeling of power can be addictive. It gives us an adrenaline rush.

In relationships, power usually manifests itself as domination. When a significant other demands submission, a partnership is lost and will not reach its full potential. Power sometimes negates God's will. It can become a power broker's God.

I have always said that two people working together are four times better than either. My definition of a partnership is when two become one in objectives, dreams, and goals. In a good relationship, power is not a problem. Power is only a problem when it is misused.

In relationships (married, parent-child, and others), sacrifice and caring (love) will generate a better relationship than power and control. Often power and control are masks for insecurity and low self-esteem. It prevents bonding and growing in a caring relationship.

"Love one another, Just as Christ loved the church
and gave himself up for her."
(Ephesians 5 vs 25)

Thought For Today: Let us keep caring, consideration, and love at the forefront of our decision-making.

Prayer for Today: Dear Lord, help us put the trials of everyday life in perspective. Guide us to inner peace. Help us find the love of Jesus. Amen

April 5 Plymouth Rock Monument
Plymouth, Massachusetts

Leadership

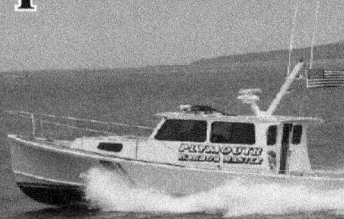

He who has compassion on them will
guide them and lead them beside springs of water.
(Isaiah 49 vs 10)

In the '60s, my engineering manager at a multi-national company ruled the roost by fear. He would lay off someone three or four times each year and warn a few that they could be next. He kept control of all projects and decisions and empowered no one. There was no compassion in the department or the company. Great things did not happen for them, and they no longer exist.

Successful leaders use a win-win philosophy that requires compassion. It seems that leaders that have outstanding accomplishments have compassion. Paul said it this way:

> "Be kind and compassionate to one another,
> forgiving one another,
> just as in Christ, God forgave you."
> (Ephesians 4 vs 32).

Yes, compassion, forgiveness, and caring are vital components of success.

Thought for Today: Today, focus on being compassionate.

Prayer for Today: Heavenly Father, we are caught up in a busy world. There is too little time and too many things to do. Pressures to make a fast decision, reaction, or remark sometimes lead to a lack of compassion. Please, help us concentrate on your place in our lives. Please help us be compassionate and forgiving in all our activities. Amen.

Pleasure Boat Heading Out
Plymouth, Massachusetts

April 6

Commitment

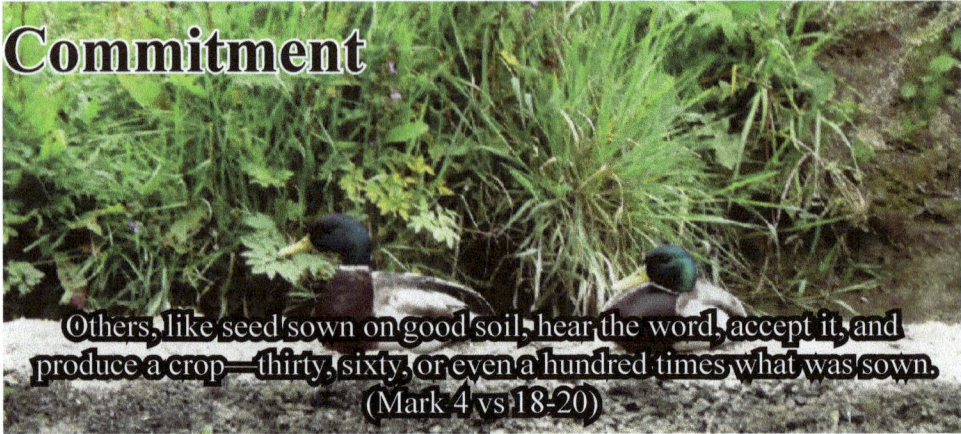

Others, like seed sown on good soil, hear the word, accept it, and produce a crop—thirty, sixty, or even a hundred times what was sown.
(Mark 4 vs 18-20)

"The Parable of the Sower" hits home with this story and again fits into another phase of our life. As a young family of six recovering from a divorce and trying to restart our lives, there were many times when the pursuit of wealth took precedent over spiritual commitment. We certainly made some interesting decisions.

We started our business in 1975, and our cash flow increased significantly over five years. It is embarrassing comparing the percent increase in cash flow with the growth in our church pledge. We avoided committee assignments but had time to attend all the kids' activities. Beyond financial commitments, our spiritual commitment was often weak regarding giving time.

One day while waiting for a tennis match with a good friend and dedicated Christian, we talked about our schedules. Ken commented that I was not saving enough time for the Lord. He promised to pray that my business activities would not cause too much harm. He even suggested that I fit in my long training runs (2 hours) on Sunday before church rather than during church. His comments and prayers worked.

God allows us to learn, grow, and forgive. The "I wish I had known that when..." syndrome is part of his reward. The return on investment in God's work is life's true reward.

Thought for Today: Let's review our calendars and ask, "Have I saved enough time for the Lord?"

Prayer for Today: Gracious Lord, the world is very busy and tense. We pray that we keep you involved in our lives today and in the futture. Amen

Mallards on the River Nene

Stress

Do not be anxious about anything, but in everything,
by prayer and petition, with Thanksgiving,
present your requests to God.
(Philippians 4 vs 6)

Stress has become part of our lifestyle. We often go through our week wound up like a rubber band that has been twisted tighter and tighter. However, please recognize that the rubber band eventually breaks when wound too tight or stressed too long; it snaps. We are a higher life form than a rubber band, but we may snap when overstressed.

We all need a way of unwinding during the most stressful times. There are many ways to release stress. Mine is by writing devotions for fellow Christians. Other ways are exercise, meditation, chatting with a friend, or reading. Paul's writings to the Philippians 4 vs 8 & 9 suggest that Faith is a tool to help us.

"Finally, brothers, whatever is true, whatever is noble, whatever is right,whatever is pure, whatever is lovely, whatever is admirable— if anything is excellent or praiseworthy—think about such things. Whatever you have learned or received or heard from me, or seen in me— put it into practice. And the God of peace will be with you."

Thought for Today: Let's focus selfishly on ourselves and feel God's peace and presence in our lives. When the "stress monster" wants to control our lives, read this passage, and let "the peace of God" control our lives.

Prayer for Today: Heavenly Father, the world seems to be a breeding ground for stress. There is always something to worry about; terror, hate, employment troubles, stock market woes- even severe weather. We pray that we may keep you and peace in our thoughts, that we have the presence of mind to make wise choices and release our stresses to find tranquility. Amen

Swans on the River Nene
Peterborough, Cambridgeshire, UK **April 8**   **Page 103**

In The Spirit

Then you will know which way to go since you have never been this way before.
(Joshua 3 vs 4)

Many of us experience challenges in our lives that we would just as soon not meet. In the story of Joshua, he was asked to take over from Moses and be a leader. He had never been a leader and doubted his capability. He was told, believed, and successfully led because of his potential as part of his Spirit.

A friend who works rehabilitating youth when released from jail told this story. A client he was working with had trouble surviving, so he stole again to be returned to prison and have a roof over his head. That was a step he knew would work, and he had the skills to implement it. Thus, he was successful.

As Christians, how do we transfer our spirit to those who need help? How do we let them find the talent that the Lord gave them?

"Not by might nor by power, but by my Spirit,"
says the LORD Almighty."
(Zacharias 4 vs 6)

Thought for Today: Help someone take a small step forward, someone at work, at home, or someone we have not met yet.

Prayer for Today: Dear Lord and Father, today we give thanks for having your Spirit within us. We pray that we may share it with someone who is in need. Amen

Personal Prayer

Let us, therefore, make every effort to do what leads to peace
and mutual edification.
(Romans 14 vs 19)

As we watch the news, read our newspapers, and study life around us, we see a lot of stress and confusion. The media presents us with more negatives than positives. We might wonder how to overcome these challenges and bring peace to the world.

Consider what our contribution to peace will be. We cannot go out tomorrow, solve the world's problems, and create "World Peace." However, we can start to be at peace every day and stay that way. Stay within ourselves through prayer to maintain our internal peace.

Our contribution to the world can and will start within us. We know that the Lord is with us, we need to let Him in, and others see the results. As Paul stated to the Romans, "We who are strong ought to bear with the failings of the weak and not to please ourselves. 2 Each of us should please his neighbor for his good, to build him up." (Romans 15 vs 1 & 2).

Thought for Today: An old expression suggests aggressive reactions: "When the going gets tough, the tough get going." That is always an option. Today for us, let's think about this: When our going gets tough, let's start to pray and be at peace". Demonstrate a better way.

Prayer for the Day: Heavenly Father, today we pray for gentle solutions to our problems. When things get tough, we pay that we may peacefully resolve the issues the way Jesus did. Amen

The Lilac Walk
Minnesota Landscape Arboretum   **April 10**   **Page 105**

Style Change

but whoever listens to me will live in safety and be at ease, without fear of harm.
(Proverbs 1 vs 32,33)

The more we change, the more we seem to stay the same (adapted from Alfonse Karr). When we focus on our spirituality, we can live "... without fear of harm." Negatives build in our lives when we lose focus and create a slippery slide.

The concept of putting one's self-first for part of each day is key to maintaining sanity and personal growth. It is essential to take time to grow every day to be a good parent, employee, and friend. How do we do all we need to do and meet our obligations? The answer is priorities and including the Lord on the list. When we do not have time for God, it is a sign of over-commitment, reacting to our "to do" lists rather than planning our day.

Pat McNamara, a former Olympian from Minneapolis, once advised me that if I was going to stay in shape, I had to give fitness a priority part of every day. Make it a calendar item and follow Nike's advice, "Just Do It." The same applies to faith. Schedule a time to listen to the Lord's message so we "...will live in safety and be at ease, without fear of harm."

Thought for Today: Recognize the internal conflict in our lives; between our over-committed "to do" lists and the time required for personal growth. The concept is simple, we all want to be better in spirit, mind, and body but do not have the time. Let's try placing the Lord first for a few minutes and feel the difference.

Prayer for Today: Father, you are at the top of my list today. I look forward to the peace that you will bring. Amen

Observation Deck

Leasr To Receive

I thank my God every time I remember you.
(Phillipians 1 vs 3)

When people meet, they often ask, "How are you?" A typical answer is OK, fine, good…etc. That answer raises the antennas of a counselor, but most are relieved because now we can change the subject and move on. We all feel better giving than receiving.

On a Friday in January 1998, I was diagnosed with cancer and was aware that surgery was a good solution. That Sunday, June and I greeted for a church service. Most people greeted me with, "Hi, how are you?" and did not want to hear my answer. God forgive me, but I lied a lot that morning.

The point is that in 1998, we needed to take from the church more than we could give. We needed prayers to cover fear and June's tears. The kids and grandchildren also needed spir-itual support. The support was for most of 1998 and was available through our Christian commu-nity. The good news was that "…He who began a good work in you will carry it on to comple-tion…."

We are welcome, and it is OK to take and receive. In 1998, God blessed the Pickering family; we accepted the support and prayers from our friends in Christ and received the benefits available to all. We must remember, "In all my prayers for all of you, I always pray with joy."

Thought for Today: Today, let us recognize when we need support. Call a friend in Christ and ask for help if there are any awful moments. The friend will be grateful. Let us stop and pray about it.

Prayer for Today: Dear Lord and Father, we offer our prayers for peace and understanding. We pray somehow that we, in some way, can contribute to spreading your love throughout the world. Amen

Green Heron Pond
Minnesota Landscape Arboretum **April 12** Page 107

Control

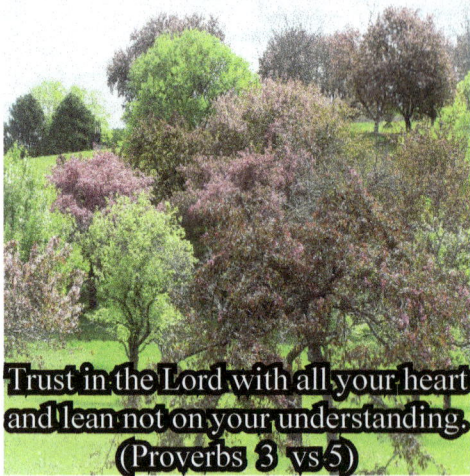

Life tests our faith in many ways. We go through valleys before we experience peaks, the good times. We find it easy to take the credit for the recovery. After all, we generally "take control" and work through problems. That's the human way.

Several years ago, our pastor presented us with a pin, Christ's feet. The pin is symbolic of footprints in the sand, serving as a reminder that we never walk alone. We often think of God as a "Macro" rather than a personal assistant. When in control, we may not be aware and feel God's presence.

Trust in the Lord with all your heart and lean not on your understanding. (Proverbs 3 vs 5)

Life tests our faith in many ways. We go through valleys before we experience peaks, the good times. We find it easy to take the credit for the recovery. After all, we generally "take control" and work through problems. That's the human way.

Several years ago, our pastor presented us with a pin, Christ's feet. The pin is symbolic of footprints in the sand, serving as a reminder that we never walk alone. We often think of God as a "Macro" rather than a personal assistant. When in control, we may not be aware and feel God's presence.

Too many outside factors play out in life to have "full control." When we feel in "full control," we are misleading ourselves. We need always to have the trust that our faith teaches. With God as a partner, it is easier to get through crises. He is always our partner.

Thought for Today: Today, really control the ball, keep our problems in our grasp, and handle it all. Then look back and thank Him for the help.

Prayer for Today: The world seems out of control. We doubt what God us playing with all the ills that exist. Economic struggles, terrorism, and world poverty dominate our lives. It is hard for us to show the needed love. We pray for guidance on trusting you more, doing your will in tough times, and being a good follower of Christ's teachings. Amen

April 13

Flowering Fruit Trees
Minnesota Landscape Arboretum

Joyfull

Shout for joy to the LORD, all the earth.
Worship the LORD with gladness;
Come before him with joyful songs.
(Psalm 100 vs 2)

The Psalmist who wrote this knew what Christianity was all about. We are told to be happy, enjoy our loves, and sing it out loud! Can we do that every day?

Each day is unique, and some are awful. Our day was bright under the clouds. We have not seen the sun in four days and had drizzle, hoar frost, and ice. Bah, humbug to a joyful noise. However, it is Sunday morning, so we went to an early church service and communed with friends in the chapel with our pastor. It was a joyous time. Then, we had breakfast together and discussed our weekly plan, including a pool party with the youth and several visits with old friends.

Gloomy is a mindset. Keeping the Lord in your life can turn a day bright and make it easy to make a joyful noise.

Thought for Today: When you are feeling down and out, think about the joy of your faith.

Prayer for Today: Dear Lord and Father, today we pray that we can keep our focus on the joys of our faith and that we may share those joys with those around us.
Amen

Flowering Crabapples
Minnesota Landscape Arboretum   **April 14**   Page 109

Peaks and Valleys

Therefore, since we have been justified through faith, we have peace with God ... And we rejoice in the hope of the glory of God.
(Romans 5 vs 1)

Life is full of peaks and valleys. It is very human to take credit for the high and blame something else for the valleys. It is hard to identify with our own "piece of the action" when there is pain. It is often hard to appreciate the lessons learned through the suffering process.

Usually, people that visit our churches come through crises. Divorce, illness, grief, loneliness, etc., are common reasons for a visit. A greeter rarely meets someone who had such a great week they came to thank God. We look to our faith more often when in a valley than at a peak.

However, one of the beauties of our faith is that we recognize God's role in helping get us to the next high and His role in getting us to the final peak. Each up-turn gives us a reason for more robust faith. The lessons learned in the valleys give us the "... perseverance, character; and character, hope" that carry us throughout our lives.

Thought for Today: Recognize if we are in a peak or a valley. Recognize the lessons we are learning if it is a "valley" and give credit to those things that helped make it a "peak." Either way, give thanks to God.

Prayer for Today: Heavenly Father, we are in a confused world. Many people are concerned about their future in tough economic times. War, fear, and terror seem to dominate the news. Indeed, many need a "peak" to help them out. We pray that through your Son Jesus, we all may find a peak and a way to share 6our love with someone. Amen

April 15   Palma Cathedral
Mallorca, Spain

Setting Examples

Who is wise and understanding among you?
Let him show it by his good life,
by deeds done in the humility that comes from wisdom.
(James 3 vs 13)

One of my recurring themes is that we are all ministers of the Gospel. Our Church congregations hire ordained ministers to lead, teach, and guide us on our spiritual journeys or catch ourselves in the Sunday-only mode.

A very dear friend of June's and mine is in spiritual crisis. For whatever reason, faith has left, and bouts of depression have occurred. It is probably not coincidental. There is a strong tie between our faith and our inner peace for Christians. When our faith is doubtful, we take control of things. We forget to "Let go and let God."

As Christians, we need to demonstrate our inner peace to others. Show our caring spirits and our love. Not on Sunday but every day in every activity. Our ministry needs to be subtle, persistent, and very public. When we function in a very Christian way, people in doubt will come to us.

Thought for Today: Let's demonstrate our inner peace to all we meet. Let us look for an opportunity to talk about our tranquility and faith. Let us offer to share with others.

Prayer for Today: Dear Lord, many significant events are masked by tragedy. We need to end hate and hateful decisions; we pray for world peace. Today, we pray that we may somehow find a way to contribute as Christians. Amen

Avenida de Gabriel Roca
Mallorca, Spain

April 16

Page 111

Enough Is Enough

Unless the LORD builds the house,
its builders labor in vain.
Unless the LORD watches over the city,
the watchmen stand guard in vain.
(Psalm 127 vs 1)

The competitive nature of our society has generated a workaholic mentality. In the 1960s, we occasionally met someone who worked a fiftty hour week, and in some families, both the wife and husband had full-time jobs, but they were not commonplace. People work way too much. They are on the internet daily, attached to cell phones, and then overloaded with our sports and recreational commitments.

In "When I Relax I Feel Guilty," Tim Hansel wrote the following regarding our present state.

"We are called to be faithful, not frantic. If we are to meet the challenges of today, there must be integrity between our words and our lives and more reliance on the source of our purpose.

In the Christian sense, running here and there volunteering is now required to be considered a dedicated, sacrificing, spiritual Christian. Perhaps the seven deadly sins have created another member- Overwork.

We must remember that our strength lies not in hurried efforts and endless long hours but our quietness and confidence. The world says today that enough is enough.

Thought for Today: Slow down, take a break.
Prayer for the Day: Dear Lord, we thank you for our many blessings. Through you, we have enough. Amen

April 17 Minnesota Landscape Arboretum
Chaska, Minnesota

Spring

I will send rain on your land in its season,
both autumn and spring rains,
so that you may gather in your grain,
new wine and olive oil.
(Deuteronomy 11 vs 14)

Spring is a beautiful time of the year. Long warmer evenings replace short winter days. Spring bulbs emerge from the ground with green sprouts, and color returns to the woods, parks, and yards. It is a time when the wonders of God bring peaceful thoughts to us all.

We also live in a world of protests, shootings, and fear. Terrorism, anger, illness, and other crises fill our world alongside the wonders of spring. Where is our "peace on earth"? Spring shows us how close it is and that God is trying to bring it to us. What is our best way to participate in having a peaceful world?

The message in another hymn,"...let there be peace on earth and let it begin with me." gives us a hint. If each of us does our part, we can influence the world.

John F. Kennedy put it like this. "One person can make a difference, and every person must try."

Thought for Today: We encounter negativity, anger, frustrations in the workplace, and frustration in our lives. We can choose to be anxious or at peace. Let peace begin with each of us. This week let's demonstrate Christian love and our quiet side.

Prayer for Today: Heavenly Father, we see violent negativity worldwide and have very little control over it all. We pray that we may lead by the example of Christ, and that our living example may contribute to a better world. Amen

Minnesota Landscape Arboretum
Chaska, Minnesota
April 18

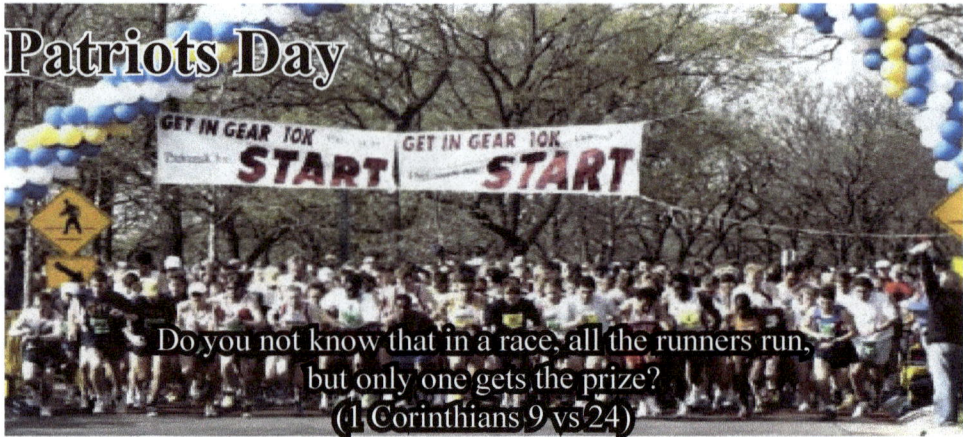

Patriots Day

GET IN GEAR 10K START **GET IN GEAR 10K START**

*Do you not know that in a race, all the runners run,
but only one gets the prize?
(1 Corinthians 9 vs 24)*

In Massachusetts, April 19th is Patriots Day. That gave me two choices to write about today; Paul Revere's ride or the Boston Marathon. There is a similarity, and it is not direction.

The marathon involves over 30,000 participants; one woman and one man will make a six-figure paycheck and win. As many as twenty others will receive appearance money and have good paydays. Most will receive personal gratification and a well-tuned engine for their body from the training and recognition for a great effort. They do it out of the passion that endurance athletes have and the feeling of accomplishment.

In 2013 two young terrorists interrupted things a bit at the finish line. That was a sad day for all involved, and it infuriated Americans and the free world. It demonstrated a world war in the process; we need to function normally through it.

In 1775, Paul Revere, William Dawes, and Sam Prescott raced out of Boston with a message that the British were moving out. Their message to the people of greater Boston was the call to arms. Unfortunately, Paul did not get very far because he was picked up in west Cambridge by a British patrol. However, he did get the poem named for him. Dawes and Prescott did not rhyme as well. They were on a mission to benefit humanity, were unselfish, and are American heroes.

Being fit is a matter of spirit, mind, and body. Life is not a sprint. It is a marathon. We must race it and live it with our eye on the ultimate prize promised through our faith: "…a crown that will last."

Thought for Today: Let us focus on our race for the prize; take a step closer to perfection.

Prayer for Today: We pray for the safety and success of the many runners in Boston. May they be blessed with great memories. Amen

April 19 Get In Gear Race Start
Minneapolis, Minnesota

Infants

Brothers and sisters,
I could not address you as people who live by the Spirit
but as people who are still worldly—mere infants in Christ.
(1 Corinthians 3 vs. 1)

I confess to you that I cannot quote a lot of scripture; I do not know a lot of biblical history; I have never visited the holy land; sometimes, I skip my Friday bible study to play golf or work out. At best, I am an infant in Christ.

That is good because it leaves plenty of room to grow, to keep trying, and a reason to keep writing. There is growth ahead when we do the right things. Our life is a spiritual journey without limits or an end. That's an excellent thought.

As a young engineer, my mentor used to quote Aristotle, "The more you know, the more you know you don't know." It is true with our faith. The more we learn, the more the mystery and the higher our thirst becomes. That may be the best part of it all.

Thought for Today: Recognize the opportunity to grow in the Spirit, that we are in our infancy and have room for exciting growth!

Prayer for Today: Heavenly Father, we are grateful for your presence in our lives and the peace brought to us through faith. We will face challenges today and go forth with the knowledge that you will be with us. Amen

Sunrise
Minnetonka, Minnesota

April 20

Capacity To Love

Photo By Simon Halsey

See what great love the Father has lavished on us,
that we should be called children of God.
And that is what we are.
(1 John 3 vs 1)

Are we made in His image? Are we the children of God? It is hard to think of ourselves like either when trudging along through life. We are taught to be humble. Being a child of God is easier to swallow than being in His image.

When my first child was born, it amazed me how much love I felt in my heart. Karen meant more to me than anything I had ever experienced. It was unbelievably good.

When my wife was pregnant with my second child, I was anxious and feared that there would not be enough love in my heart, certainly not to the same extreme. I couldn't believe that I could feel the same way.

Back to the two questions- the answer is yes. There was plenty there, and for the third and the fourth child, the first grandchild, and through the ninth grandchild. God's never-ending capacity to love, and we have the same power in that sense.

The word is "Love your neighbor as yourself," and we have the God-given capacity to do it.

Thought for Today: Today, let us recognize our capacity to love, care, and respect everyone we meet.

Prayer for Today: Dear Lord, we have love in our hearts that you have shared with us and pray that everyone can find this love and that we can take a step forward to world peace. Amen

River Nene, Peterborough,
Cambridgeshire, UK

April 21

Our Fortress

Photo By Simon Halsey

God is our refuge and strength,
an ever-present help in trouble.
(Psalm 46 vs 1)

A friend and spiritual mentor wrote the following poem.

Psalm Forty-Six
By George Ewing

With the rising sun, God starts our day
We check our schedules and are on our way
In our hearts, we may feel a twinge or a prod
Be still, and know I am God!

The phony games of life we choose to play
We do not seek to know God's will for our day
Strange voices about Jesus may seem very odd
Be still and know that I am God!

Now, as I kneel before the cross
Has life passed by, leaving me at a loss
Then Jesus' arms pick me up from the sod
Be still and know that I am God!

Thought for Today: God is our rock, fortress, and love.

Prayer for Today: We thank people like George for their contributions to our lives by helping us remember You. Amen

River Nene, Peterborough,
Cambridgeshire, UK

Strongholds

"The weapons we fight with are not the weapons of the world. On the contrary, they have divine power to demolish strongholds."
(2 Corinthians 10 vs 3.)

Life contains issues that dominate our thoughts and distract us from our spirituality. Distractions with a stronghold on us, "strongholds," block us from being Godly or spiritual. They may be destructive or even exciting and positive issues. On the surface, they may be perfect for us.

In our case, the Pickering family had some very successful years and a good life. We owned and ran three businesses, traveled, and raised four children. Those were also triathlon years, and June and I kept very fit. (I just looked at some old photos and wondered how we ever looked like that.) Some people, including my pastor, talked with me about possibly being OCD. That could never have been true, making money, having fun, having great family trips, etc., and we did go to church. That is the American way. We were victims of a positive stronghold.

There were some negatives. In the early '80s, a recession caused business stress that dominated our thoughts. Another time when there were two kids in college, and our primary business had issues that caused us to hedge our bets and start a second business.

Positive and negative issues in our lives can be overwhelming. When these strongholds take over, a spiritual focus will level the field. In our case, we knew that we needed help and emotional support. So we prayed a lot and meditated about the Lord's role in our lives. We made it with the help of spiritual growth, and so can you.

Thought for Today: Today, let's recognize our strongholds and pray for release. We can take a break from them.

Prayer for Today: Dear Lord and father, today is the day you made for us to enjoy. We simply thank you in our prayer. Amen

April 23 East Lake Waushakum
Sterling, Massachusetts

Strong Defenses

The weapons we fight with are not the weapons of the world. On the contrary, they have divine power to demolish strongholds.
(2 Corinthians 10 vs 4)

Today is confession time after yesterday's meditation. This message is on recognizing strongholds, things that have strong control over our lives. Yesterday was about positive and negative strongholds in our life experience. Today I will mention some of the things we did that should have been keys that somebody needed some additional prayer.

A. We often spent more money on vacations than we gave to the Church.
B. We would skip Church when I needed a long training run for my next triathlon.
C. Getting up on Sunday morning, working before Church, and then skipping Church to finish.
D. Lack of bible study in our lives.

It is positive to stay fit, but maybe I could have run early or after Church. Family vacations are expensive, but the Church needs support, or it will not exist. Respect for the Sabbath leads to a more peaceful life; we figured that out relatively early. Being involved in support of the local Church and attending a weekly study can keep you at peace and has many rewards.

Keeping things in perspective and having family and personal priorities leads to inner peace in our lives. They will help us keep the spirit in our lives.

Thought for Today: Think about our distractions and pray about them; keep the Holy Spirit in all our activities.

Prayer for Today: Dear Lord and father, we pray for personal peace and that we may contribute to peace around us through our tranquility. Amen

Idols

Therefore, fear the Lord and worship Him in sincerity and truth. Get rid of the gods your ancestors worshiped beyond the Euphrates River and in Egypt, and worship the Lord.
(Joshua 24 vs 14)

Living here in Minnesota, it is understandable to appreciate the warmth of the sun and fire. It is hard for me to relate to the ancient Gods and idols like Ra, the Sun God; Bacchus, the God of wine and revelry; Aphrodite, God of beauty and sexuality; and a lengthy list of others. Years ago, I appreciated Bacchus' influence on my youthful life and Aphrodite's contributions. Although they were often strong influences, they were not God-like.

Growing up in Boston, Ted Williams of the Red Sox and Bill Russell of the Celtics come to mind because they are often considered heroes. My dad had a fantasy about the Olympic swimmer Johnny Weissmuller, so my brother Wayne and I became swimmers. As a national populace, we tend to put a lot of emphasis on our sports heroes. However, it is wrong when that emphasis approaches worship status.

We need to recognize where our real bread is buttered; who will never desert us; who will always be with us. We do not always have sunshine, wine, and beauty; we always have the Lord. We are blessed.

Thought for Today: Today, we will read and hear about our heroes. The games of summer are approaching, and basketball and hockey playoffs are beginning. For today when we hear or read of them, let's take a minute to review our commitment to the Lord and His never-ending commitment to us.

Prayer for Today: Dear Lord, today we give thanks that you are with us; to nurture, support, and help us through our every need. Amen

Frozen Chosen

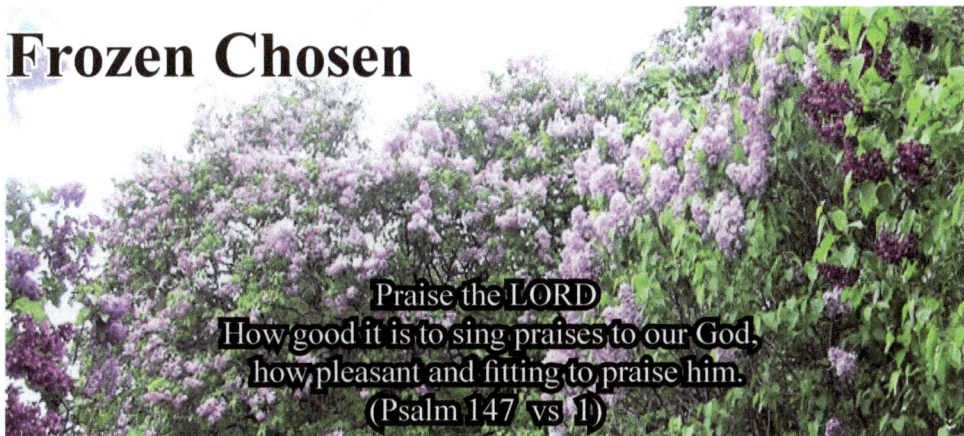

> Praise the LORD
> How good it is to sing praises to our God,
> how pleasant and fitting to praise him.
> (Psalm 147 vs 1)

Beth Moore recently talked about evangelism, sharing our faith, and singing praises. Not only during Sunday services but all week long. That is evangelism, an invitational ministry, a welcoming format. In our small Methodist church, we are far from being evangelists. The young families are too busy, and the older generation seems too tired. A term that I like is that we are the "frozen chosen."

Twenty years ago, we had a gospel group come to our church for what they thought would be a rousing concert. We enjoyed the music, but foot-stomping was not an apt description! The leader did all he could to get a group of Methodists to stomp their feet and clap their hands.

Several years ago, a group complained at a worship team meeting because people often applauded when our quartet or a soloist finished a piece. They requested that we put a notice in the announcements asking for no such show of pleasure or appreciation. As a team member, I stated that if the applause were outlawed, they would have to deal with me standing upon a pew shouting "halleluiah-Amen!" Our pastor said, "Pass the motion. I want to see that!" I was blessed, and the motion failed. We still applaud. We make decisions every day as to how we will interact with others. Today we will decide whether we will be inviting Christians or members of the frozen chosen.

Thought for Today: Let's mention our faith or our church to show someone why we are who we are. Let's take our faith public at least for a day.

Prayer for Today: Dear Lord, the world is blooming into spring, and your wondrous work abounds, but there is strife and war. Today we pray that we may contribute to peace around the world. Amen

Happy Landing

Blessed is the one who perseveres under trial because,
having stood the test,
that person will receive the crown of life
that the Lord has promised to those who love him.
(James 1 vs 12)

We all hope for an easy life without illness or discomfort, always having a job, a life partner to share things with, and the list goes on. In other words, we want to be born to live happily ever after. Perseverance is life, we need to persevere in many ways, and the easiest way is through meditation, prayer, and having the faith that the Lord will bring us through our lives.

If we were, we would not build character or learn. As I write this in beautiful Minnesota, we are nearing the end of what has been a record-breaking winter. A year ago, there was green grass and no ice, and this year we are sitting on 15 inches of dirty snow with two storms scheduled for the next five days.

It is an excellent example of why trials are in our lives. They cause growth and appreciation of the good times. In the instance of our Minnesota weather, in 1974, our real estate agent talked about our beautiful summers and said they were worth the wait. Praise be to God. We need help this year! We will get through it, and when spring comes, it will be later than usual and appreciated more.

There is a church that I drive by that posts a weekly slogan that describes it very well. I do not know the author, but it said that life is not about having a bumpy flight. It is about having a smooth landing!" The best part will be the landing! We need to keep our faith to persevere on our bumpy ride.

Thought for Today: Today will be the first day of the rest of our lives. Let us be spiritual and use it well.

Prayer for Today: Dear Father, we are experiencing a very bumpy ride. Today we give thanks for having the spirit and will to get through it all so that we may experience the landing. Amen

Hollicombe Beach
Torque, Devon, UK

April 27

Skin Deep

> So we do not focus on what is seen, but on what is unseen; for what is seen is temporary, but what is unseen is eternal.
> (2 Corinthians 4 vs 8)

In New England, growing up on the north shore of Boston, there was a lot of what my mom called "old money." She used to say that you would never know it when interacting with a family member with it. They would not be overdressed or act superior in any way. She was correct, and they did not. They spent a fortune training on speaking, dressing, and behaving so as not to stand out in a crowd.

My best friend was from an old-money family, and his dad was a great mentor and role model. Old Bert was always around to advise and unknowingly helped me throughout my life. He was a great example. Bert said, "The harder you work before you are thirty, the better your life will be after thirty." And, "No matter how hard it may be, always be honest, and you will win the battle." Bert was always dressed neat rather than gaudy and kept lean and fit.

Bert also was the first person I ever knew that mentioned bible study. He was willing to speak the Lord's word and incorporate it into his life. Bert's beauty went deep and he incorporated Sunday School stuff into his personal and business life. His beauty was not only skin deep.

As Christians, our beauty is not skin deep. We worry about how we appear, and we need a look that fits and is self-satisfying. We also need to extend our beauty deeper into our hearts through prayer and meditation.

Thought for Today: Let's look in that mirror and ensure that we meet society's specifications for being neat and trim. Then, let us take a few moments to meditate, pray, and prepare for a day of true beauty.

Prayer for Today: Dear Lord and Father, today we thank you for our beautiful lives and the opportunity to represent you and your ways. We pray that we can contribute to your loving will here on earth..Amen

Hollicombe Beach
Torque, Devon, UK

April 28

Endurance

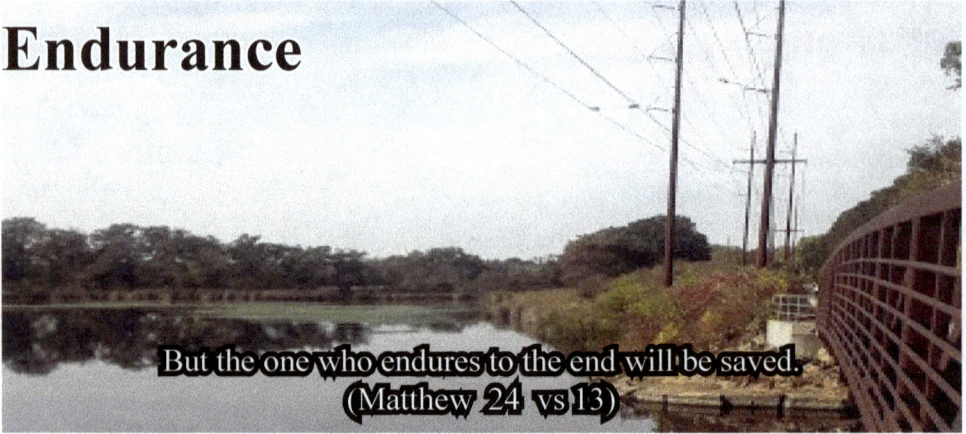

> But the one who endures to the end will be saved.
> (Matthew 24 vs 13)

"Endure to the end." I am not sure what that means because there is no end to me. June and I have spent time in twelve-step programs, and as Stephen ministers working with people with life issues, chemical demons, and mental and social issues. We dealt with anger, depression, and the "why me" syndrome. Asking the question, "What did I do to deserve this?" is useless to the recovery and spiritual growth process. Dealing with growth steps to become happy and satisfied citizens is what matters. We are all experiencing life and do not know where it leads us. That is the wondrous mystery. While here on earth, we will leave a mark, a legacy.

We recently attended the eightieth birthday party of a lady at church. She is a positive force in our congregation and the matriarch of her family. There were four generations of her family in attendance. Love, closeness, and happiness were flowing and glowing for all of us to see. Their passion will someday become their memories, her legacy.

To Christians, there is no end to some a mystery. What is not a mystery is that we will leave our mark in the memories of others; we will leave a positive legacy through our faith, spirit, and love of Christ.

Thought for Today: For today, let us go out and live our Christian lives full of enthusiasm and joy. Let us live like there is no end.

Prayer for Today: Heavenly Father, we give thanks for our wondrous lives and the many gifts you have given us. We especially thank you for the opportunity through Christ to help accomplish your will here on earth through our faith by sharing with others. Amen

Relationships

My dear brothers and sisters,
take note of this: Everyone should be quick to listen,
slow to speak and slow to become angry,
human anger does not produce the righteousness that God desires.
(James 1 vs 19, 20)

Relationships are similar to spirituality because when they are growing, they move toward perfection. We cannot become perfect in relationships, but we can approach perfection. We can never reach perfection in our spirit because we cannot be God.

Once at a marriage seminar, the instructor talked about the expectations of a wedding day and the futility of thinking that one spouse could impart change on the other. He pointed out that many marriages fail because "the other" did not adjust.

Another piece he addressed was who walked into the church and who walked out on a wedding day. As he stated, the wife's model is her dad; the husband's model is his mother. Wow, if something doesn't change, this will never work! His point was that two lovers went in, and different expectations were set in marriage.

June and I talked about this recently; without change, the growth in marriage will not occur; expecting one to change to fit will not work. We concluded that, like spirituality, both persons in a relationship need to stay the same, but the couple needs to grow together. A good analogy is the two must evolve together into something new. They need to polish their edges and fit together in a new mold.

That sounds simple. Let's pray that it is.

Thought for the Day: Today, let us look at our relationships and recognize our expectations. Let us understand how we can grow to make them better.

Prayer for the Day: Dear Lord, we give thanks for your guidance and the chance to grow in our faith. We appreciate your presence. Amen

May

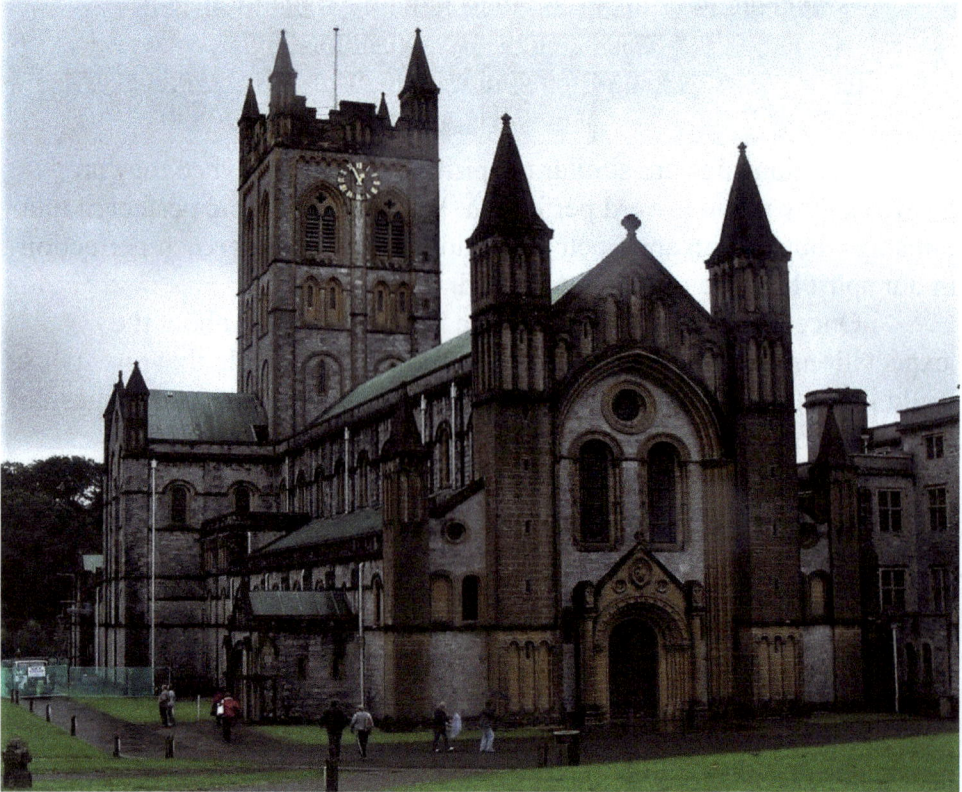

Buckfast Abby

Buckfast Abbey forms part of an active Benedictine monastery at Buckfast, near Buckfastleigh, Devon, UK. Buckfast first became home to an abbey in 1018.It was destroyed by Henry VIII in 1539. It was rebuilt by French Benedictine monks starting in 1882 and reinstated as an Abby in 1902.

Buckfastleigh, Devon, UK

Pride and Humility

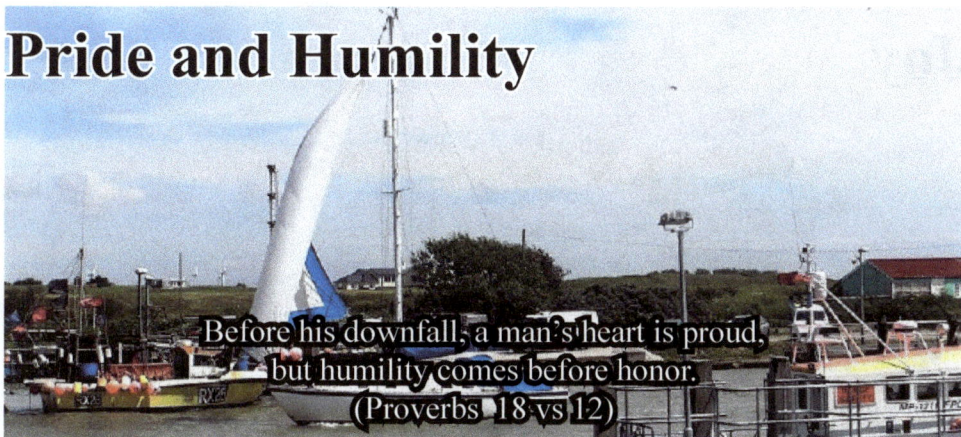

Before his downfall, a man's heart is proud,
but humility comes before honor.
(Proverbs 18 vs 12)

My mom used to use some interesting terms and expressions when describing humanity. One of her favorites was "foolhardy" when someone did something out of line. Another was, "It is better to be silent and thought a fool than to speak out and remove all doubt." Somehow, when we are proud in the context of today's text, we are not paying attention. When we exhibit false pride, it helps us grow to appreciate the realities of life.

We are often overconfident, especially when we are young. Somehow, that is God's way of teaching us. We constantly have to monitor our pride and confidence. The elders of society have knowledge and experience but are not always correct. Technology and society are changing faster than fifty years ago. Therefore many of the rules of life have changed.

In our spiritual lives, the rules have not and will not change. The ethics, love, and traditions Christ taught us will endure regardless of technology changes and cash flows. We need to take inventory of our pride and be honest. We must hold up our values to serve the Lord.

Thought for Today: Every day is the first day of the rest of our lives. The mistakes and experiences of our past are nothing more than learning
experiences and enable us to move forward with confidence. Today, let us focus on being humble and dealing with the realities of our worlds.

Prayer for Today: Heavenly Father, we give thanks for the lessons we have learned and our loves. Thank you for putting it before us through all that Jesus taught us and what we learned from the past. Amen

Rye Harbor
Rye, East Sussex, UK

Joy

The Lord is my strength and my shield. \ My heart trusts in him, and I am helped. My heart leaps for joy, and I will give thanks to him in song. (Psalm 28 vs 7)

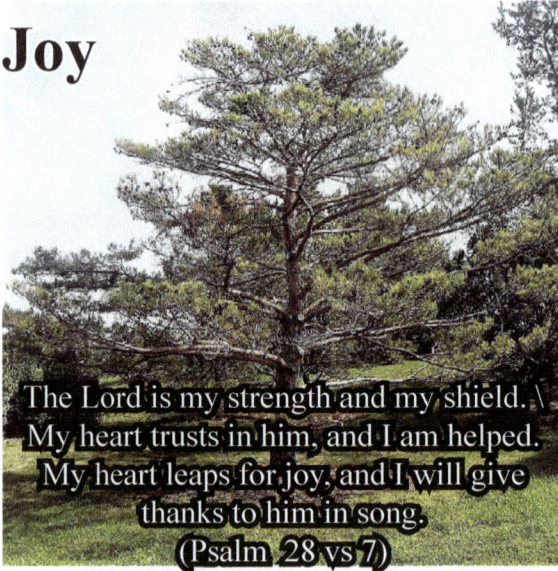

Is there joy in our lives? Let us face it, most of us have more joy (positives) than negatives. Our family, friends, and associates are sources of great joy. It is easy to see spring joy. It is spring, and the grass is green; the trees are budding with leaves, and spring flowers are showing their colors.

Many today have a problem seeing the joys in their lives. There are issues caused by COVID 19 that have changed our lives. Even so, there are always positives. Keeping the Lord in our lives through prayer when we are down is vital. As Paul said to the Romans (15:13), "May the God of hope fill you with all joy and peace as you trust in him, so that you may overflow with hope by the power of the Holy Spirit."

Our surroundings and lifestyles create our physical and emotional joys. Absolute joy comes through our Christian beliefs. This belief gives us the "strength" and "shield" mentioned by the Psalmist.

Thought for Today: Let us keep joy at the forefront of our thoughts. When challenged with life, let's use our shield - the Lord.

Prayer for the Week: Heavenly Father, many of our friends, are fighting battles. Illness, unemployment, unwanted career changes, and many others. We pray for them to understand your strength and love. We pray that they may find the joy only available through trust in you. Amen

May 2   Japanese Red Pine
Minnesota Landscape Arboretum

Happiness

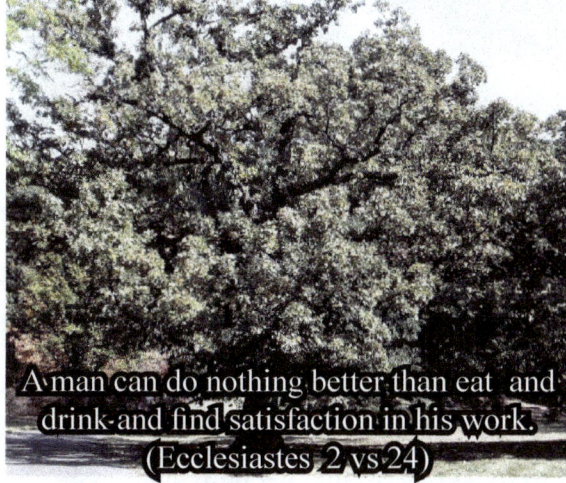

A man can do nothing better than eat and drink and find satisfaction in his work.
(Ecclesiastes 2 vs 24)

Recently my granddaughter was picked up at 6 pm and taken past McDonnell's for a happy meal on the way to buy a mother's day gift for mom. How many of us rush through the drive-through, curse the length of the line and the fact that we will be held up ten minutes waiting for lunch? I certainly have done that.

What are the hustle and bustle all about? The pursuit of "things" and "stuff"? We are all working our hearts out and often have too little time to consider what matters. Yes, it is easier at my age (81) to say slow down and smell the roses, but I pray you can.

Thought for Today: Look at our pursuits and find the time to meditate; understand where God fits into the puzzle that is our life. Let us be sure that our puzzle does not have a piece missing.

Prayer for Today: Dear Lord, please help me locate what you want from me today. There are many spring options: The celebration of mother's day, a round of golf, opening of fishing, and others. Somehow help me keep you in this puzzle so that no pieces are missing. Amen

Ministers

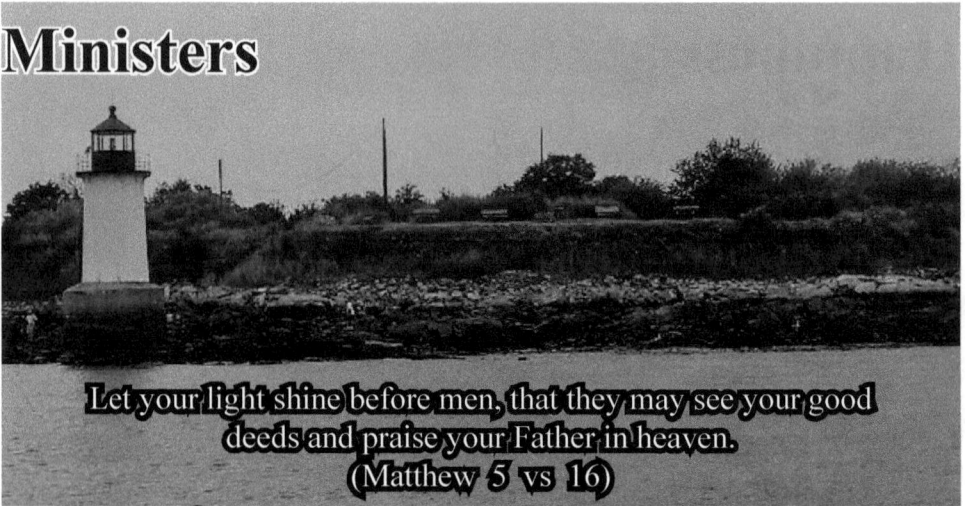

Let your light shine before men, that they may see your good deeds and praise your Father in heaven.
(Matthew 5 vs 16)

My pastor says that we are all ministers in some way. Is that true? The term closet minister applies to most Christians. We help, lead by example, attend services to learn more, and silently minister to those around us. Sometimes we do not know we are ministering.

In every Sunday service, takers, givers, and silent ministries occur in many ways. Several years ago, a young single couple acted in a very special way, holding hands, whispering in each other's ears, and an occasional peck on the cheek. Usually, that would be inappropriate. The pastor announced their pending wedding during that service.

After the service, the conversation was about how neat that was to have that level of enthusiasm for each other. That couple, without intent, set an example for older couples. They were ministers. "In the same way, let your light shine before men, that they may see your good deeds...".

Thought for Today: Be thankful for those around us, at peace, and demonstrate our passion and love for others. Spring flowers have burst into color; warm weather makes us feel great, so let's utilize our spring spirit to demonstrate our faith.

Prayer for Today: Heavenly Father, you have blessed us with many friends. We are surrounded and cannot avoid them. We are blessed at work, on the streets, and at home. Today we pray for that they all recognize the beauty of Christian friendship. Amen

Footprints

"I come to the garden alone,
while the dew is still on the roses,
and the voice I hear falling on my ear,
the son of God discloses.
and he walks with me,
and he talks with me,
and he tells me I am His own,
and the joy we share as we tarry there,
none other has ever known."
(In the Garden, C. Austin Miles)
(Methodist Hymnal No. 314)

The overwhelming support we have as citizens of faith is the most significant advantage of being Christian; it is terrific. Since birth, I have been an early riser and, as an endurance athlete and golfer, spent a lot of sunrises alone running a trail or walking a fairway "…when the due is still on the roses." The silence of the dawn, broken only by early doves and robins, is peaceful. There are times I often catch myself humming this tune.

In the Garden is an excellent reminder that God is with us and we are never alone. I would often be humming it on my way to a tough meeting or hospital visit.   It is good to remind yourself that you are never alone if you let Him join you.

Most days, my coat had a lapel pin from "Footprints in the sand," a pair of feet. It served as a reminder of the support and encouraged conversation about walking with Christ.

We are blessed.

Thought for Today: Remember that we are never alone and enjoy His presence as we walk through our lives.
Prayer for Today: Heavenly Father, we are certainly glad that you are here for support. The world around us is confusing and difficult to understand. However, we thank your role in our everyday lives and the help you give our friends and families. Amen

Shrub Rose Garden
Minnesota Landscape Arboretum   **May 5**   Page 131

Young At Heart

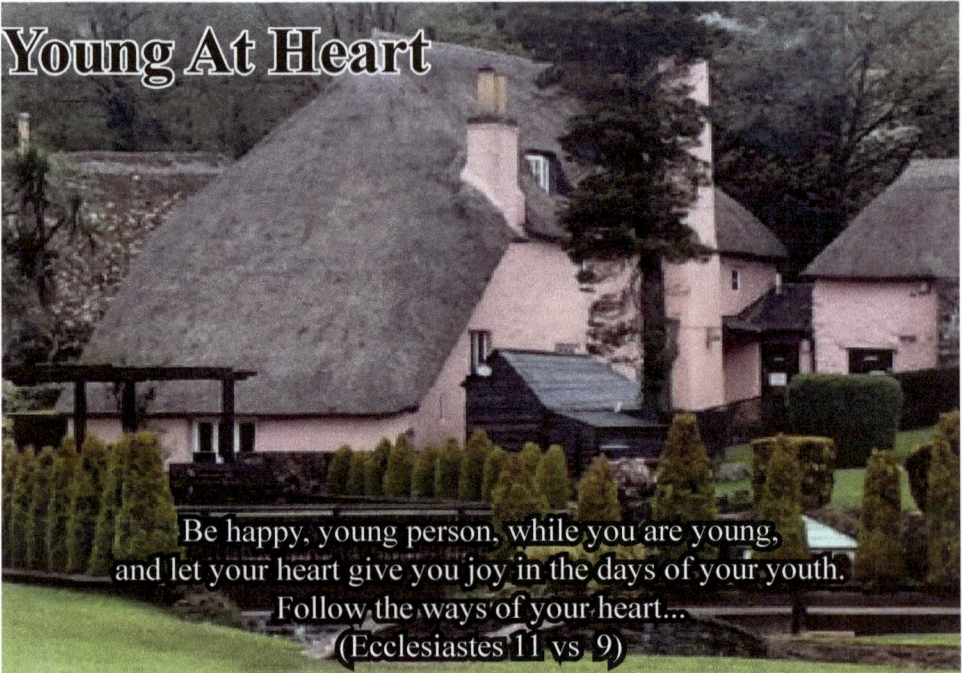

Be happy, young person, while you are young,
and let your heart give you joy in the days of your youth.
Follow the ways of your heart...
(Ecclesiastes 11 vs 9)

Some people seem at peace. They avoided the rat race of life and found the happiness most were seeking. The interesting fact is they cross all socioeconomic boundaries. The common thread is always their faith. They believe things will work out.

The strong message here is that the things that bring peace, serenity, and happiness to our lives are found in spiritual growth and can be found in yours.

Thought for Today: Today, avoid the rat race by praying for serenity and doing what we need to obtain peace.

Prayer for Today: Dear Lord, thank you for the opportunities before us. We pray for serenity, love, and the chance to promote peace in our community. Amen

May 6 Thatched Cottage
Cockington Village, Devon, UK

Faith and Forgiveness

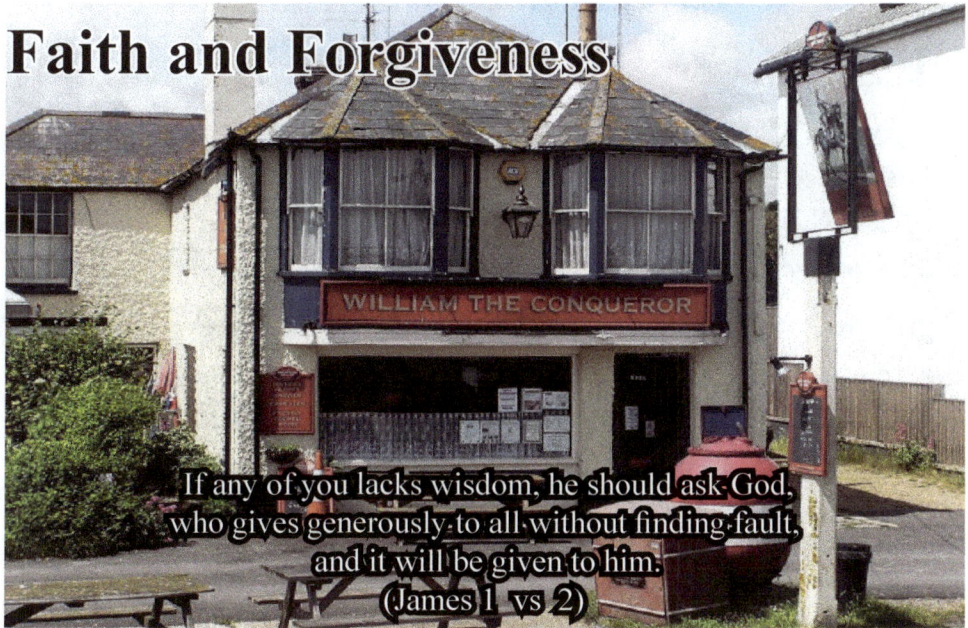

> If any of you lacks wisdom, he should ask God, who gives generously to all without finding fault, and it will be given to him.
> (James 1 vs 2)

Faith seems to be a constant challenge to us. Yes, sometimes we need to understand where God is in our lives. We can doubt that He is with us; we challenge his input and knowingly violate His rules and submit to temptation. Does this make us bad people?

The answer is a resounding NO. As we look back at our lives, we often see a trail of mistakes, moments, or events that we would like to edit or replay. Surely we know that reliving life is not an option. But, feeling guilty or bad about these things can cause a faith crisis or low self-image and harm our future.

This week, at a bible study, we talked about letting go of past discretions. When we learn to forgive others, we find it easier to accept the forgiveness we receive from God. Others forgave us long ago, and somehow as adults, we seem to hold on to past errors.

Thought for Today: When we are swamped, it is difficult to feel God's presence in our lives. Today, let us all try to take time to understand and appreciate His contributions.

Prayer for Today: Dear Lord and Father, today we give thanks for the knowledge that we are forgiven through the grace given us through Jesus. We pray that somehow we can find a way to forgive ourselves for our sins. Amen

William The Conqueror Pub
Rye Harbour, Ease Sussex, UK   **May 7**

Spring

"In the bulb, there is a flower,
in the seed an apple tree;
in cocoons, a hidden promise:
butterflies will soon be free!
In the cold and snow of Winter
there's a Spring that waits to be,
unrevealed until it's season,
something God alone can see."
(Hymn of Promise, Verse 1, Natalie Sleeth, 1986)

Spring is s glorious time of the year. The northern hemisphere goes into the transition to Summer. It is a time when the resolutions from the new year are long since successful or forgotten. A time of vacation planning, garden planting, and the anticipation of the beauty of the warm season. A time of hope led by the visible evidence of God's presence around us.

Spring is a time for reflection and review of our dark side. A review of the negative forces in our lives. This is Spring, and we need to recover the "...hidden promise..." in our personal lives "... that God alone can see."

Through our faith and belief, our Lord will share the pleasures of life with us.

Thought for Today: It is Spring. Take special notice of its wonders. Smell the flowers and enjoy the showers. Let us share these positive feelings with others and encourage positive feelings around us.

Prayer for Today: Heavenly Father, we pray for an end to senseless killing and the guidance to understand this violent world that surrounds us that somehow through your divine guidance, killing, hate, and violence may end. Amen

May 8   Shrub Rose Garden
Minnesota Landscape Arboretum

Promise

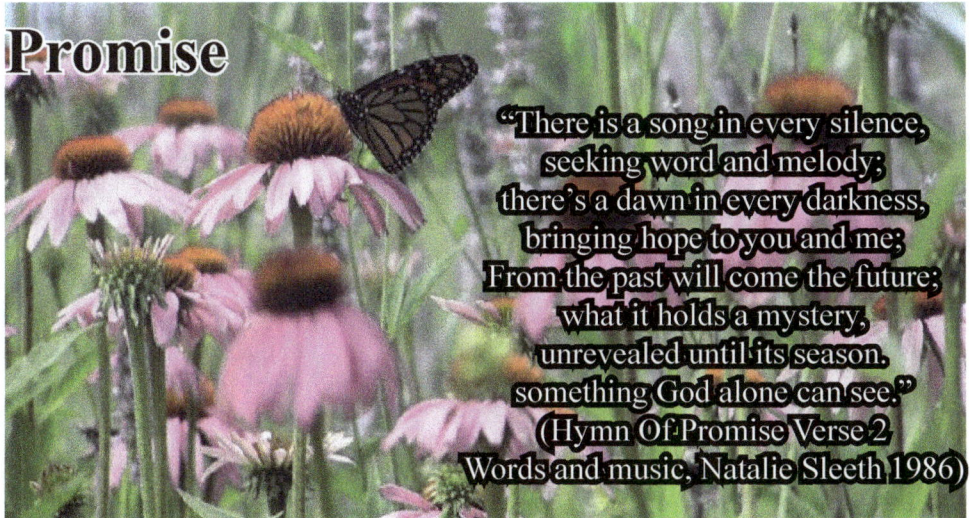

"There is a song in every silence, seeking word and melody; there's a dawn in every darkness, bringing hope to you and me; From the past will come the future; what it holds a mystery, unrevealed until its season, something God alone can see."
(Hymn Of Promise Verse 2 Words and music, Natalie Sleeth 1986)

A recently retired pastor listed this as one of his favorite hymns. It is easy to see why. We put our lives in God's hands, he knows and loves us, and we know we have a future through our faith. This verse talks about times when life is too quiet- when we need to talk. It mentions the dark times and assures that there will be light and better times; the past, which we are not always proud of, will become a bright future through Him. It points out that we do not know or predict what He has in store for us.

A case in point is a good friend called me in prayer. He has worked for a company for 18 years and was undergoing the job stress typical in today's world. We met this week, and he was now OK. Management, led by a Christian friend, solved his problems. They met with him to discuss his future and told him that they valued him as an employee and wanted to ensure he was comfortable.

Ask yourself if God was at work here.

Thought for Today: Some days are brighter than others. The symbol of a gray or sunny day is easy to understand. Our lives are like that. We know that brighter days will follow the dark ones through our faith. This week let us focus on the cheerful times.

Prayer for Today: Heavenly Father, there are many dark areas worldwide. Today, we pray for the understanding that you are with us through dark times and that we can appreciate the light at the end of the tunnel. Amen

Butterfly
Minnesota Landscape Arboretum

Follow The Way

Do not conform any longer to the pattern of this world,
but be transformed by the renewing of your mind.
(Romans 12 vs 1)

Society does not fit the biblical model we are taught and often desire. Truth, honesty, integrity, love, and many other virtues seem rare. Often, we join in and need correction in our human desire to "fit". It is normal to err and join in. It is also forgivable.

In a discussion last week in a business environment, we reviewed several long-term, successful people in business. We compared the successful men with some that were sinking fast or already out of business. Those with long-term success functioned like they had read Paul's message to the Romans. They were not always right but always seemed to grow and strive for excellence. Fairness was their trademark; perpetual growth appeared to be a trait.

They earned the respect and trust of those around them and were not "sharks" but win-win businessmen. They incorporated their Christian beliefs into the challenging world of doing business. That is truly doing God's will.

Thought for Today: Stand up and be counted; demonstrate our faith in circumstances where we would not normally do so. Demonstrate that we are considerate and Godly in our daily activities.

Prayer for Today: Dear Lord, our world is distracting and volatile. We all have too much to do, too many commitments, and too many fears. Throughout all of this, we pray for peace. We pray for our internal peace and the ability to demonstrate the value of peace to others. Amen

Letting Go

Bear with each other and forgive whatever grievances you may have against one another. Forgive as the Lord forgave you. (Colossians 3 vs 13)

At a meeting discussing our sixtieth class reunion, our discussion led to many things in our youth that we were not proud of; behaviors or incidences on our conscience. Each contributed to our development, and they did not make us bad people. At the time, school authorities, neighbors, parents, and friends did not appreciate us. James 1 verse 4 says, "Let perseverance finishing its work so that you may be mature and complete, not lacking anything." Our memories are part of the perseverance equation that makes us what we are.

Letting go of past discretions is a challenge. Others forgave us long ago, but somehow we seem to hold on to the past. As we work through our faults, life goes on, and God works his miracles in our lives. When we lack wisdom, he comes through for us.

Thought for Today: It is often difficult to feel God's presence in our lives. Today, let us all try to understand and appreciate His contributions.

Prayer for Today: Heavenly Father, thank you today because we are not what we were. We have sinned along the way and are grateful for the Grace and forgiveness we receive through Christ. Amen

Stewardship I

Honor the Lord with your wealth,
with the firstfruits of all your crops;
then your barns will be filled to overflowing,
your vats will brim over with new wine.
(Proverbs 3 vs 9,10)

Money is a challenging subject. How do we fit the pursuit of money and quality of life into our Christian values? Undoubtedly, the competition for wealth is a God-given right and necessity that goes back to the beginning of time. The operating style in which we pursue wealth and what we do with our wealth can be compatible with God's will. Working with others, servicing others, and meeting others' needs generates money and wealth. What we do with that money and wealth makes the difference.

Do we pursue wealth in a manner that helps society, or do we take advantage of others to obtain wealth? That is always a gray area that we must have clear in our minds. If in your heart, you are competing in this society with the Lord first in your mind, you are on the right track.

Thought for Today: Today, ask if we contribute to society and others; think about how much of our efforts and time we contribute to God's work.

Prayer for Today: Heavenly Father, please help me understand this complex life. The bible says to give it all away and trust in the Lord, while our social system seems to demand accruing wealth. People who give are happy and at peace within our society. Amen

View from Broadsands Beach
Paignton, Devon, UK

Stewardship II

> Honor the Lord with your wealth,
> with the firstfruits of all your crops;
> then your barns will be filled to overflowing,
> your vats will brim over with new wine.
> (Proverbs 3 vs 9,10)

In the follow-up to yesterday, here are two examples. First is a Minnesota entrepreneur who built a company that became the largest of its kind in the world. He made tens of millions of dollars. In doing so, he created wealth in the families of his employees, jobs for thousands of people around the world, and in recent years has gifted millions of dollars to schools for technical education facilities. He handled his monetary success in a way that made the Lord smile.

Another example on a larger scale was Charles M. Schultz of "Snoopy" fame. Throughout his life, he brought pleasure to millions. In his community, he contributed generously and to millions' benefit. He used his God-given vision and talent to help the world and rewarded his "barns overflowing."

In summary, it is not harmful to pursue wealth, and it is a necessity. Dating wealth by contributing to society and the art of giving back first rather than last makes the difference.

Thought for Today: As we go through the day, ask if we contribute to society and others and how much of our efforts and time we contribute to God's work.

Prayer for Today: Heavenly Father, help me understand this complex life we live. The bible says to give it all away and trust the Lord while our social system demands wealth building. We pray that we can understand your place and keep you at the forefront of my heart. Amen

Temptations

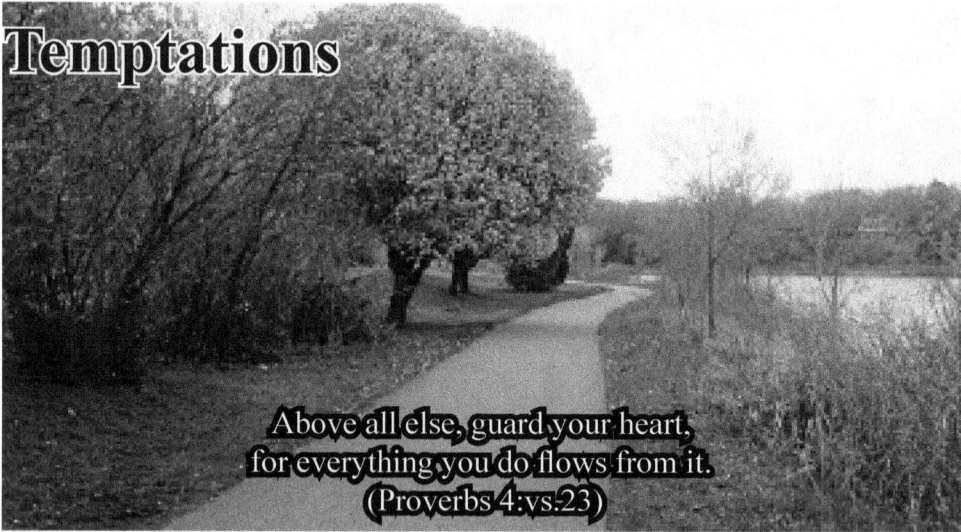

Above all else, guard your heart, for everything you do flows from it.
(Proverbs 4:vs.23)

Here we go again on being good, not succumbing to temptation. We sure get tired of that, don't we? In twelve-step programs, there is a lot of talk about the goal of spiritual growth rather than spiritual perfection. That means we will never be perfect. Are you OK with that?

This proverb goes on and on about being good by mentioning, "…guard your heart, your lips, look straight ahead, etc." I did not print it all because we all know that.

I ask but do not want to know your specific temptations and intend to share mine. The bad news is we all have them. The good news is that the Lord is with us. Purity, ethics, commitments, and standards begin in our hearts.

"For where your treasure is, there your heart will be also."
(Mathew 6 vs 21)

Thought for Today: We need to be the best we can be each day. Today we will make choices; make them from our heart- in purity with ethics, commitments, and high standards

Prayer for Today: Thank you, Lord, for your presence and guidance in our lives. We pray that we rise above our temptations and r epresent your will here on earth. Amen

May 14   Lake of the Isles Walking Path
Minneapolis, Minnesota

Maturity

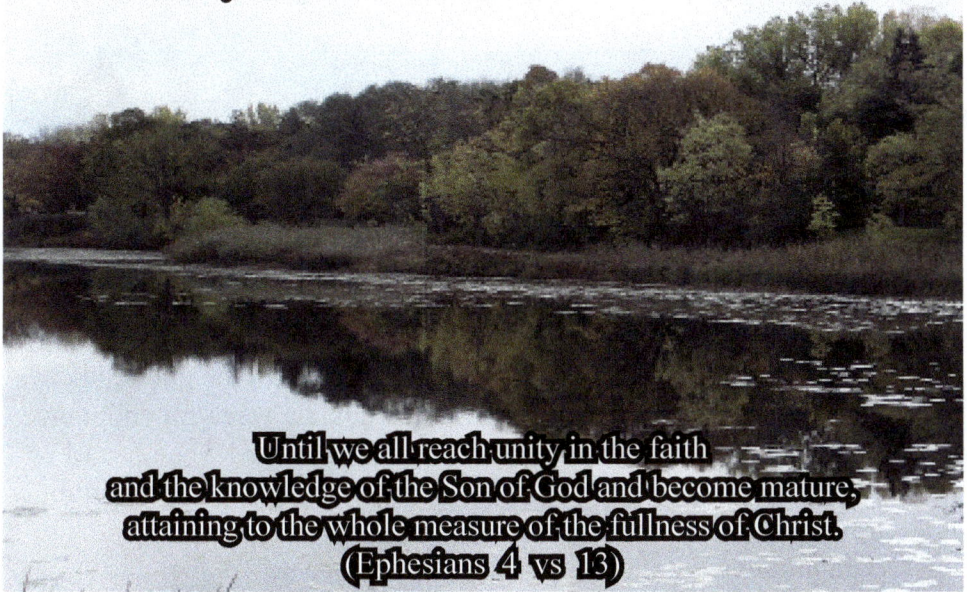

Until we all reach unity in the faith
and the knowledge of the Son of God and become mature,
attaining to the whole measure of the fullness of Christ.
(Ephesians 4 vs 13)

The piece of the twelve-step programs that I like best describes that our goal is spiritual growth rather than spiritual perfection. That lets us off the hook regarding being perfect, which we cannot attain. It removes a lot of guilt.

Yes, we always need to grow in spirit, work on it daily, and measure our progress. Some say we must measure against "…nothing less than the character of Christ." The question we have is, what is our standard?

Hmmm, that is a problem because we cannot attain perfection. That does not diminish the dream of being Christ-like. So what seems to be a problem is a gift. When faced with options and choices, we need to ask; What would Jesus Do? Then we need to do it to ensure our growth.

Thought for Today: Today, let's be loving and forgiving in all of our activities.

Prayer for the Day: Dear Lord, we pray for guidance and the ability to be more like Jesus and do your will. Amen

Lake of the Isles
Minneapolis. Minnesota
May 15
Page 141

Finishing Again

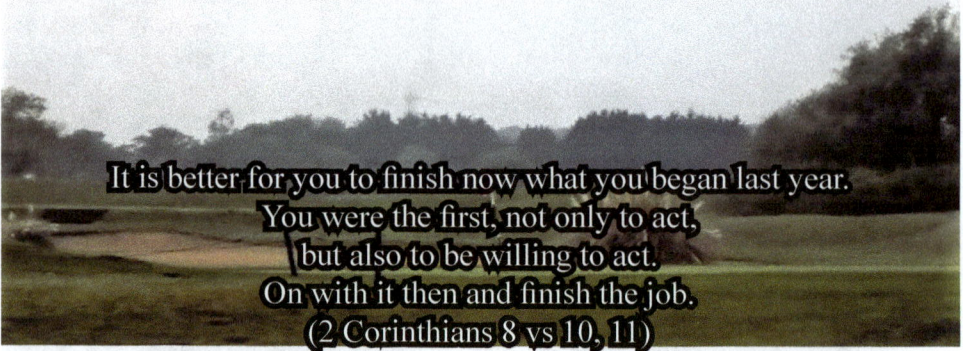

It is better for you to finish now what you began last year.
You were the first, not only to act,
but also to be willing to act.
On with it then and finish the job.
(2 Corinthians 8 vs 10, 11)

In the spring, my thoughts gravitate toward the good old days when my friends and I trained ten to fourteen hours a week for endurance events. The camaraderie of the group, the support offered when one of us was having a bad day, and the feeling of spirituality in the early mornings as we traveled on our way was priceless.

As an unranked runner but former elite master's swimmer and triathlete, sometimes finishing a running event near the bottom of the pack was more rewarding to me than a swimming or triathlon trophy. Trophies are nice mementos but, over time, become unimportant dust collectors.

In the early '80s, my friend Billy and I ran a half marathon. He finished a good half hour ahead of me and felt great. I was unprepared and had severe problems. The following year, Billy was again a half-hour ahead of me, but I had trained well and met my expectations. I fondly remember that day and have that finishing picture on my office wall reminding me that being at the bottom of the pack is not bad when you are at the top of your game. The goal is personal, to be the best YOU can be. Neither of us won that event or our age group. Both of us were proud winners because we finished. Life is like that- when we finish what we start, we win.

Thought for Today: It is spring, a time of renewal. God brings us flowers, green grass, and warm temperatures. It is easy to be busy enjoying it all and put a few issues on the back burner of life. Today let's identify what we need to finish, who we need to help, and who needs our prayers to visit. Let's complete the tasks that the Lord has put before us.

Prayer for Today: Heavenly Father, we need your guidance on using your love to succeed find a way to contribute so that we somehow finish the race for peace and security. Amen

Page 142   **May 16**   Traditions Golf Course
Pytford, Surrey, UK

Play Christ's Way

Therefore, welcome one another
as Christ has welcomed you, for the glory of God.
(Romans 15 vs 7)

We are faced with decisions every day regarding our relationship with others. Sometimes there is aggressive behavior. In business, there is a competition to get to the top; in school, the head of the class; in sports, to be number one, etc. It is the way it is.

When growing up, I was taught that winning is not everything. It was how you played the game that mattered. In the seventies, I attended a business management seminar sponsored by Green Bay coach Vince Lombardi. The emphasis was on detail, being service-oriented, and planning. Over the years, the operating principles learned at that seminar have made my life very successful. They taught us to have a game plan and work it but alter it as needed.

To play by the rules takes faith in yourself and God and love and caring for people. Two recipients of my weekly messages are Christian CEOs, and how their companies behave matters to them. Christian ethics takes strong faith. No matter where or who we are, fairness and love of others are crucial to success.

Then how do we deal with the aggressive ones? the inconsiderate neighbor? Cut-throat businessman? The ones that bend the rules? We need to pray for and love our competitors in life. John quotes Jesus in chapter 15 vs 17, "This is my command, Love each other."

Thought for Today: This week, let us practice unconditional love in our lives. If confronted with opportunistic or aggressive behavior, let us find a way to positively and lovingly through the situation.

Prayer for Today: Dear Lord, let me reach out to people this week. Help me understand them and care about them. We pray that we can improve ourselves and our surrounding world through our faith, Amen

The Navigator

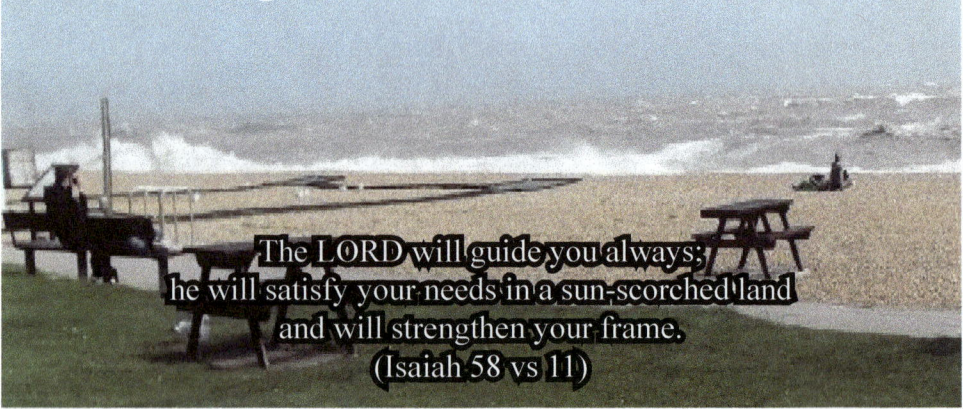

The LORD will guide you always;
he will satisfy your needs in a sun-scorched land
and will strengthen your frame.
(Isaiah 58 vs 11)

Sometimes waking up in the morning, we do not have a plan. We can be energized and happy or stressed and depressed. It is possible to adjust our thoughts to the spiritual side, open windows to our minds, and allow God's fresh breeze to liberate us when we are down. I am waiting for the breeze.

When waiting, there seems to be a need. Mine is for with strong coffee, sugar, and perhaps some Ibuprofen. That is not a good solution. It has a physical and temporary lift, but the need is better met spiritually.

We often forget that God is with us and take control. Today the breeze that arrived came through Isaiah 58:11. Using the driving analogy, I put God in the back seat with the kids and the dog rather than beside me as the navigator.

Allowing or recognizing God as our navigator will take us places we will not get to on our own.

Thought for Today: Today, there will be stress, difficult decisions, and times of anguish. Focus and remember that "God is with us." We must let Him lead, pray over the tough choices, and focus on following His will.

Prayer for Today: Heavenly Father, we pray to understand our immediate world and area of control. Our world is not well organized today. We pray that we can find a way to contribute. Amen

May 18 Pelham Beach Surf
Hastings, East Sussex, UK

Impact Play

I would rather be a doorkeeper in the house of my God
than dwell in the tents of the wicked.
(Psalm 84 vs. 10)

Faith is something that seems to be swept under the rug in sports. The Fellowship of Christian Athletes sends out a daily meditation that tends to be sports-based. It often comes from a member and is relative to an event that I watched. Two of my favorite members played or grew up here in Minnesota, former Viking Chris Carter and pro golfer Tom Lehman. Tom and Gerhard Langer used to lead bible studies when they were on the PGA tour together. I thoroughly enjoy hearing from them as they share their glory with the Lord.

Yesterday I received this passage in what they call "Impact Play." I like the name because daily reading affects your life. Psalm 84 did that yesterday.

As I read my emails, there was an urgent request for someone to usher at two special services this week. I had just replied that I did not care to participate. The following email was the "Impact Play" with the wording "…I would rather be a doorkeeper in the house of my God than dwell in the tents of the wicked." Oops, does that mean that I should change my mind? Is there a message here somewhere?

Pro golfer, Tom Lehman said that good things seem to happen when he keeps the Lord in his life. He noted that it was hard to do when lining up a fourth putt. Meditation puts the Lord closer to the forefront of our mind and makes the day better.

Thought for Today: Let's pay attention to the Lord's involvement in our life.

Prayer for Today: Dear Lord and Father, today we thank you for the beautiful lives you have given us. We pray for peace, friendship, and the ability to contribute to your will. Amen

Run For The Prize

> Do you not know that in a race, all the runners run,
> but only one gets the prize?
> Run in such a way as to get the prize.
> (1 Corinthians 9 vs 24)

For years I was involved in two running races because somehow I felt it was contributing to society. I also enjoyed it because of the people met, supported, and helped. They were primarily friends involved with being physically fit, the best they could be.

This year's spring race was special. My daughter Karen and I decided to walk or jog the 5K. My granddaughter heard and signed up with her son and created a four-generation family event. It poured with rain, and a cold wind blew. We never noticed.

This was the forty-fifth time "Get In Gear" was held and my first time as a participant. As a former board member, the experience of participating gave me a greater appreciation for the work and efforts of the volunteers.

Thought for Today: Today, we will be running through our lives. The regular schedule will keep us busy. Many will fall short of the goal; some will accomplish our goal. We will be winners if we follow the rules and compete in our lives as models of winners, as people of faith.

Prayer for Today: Heavenly Father, today's life will fly by again. Things move very fast in today's world. It is easy to forget principles when under pressure. We pray for the guidance and judgment to follow your will in our daily activities that we lead by example and make those around us glad we were with them. Amen

Looking Forward

Not that I have already obtained all this, or have already been made perfect ...
(Philippians 3 vs 12)

Keeping your eye on the prize, the good life, and focusing on the positive events and memories is life's biggest challenge. In my mind, a long-term marriage, career, or presence in any group (specifically a church family) is the most formidable challenge placed before us by the Lord. However, what He asks is to stick it out, focus on the positive experiences, and learn from the negatives.

No one is perfect. All the greats of history made errors and remember them, as do all of us. The other side is that everyone has had successes and done good deeds. A life focused on success feeds upon itself and leads to more success and happiness. The reverse is also true.

"Forgetting what is behind and straining toward what is ahead,"

Thought for Today: Today, let us become more open in our relationships- with our significant others, family, and friends. Let us look at our resentments, possibly share them and resolve them.

Prayer for Today: Dear Lord, today we pray for the courage to be open and honest in our daily lives and relationships. We pray that we may become closer and press on toward the prize together.
Amen

Talking Faith

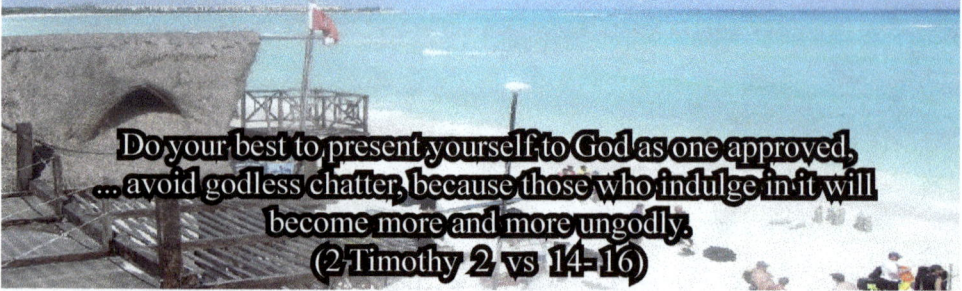

Do your best to present yourself to God as one approved, ... avoid godless chatter, because those who indulge in it will become more and more ungodly.
(2 Timothy 2 vs 14-16)

Paul is asking Timothy to guard the gospel during a time of persecution. So what does it have to do with modern Christianity? We are part of the world's society, so what is there to guard?

How about guarding our faith against the "Godless chatter" that surrounds us daily? We read, hear, and sometimes participate in it. It exists in our print and broadcast media and our personal lives, and we can quickly become wrapped up in it.

Groups of caring Christians always want to help. It is natural to be concerned with society's un-Godly issues. Thus, Bible studies, church volunteer groups, and services may sometimes slip into the chatter mode.

Today, our reality is that less than half the people we deal with are practicing Christians. Therefore, we need to guard the gospel with our behavior; by listening to others, paying close attention to their needs, and speaking out in a loving and Godly way.

Thought for Today: Today, we will hear some Godless chatter; recognize it, correct it when we can, and keep it in perspective.

Prayer for Today: Heavenly Father, we thank you for all the things reborn in the spring. Flowers, leaves, and green grass all make us appreciate your world. We pray for the opportunity to enjoy and love each other.
Amen

May 22   Grand Coco Bay
Playa Del Carmen, Mexico

Can't Get Away

The Lord Almighty is with us;
the God of Jacob is our fortress.
(Psalm 46 vs 7)

We view life in many ways. In an over-simplification, consider these four phases: the rapid learning phase, age one to adulthood. The working or wealth-building phase is working hard to raise a family or just trying to retire. The secure phase, grown-up or, in the case of a family, an empty nester, the senior or retirement phase, winding down.

Life is certainly more complicated than represented above. Meaningful events dominate our thoughts—weddings, funerals, pandemics, and happy and sad times. There will be a sunrise and sunset every day, twenty-four hours, but we know that all days are not equal. There will be happy and sad times. The one constant is that we are never alone. God is our partner and with all of us, always.

Thought for Today: Today, let us share our beliefs with someone who needs us, who may not believe. We may find they welcome the Lord and us into their lives.

Prayer for Today: Dear Lord and Father, we thank you for always being with us this week. We pray for those who do not believe so they may find your gifts and love.
Amen

Grand Coco Resort Beach
Playa Del Carmen. Mexico

Respect

The lips of the wise spread knowledge; not so the lips of fools.
(Proverbs 15 vs 7)

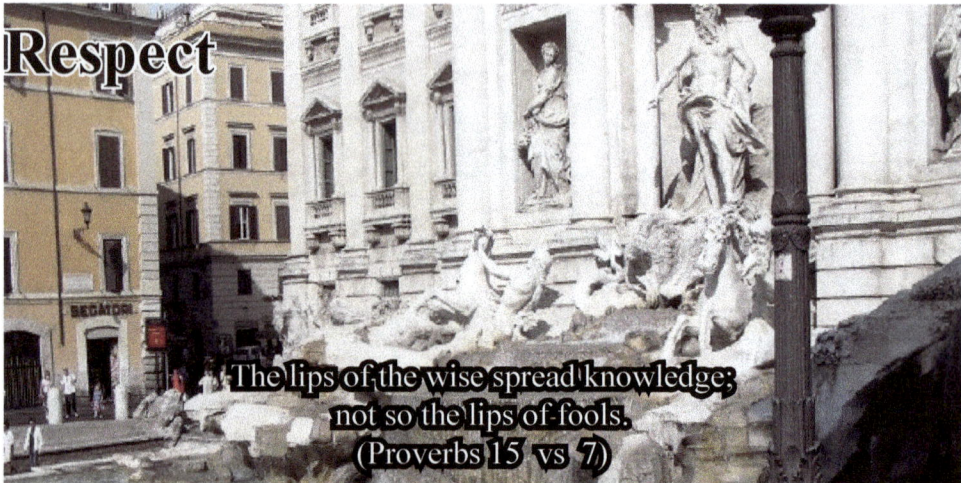

One characteristic that we all seem to want is respect. We earn respect through our interactions with other people. It is achieved both with words and actions. Saying good things without commitment and follow-through does not earn it. Actions with course words, sarcasm, and hurtful methods also will not earn respect.

From my youth, I remember two of my family's favorite expressions: "If you don't have something good to say, then say nothing." (Don't be negative) and "It is better to be silent and be thought a fool rather than speak and remove all doubt." Most of us have violated these rules more than once.

We are all born with God's blessings and a high level of respect. If we are not satisfied with the respect we have in our present lives, we need to recognize that we have not earned it yet. The good news is that we can turn it around by living our lives as our faith taught us.

Thought for Today: Today, let's focus on earning respect through our words and search out the good things to say. Sing the praises of the Lord in our daily lives.

Prayer for Today: Heavenly Father, we live in a confusing world. Hate is running rampant, and integrity seems on the wane. We pray for some understanding and a way to contribute to a solution, for a way to help. Amen

May 24 Fountain Di Trivi, Lazio, Rome, Italy

Perfect Will

Do not conform any longer to the pattern of this world, but be transformed by the renewing of your mind.
(Romans 12 vs 2)

Being as good as we can be in spirit, mind, and body is a worthy goal. Paul's message to the Romans today focuses on the mind. If you are reading this, you probably don't need it.

Television and computers seem to have replaced reading books. Before television, we would spend a lot of time reading. Whole groups of us, reading and trading books. Yes, sometimes comic books and everything from Uncle Wiggly to Sherlock Holmes. The books changed to National Geographic and Mickey Spillane as we grew older. It was a period of intellectual and physical growth.

Television replaced reading, and I went years without reading a book for pleasure. The ability to imagine myself in a story and fantasize about being the great Sherlock Holmes, Huck Finn or Superman passed me. Indeed my intellectual growth was stagnant or at least slowed down. I fit the pattern of the new television world, visual rather than intellectual.

A career change to sales saved me from being stagnant. Engineers need to work on their skills to become salespeople. The best source of information was reading books. So after a fifteen-year drought, my job forced me to read. Reading again became part of my life, spreading to both growth and recreational works. I feel blessed by this today.

Thought for Today: Let us ask: "What may we choose to do differently to "...be transformed by renewing our mind." Let us take the time to renew our commitment to intellectual growth.

Prayer for Today: Dear Lord and Father, we pray for guidance regarding love and peace. We are a nation and world out of control. As Christians, we pray world leaders find a solution to and resolve issues through love, peace, and understanding Amen

Fountain Di Trivi,
Lazio, Rome, Italy

May 25

Communication I

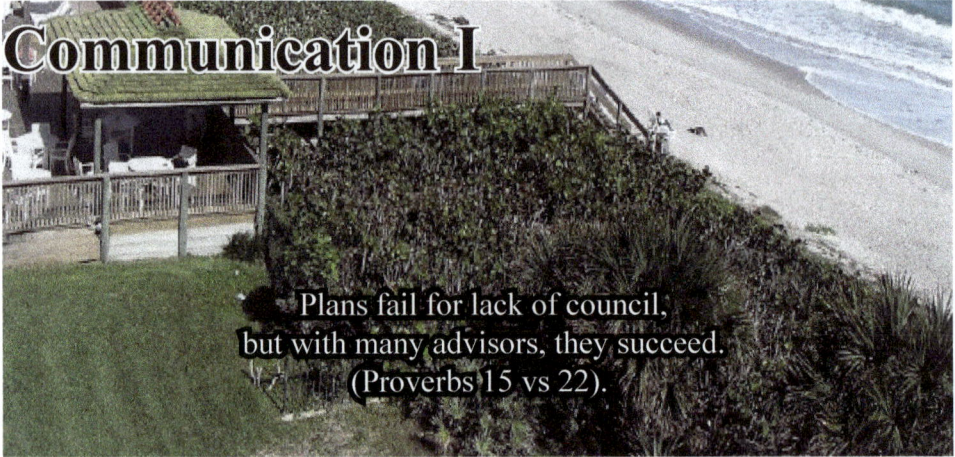

Plans fail for lack of council,
but with many advisors, they succeed.
(Proverbs 15 vs 22).

There are several proverbs regarding communication. People want shared knowledge and praise. Others seek out those who have learned the style of the good book to connect with them.

It is great to share our knowledge when asked. People who respect our expertise and experience will benefit when we share. Two heads are generally better than one when working together. We always want to remember to contribute and ask when we need support.

"He who rebukes a person will, in the end,
gain more favor than he who has a flattering tongue."
(Proverbs 28 vs 23)

Umpires and referees "Call them as they see them." We humans often want to cushion any criticism, avoid issues and hope they go away. Avoiding issues does not help, and we need to support and contribute. Loving and sensitive criticism is a great help to others, and as an aside, a relationship builder/

Thought for Today: Today, let's be more than honest. What do I mean by that? Let's focus on
being "open and honest." Expose ourselves in our communications, and the people we are with will know us better and become closer.

Prayer for Today: Dear Lord, today we pray for those that are manipulative and opportunistic in their communication style; that they may become open and honest and learn how to communicate according to the book of proverbs. Amen

Communication II

This is the day the Lord has made,
let us rejoyce and be glad in it.
(Psalm 118 vs 24)

More on communication, in our world of high stress and overcommitment, it is important to lighten up and keep a sense of humor.
"All the days of the oppressed are wretched,
but the cheerful heart has a continual feast."
(Proverbs 15 vs 15)
 This is not to say that we laugh at the expense of others. Rather we need to look at the light side.
"An anxious heart weighs a man down,
but a kind word cheers him up."
(Proverbs 12 vs 25)
 We need to relax, keep it light, and enjoy while demonstrating to others how to do the same. When we grew up, many of us viewed religion as "God-fearing" and the Bible as a set of rules. With that in mind, how do we interpret these passages?
 In life, we need to deal with negative forces. Today we are dealing with increasing basic living costs and a new normal pandemic. Society is changing, and our attitudes and actions as Christians need to be precise. Deal with the issues as best we can and demonstrate to the world that we can change and stay happy along the way through Christ Jesus.

 Thought for Today: Let's all be happy and demonstrate to those around us that our faith keeps us at peace.
 Prayer for Today: Our world is in turmoil with war and civil unrest. We pray that we can help to bring normalcy back to the lives of many through our faith. Amen

Paradise Beach,
Melbourne Beach, Florida

May 27

Respect and Love

> May the Lord make your love increase
> and overflow for each other and everyone else,
> just as ours does for you.
> (1 Thessalonians 3 vs 12)

Love and respect are the two things that abound in our faith. If we could spread this worldwide, we could save a fortune on armaments. Unfortunately, jealousy, hate, and disrespect also tend to fester worldwide. Maybe we have to learn to live with it.

The founding fathers set us up as a democracy, a free nation of free people. They also said, "In God, we trust," and then set up a clear separation between the Government and religion. We want to be free, and we Christians want our God, our friends, and peace on earth. It is a conundrum.

Our role is stated clearly by Paul's message in Thessaloníki: Our part is to grow in the Spirit, and love will come. Spiritual growth results in love and respect blossoming and jealousy, hate, and disrespect fading away.

Thought for Today: Today, we will interact with people. We will choose to see many and are glad to see them; others we would rather avoid. Let's show our Christian love and respect.

Prayer for Today: Dear Lord, today we give thanks for having friends, family, and acquaintances, the people that bring pleasure and peace to our lives. Amen

New Beginnings

Therefore, if anyone is in Christ,
he is a new creation.
(2 Corinthians 5 vs 17)

Today is the first day of the rest of your life; believe it. Every day is a new day, a chance to start over. Yesterday is past, tomorrow is the future and today is a gift from God. It is up to us how we are going to use it. We can choose to carry around our old baggage or harvest new joys. It is our choice.

We can turn bad into good. Using a golf analogy, life is match play, hole by hole versus day by day. A bad golf hole in match play does not cost you the match; it counts as one of eighteen. A bad day is painful and certainly not wanted in life and may contribute to a bad week. However, it can be a bottom, and life can be all uphill.

If you are reading this today, you are on the right track, giving yourself the opportunity for a better day. Meditation and prayer will jump start your day and open the window to the light of our faith.

Thought for Today: Let's start a new beginning.

Prayer for Today: Heavenly Father, we thank you for our many blessings, especially for a new day. We pray that we capture the joys of life that you lead us to and help someone else find them. Amen

Honor Them

> Here is a trustworthy saying:
> If we died with him,
> we will also live with him;"
> "Keep reminding God's people of these things...
> (2 Timothy 2 vs 11, 14)

Celebrate Memorial Day, and pray for all who served and went before us and those we love.

My son-in-law Rick played in the 451st Fort Snelling Army band for several years, and we would go to his parades. At each show, they traditionally played the Coast Guard, Army, Marines, and Navy military anthems while the veterans in the crowd stood and saluted. My eyes teared up with emotion when I thought about what these people had done for us.

There are places in the world where my publishing these messages would be criminal. That is not the case here. One thing that makes America great is the freedom to worship and our varied culture. We welcome all faiths to our shores.

Abraham Lincoln said it like this:
"I am nothing but truth is everything.
I know I am right because I know that liberty is right,
for Christ teaches it, and Christ is God."

Thought for Today: Today, let us remember all who have gone before us and be thankful.

Prayer for Today: Dear Lord and Father, today we thank all those who have gone before us and contributed to our lives today. First, all those who fought in our military contributed to our freedom, second to our family ancestors who built our traditions and lifestyle; and last to Jesus, who gave us grace. Amen

May 30 Azalea Trial Garden
Minnesota Landscape Arboretum

Spiritual Growth

I gave you milk, not solid food,
for you were not yet ready for it.
Indeed, you are still not ready.
(1 Corinthians 3 vs 2)

Several years ago, June and I decided that our families would not remember us as angry older people. Based on our time spent interacting with elderly people as Stephen ministers, we decided that. Since then, we have concluded that the two major causes behind the frustration are reluctance to change and spiritual growth.

The change piece is probably universal. We will grow older, we will lose some of our youthful capabilities, some friends, and have battles to fight. Consider Edmund Vance Cooke's humorous poem published in 1923:

> "This world is nothing but a bubble, don't you know,
> A mighty lot of trouble, don't you know:
> You live, you sigh, and then you die, don't you know."

My friend John says it this way, "Life is a bitch, then you die!"

The Lord wants us to be happy, cheerful, and appreciative. He has given us the tools, and we need to use them daily. The tool we have is faith and the Holy Spirit. We need to keep them in mind and in our hearts to be happy.

Thought for Today: Let's drink our milk but demonstrate that we are ready for the Lord's solid food with our happiness and spirit.

Prayer for Today: Dear Lord, today we pray for all experiencing anxiety and anger. We pray that they may find peace and tranquility through the Holy Spirit. Amen

Azalea Trial Garden
Minnesota Landscape Arboretum **May 31**

June

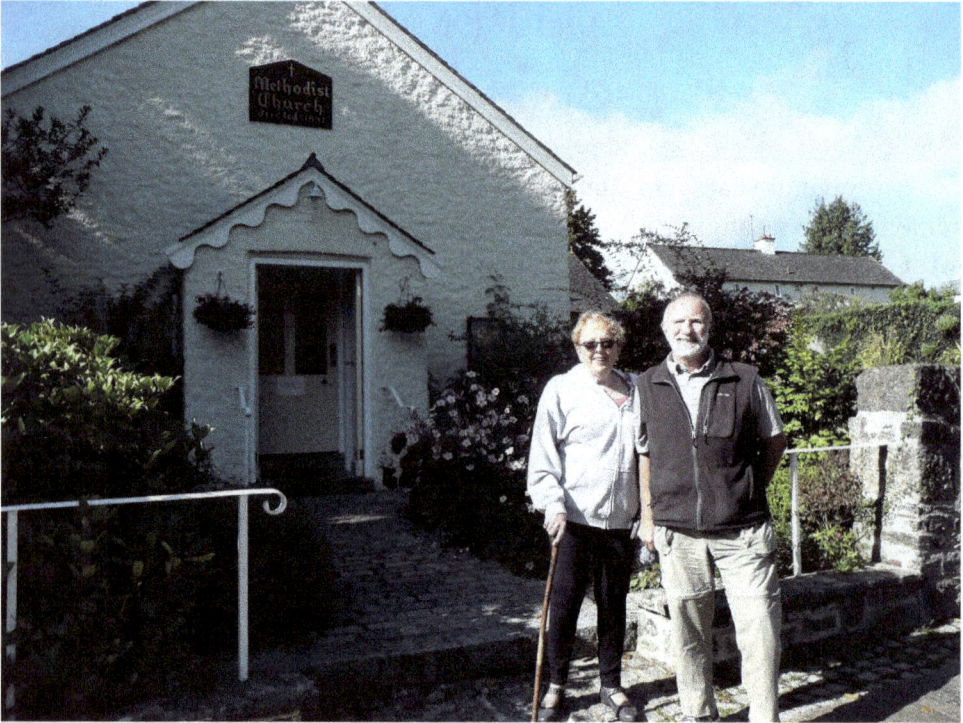

Buckfast Methodist Church

Erected in 1881, the chapel was built on what was
the main road through Buckfast village It predates the
return of Roman Catholic Benedictine monks to Buckfast
Abbey in 1882, which has since developed around the
Chapel.

Desire

Flee the evil desires of youth,
and pursue righteousness, faith, love, and peace...
(2 Timothy 2 vs 22)

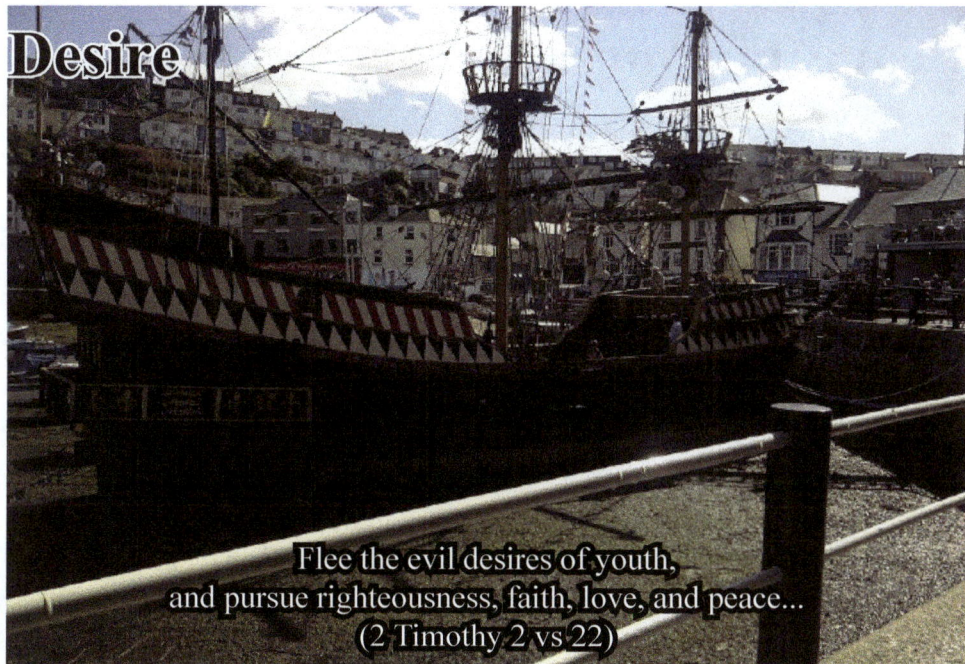

Paul sounds a lot like my mom sounded during high school. During my teen years, listening was not my strong suit. How could a ranked athlete and honor student be a bad guy? In my mind, my record justified my behaviors, and the price paid was ten years, which I refer to as my dark period. Those years were the times I spent learning how life was a two-way street instead of a one-way street that I owned.

Faith somehow stayed with me, and praying was often present when the darkness was dominant. God was with me despite my behaviors. He was always there, and I would reach out to him just as Popeye would grab for his spinach. And, just like Popeye's spinach, He always came through for me. He will also come through for you.

Thought for Today: Today will not be perfect, so keep your prayer close by and ask for support.

Prayer for Today: Dear Lord, today we thank you for the goodness in our lives and the hope and love that tomorrow will surely bring. Amen

Sir Frances Drake's
Golden Hind Replica
Brixham Sea Front, Devon, UK   **June 1**   **Page 159**

Peace Through Faith

The Lord's servant must not quarrel; instead, he must be kind, able to teach, and not resentful. (2 Timothy 2 vs 24)

Forgiveness is the way of our Christian lives. Anger and resentment are always available if we choose to hold on to them. It is easy to be vindictive and want to even wrongs. It is not possible to find peace through revenge.

In 2020 the news was traumatic about Pandemic and bigotry. Not much about love. So, what is next, and are we going to lead? Follow? or be spectators? I suggest an appropriate time for all three, but we each start with a self-evaluation and prayer.

Sociologist Anne Curtis summed it up recently, "Social change happens in stops and starts. It moves along at a snail's pace, trudging, like through molasses, then suddenly jolts forward when something big happens, often with expressions of violence (such as this). Violence has advanced social change for the millennium. We need to make some really tough decisions about our own beliefs: Saying "violence is not the answer" ignores historical context. Between the lines, we're really just saying "I am more comfortable with the status quo."

The Christian message is clear; we will find peace only when we have a strong enough faith to forgive and keep God through Jesus Christ at the forefront of our lives.

Thought for Today: Let us contribute to the process of healing and creating true equality.

Prayer for Today: Heavenly Father, we pray for peace and social justice. Let us lead the way. Amen

June 2

Lake Bde Maka Ska
Minneapolis Minnesota

Perseverance

Suffering produces perseverance;
perseverance brings character, and
character brings hope. And hope does not disappoint us.
(Romans 5 vs 3,4)

The keyword this week is perseverance. Our lives are a constant search for serenity or peace. Where does it hide, or do we hide it ourselves? We all go through phases when we are not at peace. Careers get in the way, illness occurs, and our general business disturbs tranquility.

When we are not at peace, which is in control? Years ago, during stressful times, my daughter gave me a daily meditation book and suggested I pay attention to it. Not reading the morning newspaper and replacing the news with meditation resulted in a more positive start to the day. I no longer knew the baseball scores, how Tiger did, or how many negative things occurred in the world yesterday. Meditating gave me a level of peace at the start of the day.

So, where does persistence fit? Well, peace is elusive and hard to grasp or even define. The search may be everlasting. Paul's message to the Romans is reasonably straightforward. Throughout our lives' ups, downs, and general activities, we must be persistent in our faith and keep God in our lives to find the tranquility we desire.

Thought for Today: Today, let us review our long-standing frustrations. The demanding boss, the developing teenager, the morning commute, whatever is in our lives. Let us pray for God's guidance on how we should help Him deal with the frustration. If He is involved, we will be less frustrated.

Prayer for Today: Dear Lord, I give thanks for the many blessings in my life; the good friends, the lifestyle, the rain, and flowers. There still are many issues that need attention. I pray for your guidance to work through these everyday issues. Amen

Lake Bde Maka Ska
Minneapolis Minnesota

Forgiveness

Blessed is the man
whose sin the Lord will never count against him.
(Romans 4 vs 7)

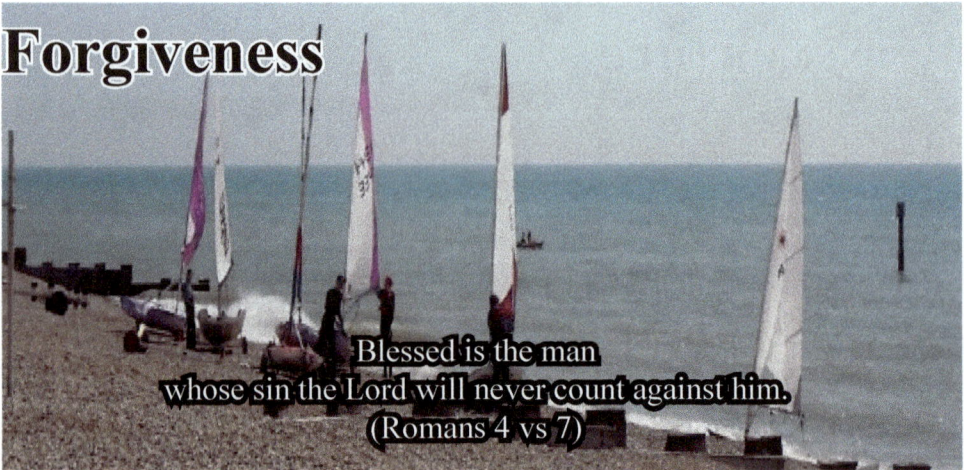

There are moments in our lives that we have erred and perhaps are not proud of that memory. When we truly believe, we will be at peace. Not because we have been perfect, but because we will know we are forgiven. That is a powerful and moving statement.

That is an interesting thought. Many twelve-step programs and clinics full of people have never let go of sorrowful memories. They are searching for peace, and it will find them when they "...turn their will and lives over to the care of God..".

For example, the expression: "Let go and let God." We are obliged to turn these memories over to God in our lives. How do we accomplish that? Perhaps through the forgiving of those who have harmed us.

Colossians 3:13 says, "Bear with each other and forgive whatever grievances you may have against one another. Forgive as the Lord forgave you". When we learn to forgive others, we find it easier to accept the forgiveness we receive from God.

Thought for Today: Let's focus on the many positive things we accomplish, the people we help, and the positive memories we all appreciate. When a negative or remorseful memory comes to the forefront, stop a moment, pray, and remember that God is forgiving.

Prayer for Today: Dear Lord, thank you for the opportunity to find grace and live in peace. Please help me focus on the positive things in my life and help me see the good in others. Amen

Love and Hospitality

"Twas grace that taught my heart to fear,
and grace my fears relieved;
how precious did that grace appear
the hour that I first believed.

Yea, when this flesh and heart shall fail,
and mortal life shall cease,
I shall possess, within the veil,
a life of joy and peace."
(Amazing Grace, Vs. 4 & 5)
(Words by John Newton, 1779)

There are almost as many ways to find joy and peace as people. It can be found anywhere at any time because we each measure it individually. Christians have the tools and knowledge find it.

However, we often let our everyday tasks and challenges disturb our peace. This past week it seemed that the traffic threatened many people's tranquility. The construction season and heavy rains slowed things down to a crawl. Frustration seemed to replace grace on the highways.

A dear friend and author, regarding traffic, wrote, "...leave early, take the pretty route and listen to good music." He is right on.

As Christians, when we find our tranquility threatened, we need to use our tool kit; prayer, meditation, and even a chat with a friend. They all will work. God did not put us here to be frustrated. Experience grace as He wants you to.

Thought for Today: This week, let us all keep grace at the forefront of our daily prayers. Let us expect the daily challenges and be ready with our tool kit. This week let's experience grace and joy every day.

Prayer for Today: Heavenly Father, we recognize that your joy and tranquility are always available, and you are always with us. This week we pray that we may keep you on our minds and thoughts as we work through the challenges of our Christian lives. Amen

Sail Boards
Bexhill On Sea, Ease. Sussex, UK   **June 5**   Page 163

Acceptance

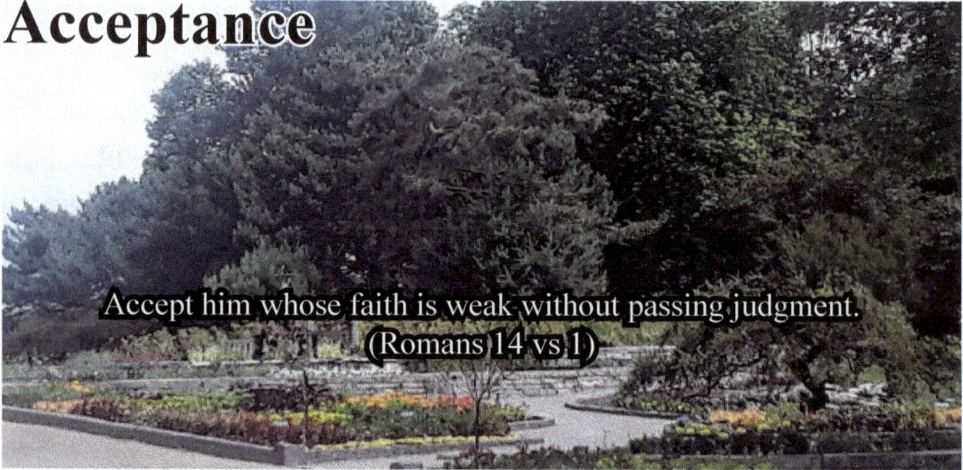

Accept him whose faith is weak without passing judgment.
(Romans 14 vs 1)

Paul's messages to the Romans make it clear that acceptance leads to peace. Acceptance is required as a piece of Christian love. In recent years, the world has been dominated by new experiences; pandemics, the American election politics of hate, Brexit and Boris, and international wars and skirmishes threaten peace. The final straw triggered long-term oppression here in my hometown based on color.

I remembered a 1961 musical by Anthony Newley and Leslie Beicusse, "Stop the World, I Want to Get Off." It was a good title, a tongue-in-cheek musical, and it is sad that it still rings a bell here in the new millennium.

On a more positive note, in 1955, Jill Jackson-Miller and Sy Miller wrote: "Let There be Peace on Earth." Wow, that would be great.

You (We) are responsible. Each of us plays a role in some way by not speaking out or speaking out. We can go either way by not making amends when we messed up or forgiving when wronged. Yep, none of us is perfect. So, let's try a bit harder; let the peace on earth begin with you.

Thought for Today: Let's focus on our contribution to peace through Christian Love this week.

Prayer for Today: Dear Lord, we pray that we may learn to love others under any conditions and that we may personally contribute to a caring and loving world. Amen.

Harmony

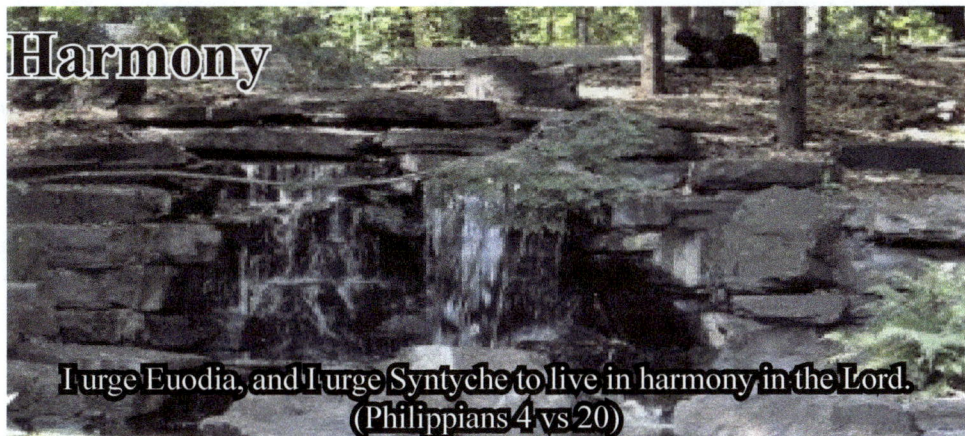

I urge Euodia, and I urge Syntyche to live in harmony in the Lord.
(Philippians 4 vs 20)

Recently, in our neighborhood, we watched as a family fell apart. There were court orders, police escorts, and all the ungodly things that go with a broken home. Respect, love, and spirituality had left the relationship. It was sad.

Let me confess that our family did not always go to church. (Sunday was a long training run and cleaning the pool.) Also, when the kids were small, church on Sunday was our only "quiet time." Somehow, there was always trust and a spiritual presence within our family that held us together.

Consider this analogy. If your car battery was dead this morning, you could put it on a charger and be able to get going. However, if your alternator was weak, your car would quit running in a few hours. Many of us use Sunday's service as our time to charge our spiritual batteries.

Families and individuals with solid spirituality tend to survive. They grow while meeting life's challenges, develop deeper friendships and learn the value of love. Somehow we all need to carry Sunday's charge throughout the week. I pray that my messages help.

Thought for Today: Somehow, we need to ensure that the weekly calendar does not overwhelm our spirituality. We cannot be too busy to love each other. We all know that is a formula for tragedy. Today and always, let us focus on positive interactions with friends and families.

Prayer for Today: Dear Lord and Father, our lives are full of distractions. Somehow, we don't have time. Children's activities, work projects, and many other issues get in the way of peace and love. Today we pray for the presence of mind to focus on your love and include it in our daily lives. Amen

Water Fall Feature
Minnesota Landscape Arboretum

Good Name

A good name is more desirable than great riches.
(Proverbs 22 vs 1)

In the 60s, when I desired to change careers from engineering to sales, I had several interviews that changed my life. On my first one, I did not know what I was doing and slid into a deep hole fast. The fellow conducting the interview let me know quickly and, for whatever reason, gave me a lecture on selling myself and dressing for success. He pointed out that the most important product I would ever have to sell would be myself and how important it was to ensure the product was high quality. He scared me to death. That was in 1964, and my next sales interview was in 1972.

In 1972 a gentleman named Warren started my second sales interview with a question, "What have you ever sold?" That question would have sent me packing in 1964. I talked about selling myself to my company to get my job, selling management on budgets and projects, and that I believed everyone was a salesman every day, whether they knew it or not. The job was mine, and it has been all uphill ever since.

From 1964 through 1972, I did a lot of product development; college courses, business books, church, and of course, by my mentor and partner, June. That first interviewer was put in my life to advise me, and the Lord gave me two ears to listen and understand.

George Washington said that one of the most precious things this side of the grave is a good reputation.

Thought for Today: Let's consider what we sell in every situation. Make sure that we are the best possible brand.

Prayer for Today: Dear Father, today, we will be working with younger, less experienced folks. We pray that we may influence them in a positive Christian way. Amen

Listening to Criticism

> Wounds from a friend can be trusted,
> but an enemy multiplies kisses.
> (Proverbs 27 vs 6)

We often feel criticized when someone tries to help us be or do better. When people criticize us is generally not out of meanness, it is to help. How we listen and consider their advice (criticism) is up to us. Most people are helpful and caring, but because of our natural pride and ego, we can hear help as hurt.

Remember growing up how often our choices were challenged? Mom, dad, uncle, or aunt? They were teaching out of love. It is generally the same if a good friend mentions something; a desire to make you better rather than put you down, help not hurt. We get to make that choice.

It is easy for us to feel wounded or hurt. Our gut reaction to criticism can be hurt and go towards anger. Verbal wounds are an opportunity to display faith, patience, and understanding; a chance for spiritual growth. This message asks you to focus on the positive point of view, to be open and receptive. Then, with each criticism, we will learn and be better people.

Thought for Today: We will be criticized and have the opportunity to react. Learn from the experience. Let us respond as Christians, emulate Jesus, listen, and pray about it.

Prayer for Today: Dear Lord and Father, we pray for simple things; our families, friends, and ourselves. We pray for understanding the world and your master plan; so that we may somehow contribute to peace and goodwill toward others. Amen

Lost Pond Trail
Minnesota Landscape Arboretum **June 9** Page 167

Smile

This message was written at a food court at Midway Airport in Chicago at 8 am after an early flight towards Boston. There are smiling faces all around; even the TSA security people seem upbeat today. The smiles are infectious, and the general mood today..

It seems most people here today read Paul's advice to the Romans and are being zealous and hospitable. It is infectious. I was not looking forward to this trip because there is much work lying ahead at mom's in Massachusetts, helping reorganize the house after my brother's passing.

I awoke in a reflective mood and have dealt with smiling, happy people for two hours. First, the TSA security people were in good spirits, then a flight attendant greeted me with an exceptional smile, a guy helped me with my carry-on when I almost dropped it, the flight out was on time, and I had a first-class upgrade. It also helps that I am writing Good News and having an omelet between flights.

Today I had forgotten my rules about praying to start a new day. Up at four, fly at six, stop in Chicago, and then on to a stressful week. My funky start has been turned around by others. Somehow, the spirit and joy of those around me have affected my mood. I can feel the spirituality around me.

Thought for Today: Today, thank those around us who support our lives. Follow Paul's advice, "Share with God's people who are in need," and "Practice hospitality."

Prayer for Today: Dear Lord, I thank those around me who have lifted my spirits. Amen

Turtles Resting
Green Heron Pond

Walk With The Lord

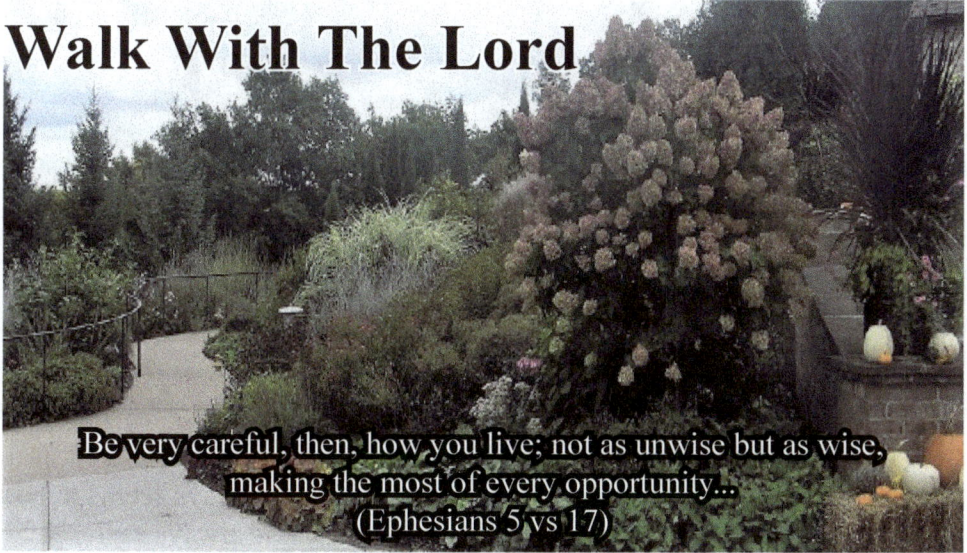

Be very careful, then, how you live; not as unwise but as wise,
making the most of every opportunity...
(Ephesians 5 vs 17)

Wow, we are sure busy. When saying, "Hi, how are you?" the reply is often followed by a calendar review. When Paul wrote this passage, he was advising an active lifestyle.

It is OK to slow down and smell roses! Many retirees comment that they do not know when they ever had time to work. A good goal for the retirement phase of life is not to feel that way.

As "qualified" retirees, June and I often reminisce about our frantic past lifestyle. Many times that seemed the craziest and most out of control have generated the fondest memories; The blessings.

Paul says in verses 17 and 18, "Always giving thanks to God the Father for everything, in the name of our Lord Jesus Christ."

Thought for Today: It seems that being busy is a good thing. As we move through our schedules this week, take time to thank God for the opportunity to be involved or engaged; stop, appreciate, and feel good about our contributions.

Prayer for Today: Heavenly Father, we live in a world of hate and fear. We pray that it will end, but it seems it is just beginning. We pray this week for some a love attack to break out. Somehow for, the world to recognize the advantages of Godly love. Amen

Garden Walkway
Minnesota Landscape Arboretum   **June 11**   Page 169

Correcting

He who rebukes a man will, in the end, gain more favor
then he who has a flattering tongue.
(Proverbs 28 vs 23)

Our faith teaches us to be open and honest with everyone. That is a tall order when it comes to correcting someone. There always seems to be a fear of the negative or the possible confrontation. It is always easier in the short term to be silent.

Proverbs 28:23 tells it like it is. We earn more respect and have a better relationship if we express our concerns promptly and honestly. In all our relationships, the ideal situation is when everyone's feelings are shared. There are justifications for holding back. Fear of disturbing our families or risking our careers is the most common. However, appropriately sharing our feelings always works out better than keeping quiet over time.

Proverbs 25:11 tells us that "A word aptly spoken is like apples of gold in settings of silver." We need to express ourselves and share those feelings under all conditions.

Thought for Today: To,day, we will be tempted to avoid issues. We need to recognize and think about that; find a way to deal with the issues that reflect our faith's teaching by being open and honest.

Prayer for Today: Heavenly Father, you teach us to be open and honest with everyone. It seems unreasonable and, at times, impossible. We pray that we can deal with problems that come our way openly and honestly as Jesus did. Amen

Positive Focus

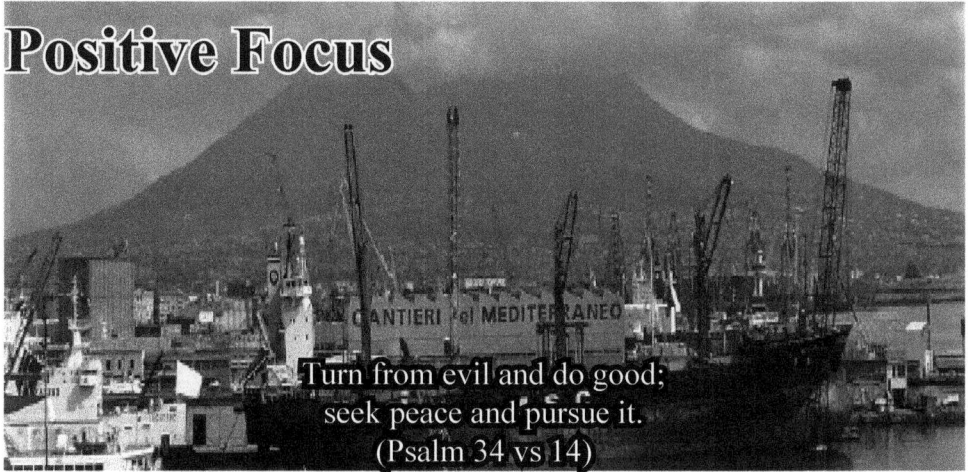

Turn from evil and do good;
seek peace and pursue it.
(Psalm 34 vs 14)

We are all challenged with issues. Lost jobs, divorce, illness, anger, fear, and resentments are typical in America and worldwide. How do we deal with the issues without destroying the peace in our life?

Challenges that threaten our livelihood and families are demanding. Some require hard decisions but get dealt with quickly; others seem unsolvable and drag on forever. The quickies are best dealt with on the spot and then go away. The long-term issues need other techniques, and the best is through our faith.

Years ago, there was a serious issue of racism in our Methodist church. There was no apparent solution, and prayer did not work for me. So I went with plan B. When prayer does not work, pray again. The second time was with my spiritual mentor. It eventually worked out the way the Lord wanted it.

I like to say that when the going gets tough, the tough start praying. Sometimes that is the only solution.

Thought for Today: Today, let's recognize tough spots or bumps and pray for a win-win solution.

Prayer for Today: Heavenly Father, we give thanks today for the ability to insert you into our life's problems through prayer. Amen

Clouds over Vesuvius
Campanian, Gulf of Naples, Italy

Perfect Peace

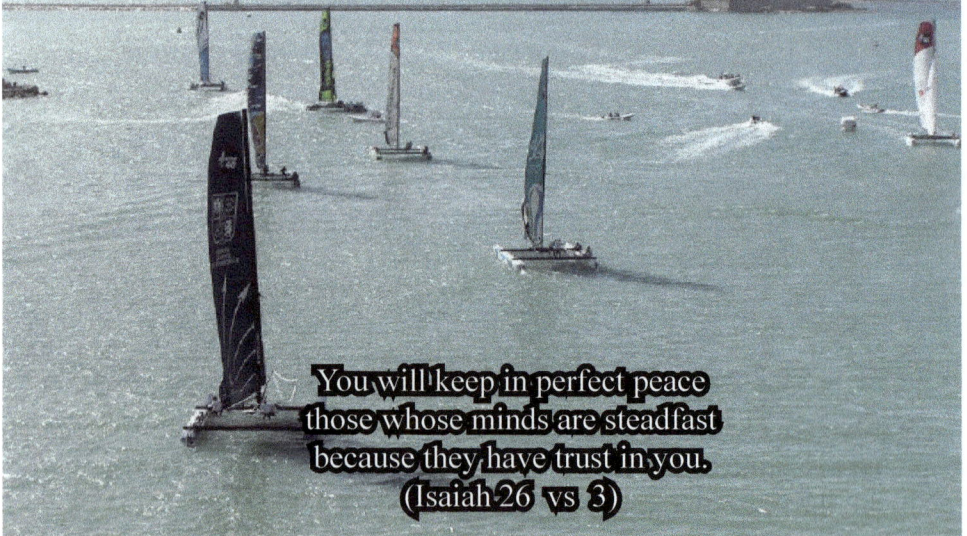

You will keep in perfect peace
those whose minds are steadfast
because they have trust in you.
(Isaiah 26 vs 3)

Peace is a direct result of faith and trust. It is essential to stay on an upbeat track and be steadfast. When situations are not what we like, we have options. One is to fear negative results; another is to focus on how we can avoid or minimize negative impact.

In life, we need to keep our eye on the sky, and look upward, and outward for positive results. Our news and media outlet rating systems have proven that bad news sells. The news about pandemics, riots, fires, and murders is essential to hear but risks dampening our positive attitudes.

As Christians, we need to be steadfast and optimistic; have a positive outlook. We need to be the leaders in fairness, equality, and displaying the social values Jesus taught us. We can help solve the world's issues when we are steadfast and trust in our faith.

Thought for Today: Let's be positive in the face of all challenges. Let's snatch peace from the grasp of negativity.

Prayer for the Day: Dear Lord, today we give thanks for the opportunity to have peace in our lives. We pray that we may focus on doing your will and that through our steadfast love, we will have peace and contribute to the peace of others. Amen

June 14   Catamaran Race
Trapani, Sicily

Tough Love

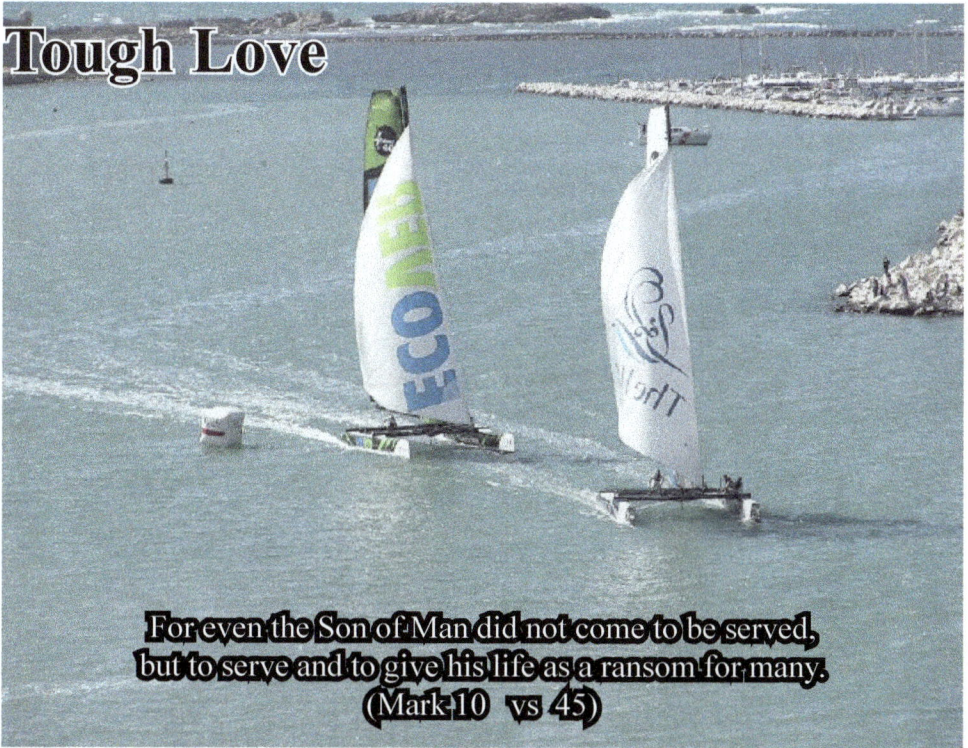

For even the Son of Man did not come to be served,
but to serve and to give his life as a ransom for many.
(Mark 10 vs 45)

Serving others has more to do with following God's will and sharing God's word than being a caregiver or a soft touch. Often he is referring to what therapists call "tough love."

That is real love and not an easy thing to do. It often means saying no or advising people of a direction they would rather not go. Each time we make a tough decision, we somehow experience spiritual growth. The results are usually very positive. We take a step up the ladder of success.

.

Thought for Today: Let's look forward to the tough decisions rather than shying away from them. Decisions made with love and faith are the correct ones. When we need to, let us think about the question, "What would Jesus do?"

Prayer for the Day: Dear Lord, we often have to advise friends, colleagues, and family to do things they would rather not do. Today we pray for the ability to recognize what is correct and the strength to do the right thing as we walk the walk. Amen

Catamaran Race
Trapani, Sicily

Live The Life

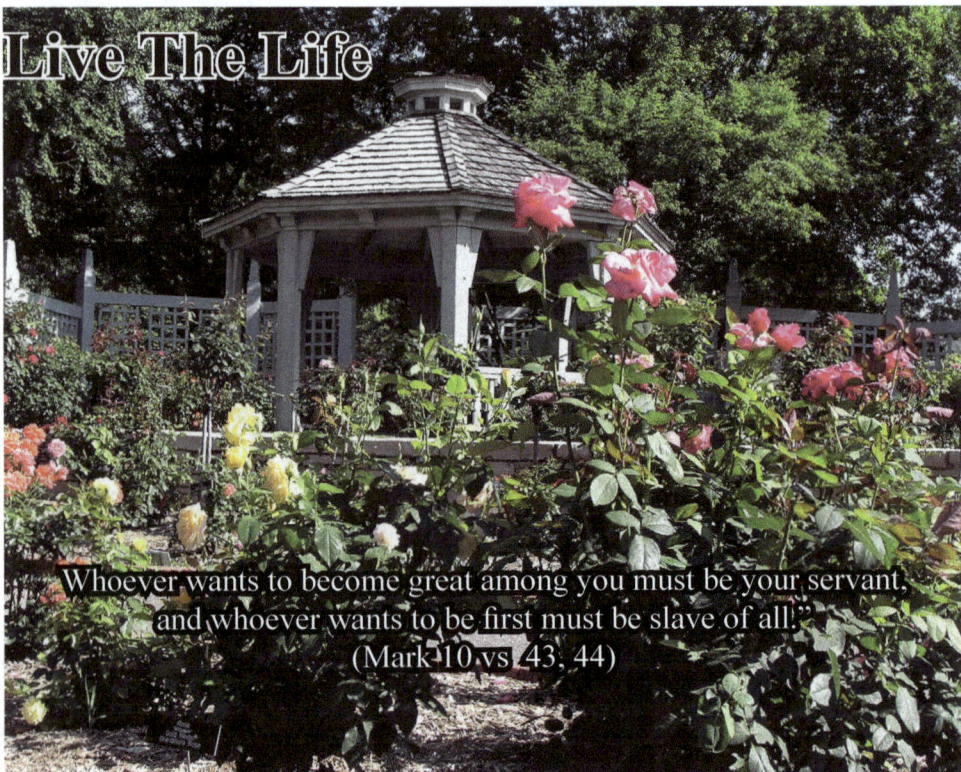

"Whoever wants to become great among you must be your servant, and whoever wants to be first must be slave of all."
(Mark 10 vs 43, 44)

Spiritual growth is an essential part of living a peaceful and rewarding life. Defining it is sometimes tricky. It is more than reading a passage. It is living the life and climbing the Christian ladder of success. Not running around preaching; it is demonstrating the lifestyle. In the above quote, Mark mentions greatness, and to be great, one must be at peace. This peace is found by walking the walk, serving others as a lifestyle.

Television Evangelist Mac Hammond defined serving others as "...meeting another person's needs when they do not believe you are serving them".

Thought for Today: Let's reach out and help someone in need.

Prayer for Today: Heavenly Father, today we feel the need to help. We pray that we recognize those in need that you have placed before us. We thank you for the opportunity to serve. Amen

The Valley

Even though I walk through the valley
of the shadow of death,
I fear no evil, for you are with me.
(Psalm 23 vs 4)

Physically healing is something we all are used to; our bumps and bruises over the years all go away in time. Recovery from surgery is a tough mental and physical battle that frequently ends in deepening spirituality. It is easy not to recognize the miracle of God with minor problems.

However, when a big one comes, it is equally easy to ask "Where are you, God?" or "Why are you doing this to me?" It is easy to lose sight of what matters when facing a life-threatening event. Often, we take time to analyze the doctor's skills and the various treatment options. Let's get technical and analytical to ensure that we get the best doctor and hospital. But somehow, let's not forget God in the process.

In 1998 when I had cancer, my impatience and outright fear chased me into the hospital in only three weeks. There was no analysis or wait and see. Just my impulsive, "Just do it" (thanks, Nike). Somehow, I threw it over to HIM with reckless abandon. That brings to mind the last line of Psalm 23, "Surely goodness and love will follow, all the days of my life, and I will dwell in the house of the Lord forever."

The Lord and physicians came through for my family and me. We all need to remember Him during times of fear and illness.

Thought for Today: Let's focus on unfortunate individuals who are ill while keeping the 23rd Psalm in mind, helping in some way when possible.

Prayer for Today: Dear Lord, many of our friends have health issues; minor, serious, and some terminal. We pray that we may find a way to help and calm their fears as they walk through their valley. May we help by following your guidance through prayer. Amen

Rose Garden
Minnesota Landscape Arboretum   **June 17**   **Page 175**

Talkers

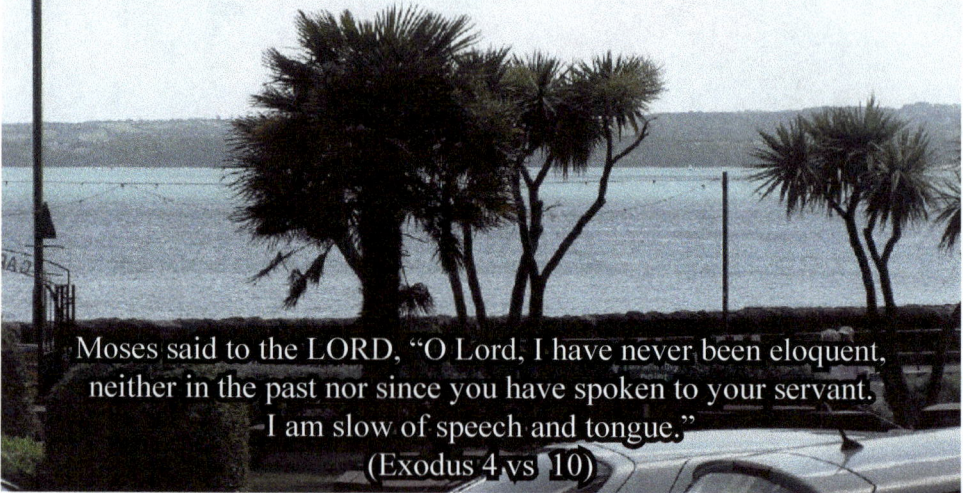

Moses said to the LORD, "O Lord, I have never been eloquent,
neither in the past nor since you have spoken to your servant.
I am slow of speech and tongue."
(Exodus 4 vs 10)

Growing up in Boston, there were what we called talkers on Boston common. They virtually stood on milk crates (soapboxes) and discussed political issues and religious beliefs. As a teenager, I considered them nut cases because no one in their right mind would do that from my perspective. Apparently, not even Moses.

Lately, I have coined the term "closet ministry"- we are there when needed, and we all do some great work. Be proud of that because God is with us in that effort. Most of us prefer to do God's work quietly and on our terms. We have the belief to do that.

Tomorrow we will talk a bit about doing more.

Thought for Today: Today, let us continue our "closet ministries." Helping others, praying for the sick, the underprivileged, serving the shelters, etc. We do that well.

Prayer for Today: Dear Lord and father, life is good for us. We have food, shelter, and love. We thank you for your abundance and the opportunity to share our faith. Amen

Trust Versus Belief

"Now go; I will help you speak and will teach you what to say." But Moses said, "O Lord, please send someone else to do it. (Exodus 4:12 &13)

More on our closet ministries.

Is that what God wants? Should we speak out more? Be Evangelical? Stand on our soapboxes?
The answer to that is a definite – YES.

God's answer to Moses was, "I will be with you." We hesitate to "talk the talk" in public. After all, the human resources department at work has a policy against it. Someone uncomfortable in the workplace may be uncomfortable. Sometimes we need to show trust and say what needs to be said. We must go beyond our belief system and trust that God wants us to speak out.

If you are reading this, you are ahead of the game. In verse 5 vs 19, Mark advises

> "Jesus did not let him but said,
> "Go home to your people
> and tell them how much the Lord has done for you,
> and how he has had mercy on you."

Thought for Today: Continue our closet ministries and share our faith. Recognize that opportunity and speak out! Let's take the risk and be Talkers.

Prayer for the Week: Dear Lord and father, we pray for the opportunity to share our faith and the opportunity to represent you in our daily lives. Amen

God Is With Us

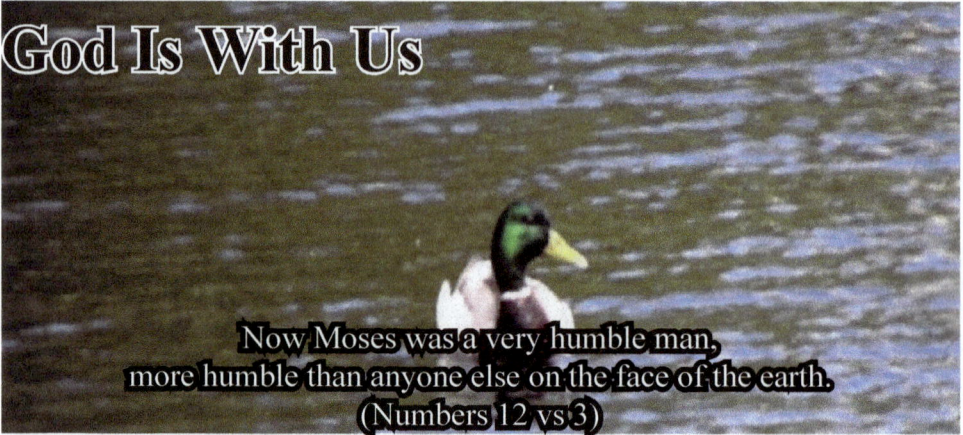

> Now Moses was a very humble man,
> more humble than anyone else on the face of the earth.
> (Numbers 12 vs 3)

Like Moses, we are not always enthusiastic about what God wants. We are a humble lot, conservative, and considerate of others' views and feelings. We are humble before God.

Many of us are leaders in the community, at work, and at church, often in roles that require strength while remaining humble. However, we need to perform tasks that require an assertive posture in our lives. That is a challenging task.

God's response to Moses was, "...I will be with you." He will always be with us.

When you feel hesitant and inferior, God says, "I will be with you."

When you wonder if you can make it another day with the job stress, He says, "I will be with you."

When you're faced with a tough decision and wondering what to do, He says, "I will be with you."

When you are experiencing great joy, God is with you.

You may be a bit reluctant, as was Moses, but we must remember that God is always with us as we go through life.

Thought for Today: We need to remember that we are not alone. Through our faith, we have help meeting our obligations. So take control of situations humbly and allow ourselves to be led through the tasks ahead.

Prayer for Today: Dear Lord and Father, we thank you for being with us. We are often confused in a world of activity. Usually, we feel that we controlled the situation when things go well. We pray that we can recognize your involvement in our everyday lives and have the forethought to give you thanks through our actions and prayers. Amen

Mallard on the River Nene

June 20 Peterborough, Cambridgeshire, UK

Finding Others

> He has shown you, O man, what is good.
> And what does the LORD require of you?
> To act justly and to love mercy
> and to walk humbly with your God.
> (Micah 6:8)

As we move through life, we meet all kinds of people. Some we warm up to; some we don't. We often cannot understand why; it has to do with behavior and operating style fitting our comfort zone.

Once when experiencing a technical problem at work, my customer and I were very perplexed. There seemed to be no reasonable explanation, and I was considered an expert. So, I called in a big gun, a fifteen-year colleague. He was not only an expert but also a specialist, a person who, for whatever reason, fit technically and personally, would help even if there were no financial gain.

After discussing and resolving the technical issue, we discussed our work schedules. As a small business owner, he starts the week with a prayer breakfast with his whole company. He needs to be on the road at 5 am and drive two hours to do this. He is not only a dedicated businessman but a dedicated believer. He is a "good fit" because he "...does what the Lord requires..."

Thought for Today: Look at our associates. Not the ones we meet on Sunday morning at church, but all others. The store clerk, barber, hairdresser, or whoever; the ones we are comfortable with; the ones that fit. Often, they will "fit" because of their beliefs and Christian practices.

Prayer for Today: Heavenly Father, we pray that we somehow find understanding through prayer and your word. We pray that somehow we solve problems rather than create them. Amen

Swans Taking Off, River Nene

Chemical Dependency

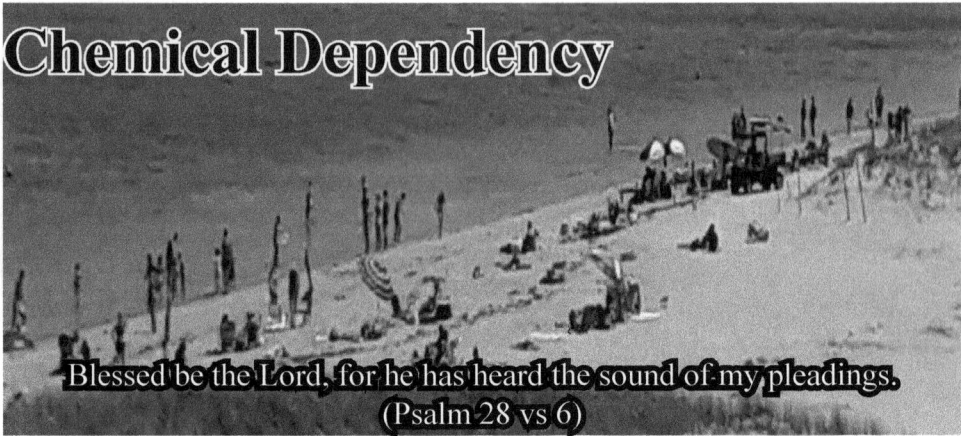

Blessed be the Lord, for he has heard the sound of my pleadings.
(Psalm 28 vs 6)

It is a few minutes before bedtime after a stressful day, and the phone rings. Often you are not in the mood to listen, but someone heard you some time ago. It is someone you sponsor and care about that has a serious issue. This story is repeated over and over in twelve-step treatment programs.

The person talks and rambles on for an hour, more or less, and you can hardly get a word in. Generally, you get to make a few suggestions of unwelcome tough love. The person was not ready to listen.

Near the end of the call, well past your bedtime, there will be a prayer, often about his issue, followed by the serenity prayer. The typical response is something like," Thanks for listening. You have helped me so much. I cannot believe that I hesitated to call you,"

Sometimes we need a set of ears to hear our problems. Sometimes the listener may be a friend. But we also have another wiser, more faithful listener- God. In Psalm 28, David cries out for help. Like David, when we express our feelings to God, we always find a patient and a willing listener. At the end of the Psalm, David expresses trust and confidence in God. We can too.

Thought for Today: God is willing to listen and help you.
Prayer for Today: Let us pray for those who suffer from the self-inflicted,and powerful disease, "Chemical Dependency." Let us pray they find honesty, openness, amd spirituality. Amen

Capd Cod Beach
Chatham Massachusetts

June 22

Life Goals

> Watch out! Be on your guard against all kinds of greed;
> life does not consist in an abundance of possessions.
> (Luke 12 vs 15)

In our democratic society, we are encouraged to compete in the workplace and elsewhere. In the 1950s, there was the term "Keeping up with the Jones." In the 1990s, that seemed to become "Leave the Jones behind." It is easy to understand why attendance and giving in church declined; no one has any time or money left. The two-car family of the 1960s becomes the two home, four cars, and a boat family of the new millennium.

This is not meant to be a stewardship message asking for more. It is intended as a caution and designed to provoke thought. One of my blessings was being raised in a household with two cars and two homes. You see, I grew up maintaining two homes with my dad and never wanted to do that again. When we moved to Minnesota, the land of 10,000 lakes and 10 million lake homes, we said no way.

In confession, June and I did have too much stuff and too many things. We downsized in 2006 and have not finished yet.

Jesus is clear in his message as reported by Luke. Happiness has nothing to do with stuff or things. Life is about spiritual growth, love within the community, helping others, being comfortable in your own skin, etc.

Thought for Today: Let's think about what we need to get through the day and contemplate what we want; understand the differences.

Prayer for the Day: Heavenly Father, today we are blessed and live in a great society. We ask forgiveness for our participation in blatant consumption We pray that we experience the blessing of learning what our real needs are and experience the true abundance of your love as we move forward.Amen

Cape Cod Sand Bar
Chatham, Massachusette

Lighter Life

For life is more than food, and the body more than clothes.
Who of you, by worrying, can add a single hour to your life?
(Luke 12 vs 23, 25)

Yesterday may have seemed like a stern message regarding our society, so on a lighter note, I do not believe that the Lord is wasteful and wants us to be ecologically sound, not waste our resources. So with my tongue in cheek, let us consider the benefit of having many things

. June and her many friends all do crafts and have rooms dedicated to their hobby; craft rooms. These rooms have years of unfinished projects; cross stitch kits, quilt squares waiting to finish, yarn skeins and thread spools awaiting the needle, and even unfinished braided rugs. When they are together, one will often comment that they know the Lord will not take them until they have finished their last project.

As men, we are not much different. The fisherman has a tackle box full of jigs and lures; he is good until the last lure is lost or the last fish caught. The gardener and landscaper can never finish until every crop has matured. The hunter has many guns, and the game is never-ending; indeed, his job will never end. We are safe, guys.

We know the above is levity and not serious. The reality is that when doing a craft, fishing, hunting, or gardening, we are quiet and at peace. The Lord blesses us through our many activities. Using our stuff contributes to our peace and compliments our spirituality. We must always be careful and remember that love and the holy spirit will bring everlasting peace.

Thought for Today: Remember our faith and commitments with joy. It is ok to have fun and laugh.

Prayer for Today: Lord, hear our prayer for the good life, one of joy, love, and abundance. We pray for these throughout the world. Amen

Lean On Me

Rejoice in the Lord always. I will say it again: Rejoice !
(Philippians 4 vs. 4)

Rejoice and celebrate, yes. But we need to fight battles, and some never end. Think about that. In the 1980s, there was so much stress and negativity in my life that rejoicing was absent. My spiritual advisor challenged me to do my meditations more often.

This morning I walked a golf course "marking" for my grandson Chris' foursome in a junior league. Last evening June, I took an after-dinner walk under a clear blue sky at 75 degrees F. (I need to specify the scale because of my Euro-readers!) This afternoon I bumped into a friend at the outdoor pool, and she is doing well after losing her husband three years ago.

As Christians, we have hope. Every day there will be challenges that require our attention. We need to accept those challenges and work through them. That is living.

Erma Bombeck wrote a book entitled "If Life is a Bowl of Cherries, What Am I doing in the Pits?" We need to focus on the good stuff , listen to Paul. and rejoice in the Lord

Thought for Today: It will be too hot outside, the air conditioning inside will be too cool, the sun will be too bright, and there may be a thunderstorm. It will not matter, so rejoice in the Lord and enjoy it. It is a present from the Lord.

Prayer for Today: Dear Lord and Father, there are many things wrong in our world; Wars, revolutions, and national and local money issues. Today we give thanks for what we have and the ability to seek peace through you. We pray for the strength and guidance to find a way to contribute to a worldwide solution. Amen

Trail Bridge, Gleason Lake
Plymouth Minnesota

Listen

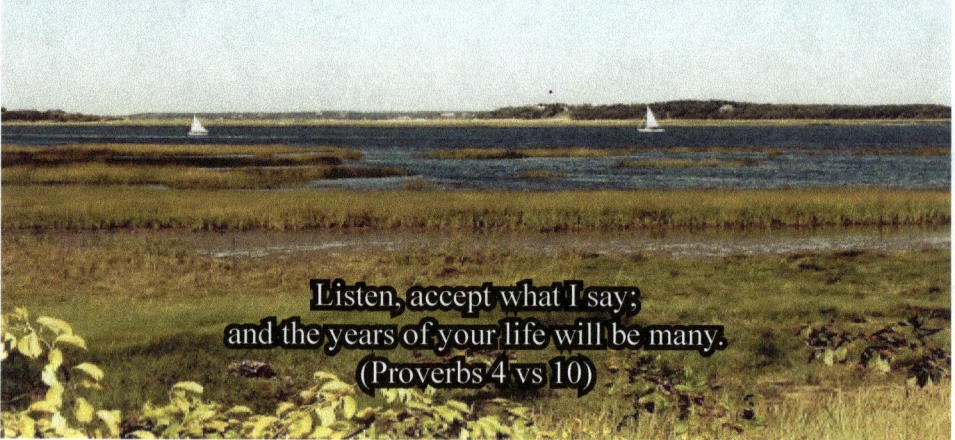

Photo by Jackie Collins

Listen, accept what I say;
and the years of your life will be many.
(Proverbs 4 vs 10)

Driving to the trail to do my morning walk, a father and son were in the car behind me. The son was wearing a headset and probably listening or viewing something on his phone. The dad had his phone up to his ear. There are parents with their children in our apartment complex but on their screens. Screens and blue tooth are an integral part of society today; we are together but separated by technology.

So, not to sound too much like an old fogey, I must admit that most of my communications today are with text, email, or social media. It is a great way to stay in touch with people and twenty-two family members. My question is, "Are we missing out on closeness...or increasing our contact?

In the ancient 1950s, my folks and I rode together a lot, and they would not turn on the radio. It was our time to talk. Often, I was getting grilled, but it was my turn to ask and question once in a while. I especially liked to quiz my mom when we were riding to school. She was a teacher and always had the inside scoop. My dad was a talker; with him was my time to listen and learn. I do not remember much about what I learned, but we sure talked. There is a closeness to a personal conversation that we may be missing.

I saw no conversation between the boy and his dad in my mirror. They were in different worlds. Sometimes my grandkids do that when I pick them up from school. Alone time is essential. Use it. With that said, the increased communication through technology makes keeping in touch easier.

June 26 Sailboats off Lieutenant Island
Wellfleet, Massachusetts

My conclusion for today is nothing. Times are changing, and people change with the times. We are parents charged with raising and mentoring the next generation. Prayerfully our love and Christian values will be passed on.

Thought for Today: Let's be communicators with those around us. Let us share our love and faith and some hints on life.

Prayer for Today: Father, we pray for future generations. That the technology making their lives simpler enhances their understanding of Jesus and his grace. Amen

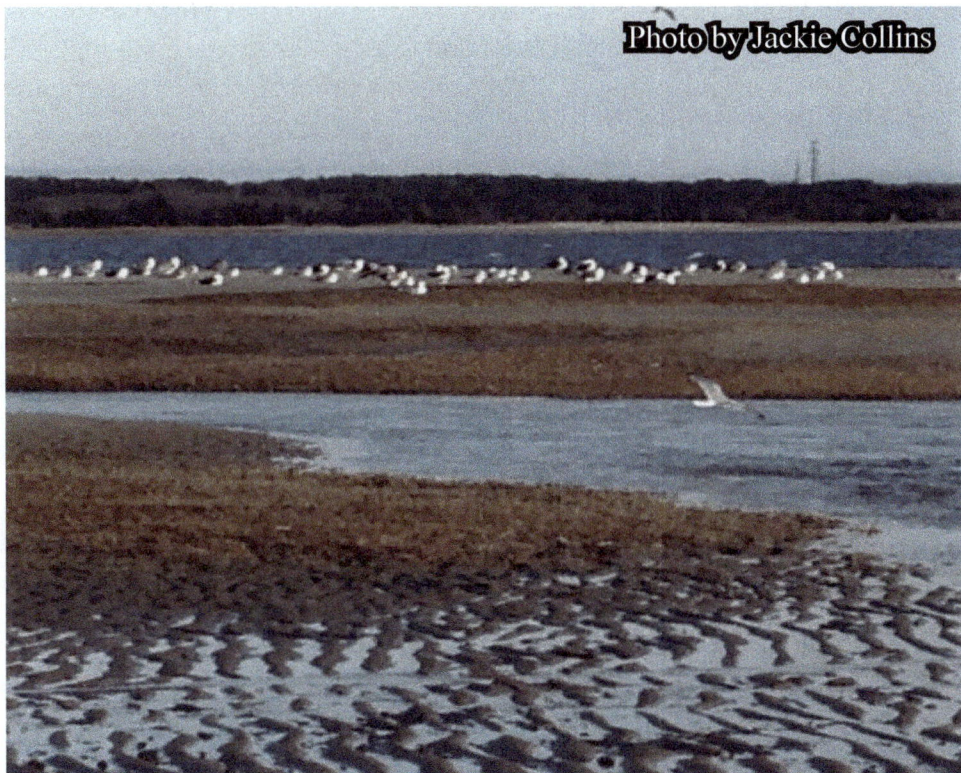

Photo by Jackie Collins

Gulls on Lieutenant Island
Wellfleet, Massachusetts

Anxiety and Faith

> Do not be anxious about anything,
> but in everything, by prayer and petition,
> with Thanksgiving, present your requests to God.
> (Philippians 4 vs 6)

Stress is becoming an American, if not a worldwide tradition, part of our lifestyle. We often go through our week wound up like a rubber band twisted tighter and tighter. However, we all recognize that the rubber band eventually breaks. When it is wound too tight or stressed too long, it snaps. We are certainly a higher life form than a rubber band, however, are we similar when stressed.

We have a way of unwinding during the most stressful times. There are many ways to release stress. Mine is by writing devotions to people that I love. Yours may be different- exercise, meditation, a chat with a friend, reading. Paul's writings in Philippians 4: 8 & 9 suggest that Faith is a tool to help us.

"Finally, brothers, whatever is true, whatever is noble, whatever is right, whatever is pure, whatever is lovely, whatever is admirable—
if anything is excellent or praiseworthy—think about such things.
Whatever you have learned or received or heard from me, or seen in me—put it into practice. And the God of peace will be with you."

Thought for Today: Today, let us focus selfishly on ourselves; feel the peace and presence of God in our lives. As Christians, we deserve peace. When the "stress monster" wants to control our lives, let's read this passage and let "the peace of God" into our lives.

Prayer for Today: Heavenly Father, the world seems to be a breeding ground for stress. There is something to worry about; terror, hate, employment troubles, stock market woes- even severe weather. We pray that we may keep you and peace in our thoughts, have the presence of mind to make wise choices, and release our stresses to find tranquility. Amen

RHS Wisley Gardens
Wisley, Surrey, UK

The Answer

You, however, are not in the realm of the flesh
but are in the realm of the Spirit,
if indeed the Spirit of God lives in you.
(Romans 8 vs. 9)

We certainly do not feel filled with the Spirit every day. (or at least I don't!) Quite often when I sit down to write these messages, there seems to be a writer's block. That says that my Spirit may need more coffee or, better, a prayer. Often it is both.

With our busy schedules today, it is easy to jump out of bed and get into our daily activities without thinking about our Spirit. That is normal, but it may not lead to a peaceful lifestyle. It is the way we achieve our material objectives.

However, we are given grace through our faith and cannot escape it. The message is clear: the solution is through the Spirit that lives in us when we feel empty or down and out. All we need to do is slow down and let it take over.

Thought for Today: When we feel stressed and overloaded, let's remember Paul's words above and take a break.

Prayer for Today: Dear Lord and father, we often cannot feel the Spirit that we know is within us. Today we pray that when we are too busy and stressed out, we will remember You are the answer. Amen

RHS Wisley Gardens
Wisley, Surrey, UK

Tough Times

Contend, LORD, with those who contend with me;
fight against those who fight against me.
Take up shield and armor;
arise and come to my aid.
(Psalm 35 vs 1, 2)

All days are not created equal. There are negative forces in our competitive society that seem overwhelming. There are career issues; many people don't awaken with enthusiasm to go to work every day. Financial issues always need to be dealt with and recreated monthly, weekly, or quarterly. The calendar always seems too crowded. Altogether it is easy to wonder where God is in all of this and ask if someone is working against us?

Early Christians had it more challenging than we do. In David's case above, most of the crowds wanted him dead. That was also the case for Paul and Silas almost everywhere they went; "But other Jews were jealous; so they rounded up some bad characters from the marketplace, formed a mob and started a riot in the city." (Acts 17 vs. 5) Being an early Christian required a strong faith dedication.

The early Christians turned things around through their belief system. We can also do that. We do it with prayer and meditation; God is always with us and available to help.

Thought for Today: Let's start without fear, stress, and conflict. If it finds us and interrupts us let's deal with it in a Godly way.

Prayer for Today: Dear Lord and Father, today we give thanks for your presence in our lives; for the opportunity, you give us when we speak to you. We give thanks for the peace you bring us. Amen

Turn Around

May those who delight in my vindication shout for joy and gladness.
(Psalm 35 vs. 27)

We learn in basic physics that perpetual motion does not and cannot exist. Something in motion will eventually stop due to outside forces unless we apply energy to keep it moving. For non-technical people reading this, a good summary statement is that there is no free lunch. If you don't believe it, take your foot off the gas.

Yesterday we read about the resistance felt by early Christians. The majority did not believe or support them, and they had some long days. Paul and Peter, and many others were martyred. Yesterday's message was entitled "Tough Times" because life will be hard at some level. In our lives, we have stress and negativity.

We need to understand that somehow negativity is an opportunity for growth. When we resolve it, we will feel better. Through dedication and prayer, and a bit of effort, we can always turn things around.

We can apply physics to our lives, congregations, and careers. We need to use our skills and efforts to keep the ball rolling in a positive way. There is no free lunch and no penalty for success. As stated above, "The LORD be exalted, who delights in the well-being of his servant."

We need to turn negativity around through our strength and faith.

Thought for the Day: We will have an opportunity to turn over a negative force; to improve our lives. Let's make it happen through our strength, efforts, and prayers.

Prayer for Today: Heavenly Father, today is the first day of the rest of my life. It will start carefree with a beautiful sunrise. We pray that you guide us and give us the faith and strength to make it through. Amen

Shrub Rose Garden
Minnesota Landscape Arboretum

June 30

July

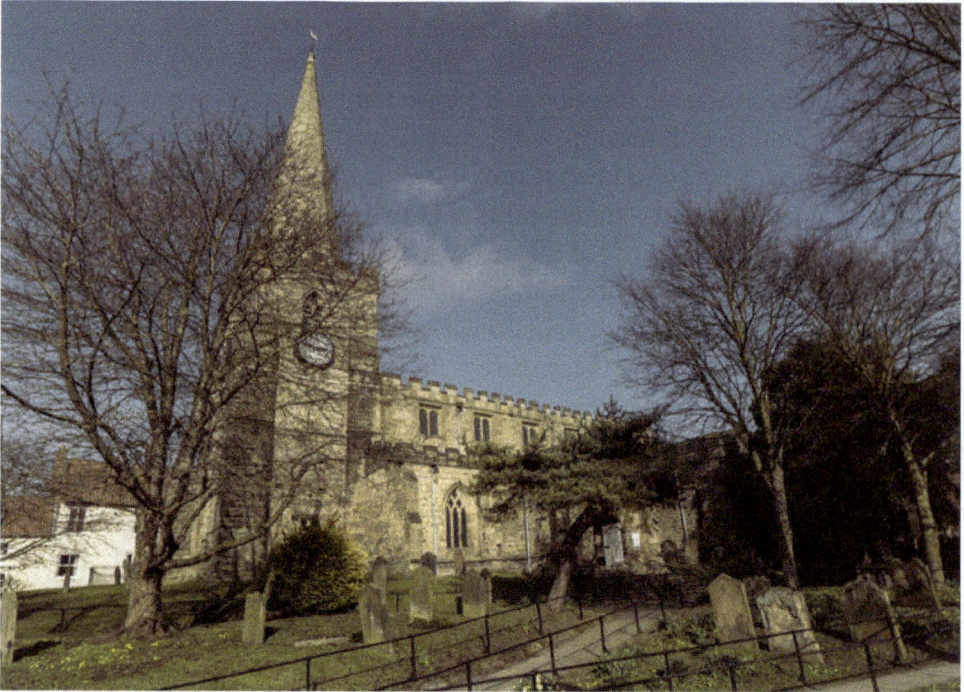

St. Peters and St. Pauls
Pickering, UK

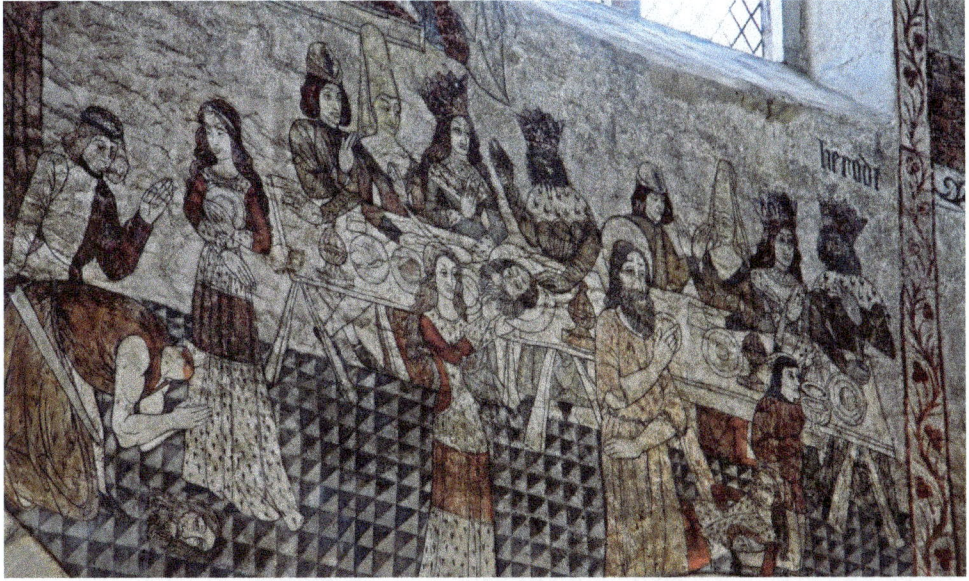

The Church of St Peter and St Paul, Pickering, is the parish church of the market town of Pickering in the county of North Yorkshire. The church sits on the top of a small hill in the centre of the town and its spire is visible across the Ryedale district. The church is part of the Church of England Diocese of York, and houses a collection of medieval wall paintings.

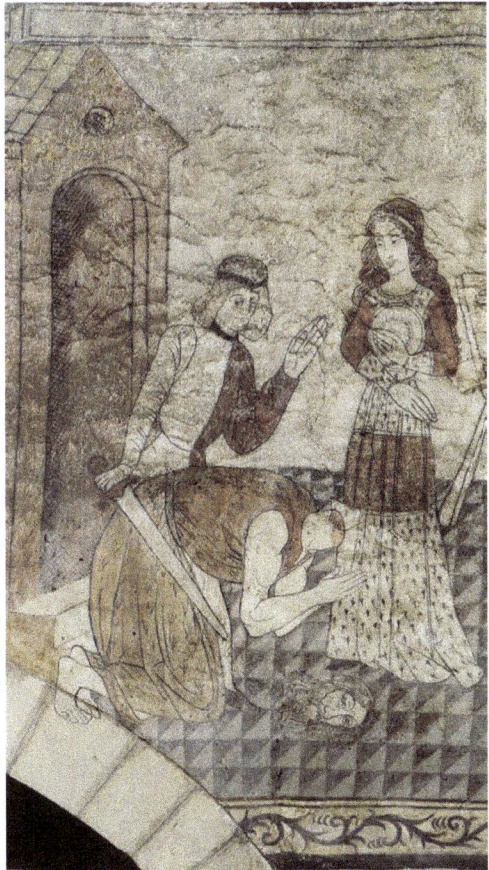

Sheep

Know that the LORD is God. It is he who made us,
and we are his people, the sheep of his pasture.
(Psalm 100 vs 3)

None of us like to think of ourselves as sheep. We are at a higher level than that and in control of our destiny. After all, sheep live in flocks, huddle together against all weather, feed on pasture grasses, etc. The Sheppard keeps his watch on them daily and has border collies to round up the ones that get lost.

Maybe we should look at ourselves as wolves. They have a definite pecking order, a family system, and work together when hunting. That sounds a little bit more human. The point to understand is that yes, we are a higher life form; we control ourselves through the power of logic, and yes, we follow our beliefs.

Today, my daughter called me regarding a 95-year-old lady that we both love. This lady is having issues with being old and probably nearing her end-of-life experience. She also does not have faith or belief in God. By not believing in a higher power (God), she de-facto appointed herself in control, which is scary when nearing the end.

Something extraordinary creates this world and our society. I prefer to believe in God and the blessing and grace we have through Jesus. These are Abe Lincoln's comments on it.

*"The purposes of the Almighty are perfect
and must prevail, though we erring mortals may fail to
accurately perceive them in advance."*

Thought for Today: Let's follow our Sheppard and do his will.
Prayer for Today: Dear Lord, today we will be making decisions regarding life, children, business, and anything else. We pray for your guidance as we go through our day. Amen

July 1 Marsh at Monomy Wildlife Refuge
Chatham, Massachusetts

Tim's Story

In the same way, we can see and understand only a little about God now, ... but someday we are going to see him in his completeness, face to face.
(1 Corinthians 13 vs 12)

I have known Tim, a devout Christian friend, for over twenty years. He trains for marathons, works in the same industry, loves music, and shares many of the same ideals that I do. I like the guy, and he had a tough spring. Here is his story.

Training for marathons is often a matter of working through ever-increasing pain thresholds. Everyone experiences them in their way and many different ways. Tim used to experience pain in the lower stomach/colon area. I used to think he ate incorrectly. The pain grew unbearable this year, so Tim searched for the reason. He did not have much success, and in February, he became very ill at a business meeting.

Finally, a doctor identified a blockage in his colon and prescribed surgery. However, there were several more tests and some misdiagnoses over several weeks, and Tim lost weight and became very weak. He described himself as "in a black tunnel with no light at the end." He was dying and did not know why. And yes, he did ask God why.

He had some major surgery and spent 13 days in the hospital recovering. He had been close to death. During this process, Tim realized God was with him and in control rather than the medical community. What a blessing and excellent result. The Lord is with all of us.

Thought for Today: Let's focus on the unfortunates around us that are ill and keep the 23rd Psalm and Paul's message to the Corinthians in mind. Let us see if we can contribute to helping in some way.

Prayer for Today: Dear Lord, many of us are ill, some are minor, some serious, and some terminal. We pray that we may find a way to help and calm their fears; help them understand that you are with them through it all. May we help by following your guidance through prayer. Amen

Sand Bar
Chatham. Massachusetts

Commitment

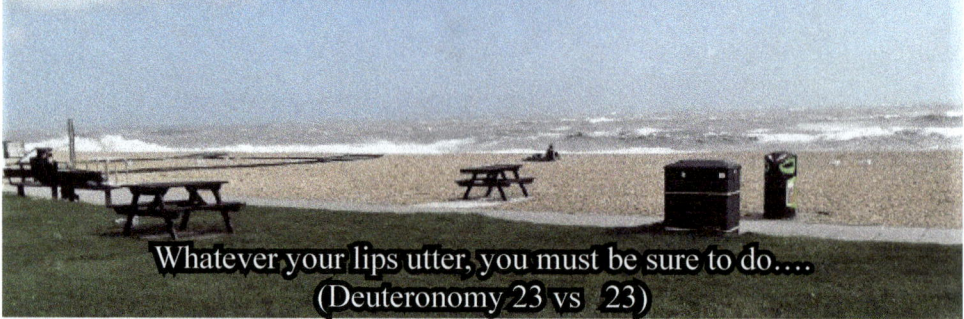

Whatever your lips utter, you must be sure to do....
(Deuteronomy 23 vs 23)

Reliability breeds success. People who are successful in life keep commitments. They say it and do it, even after having second thoughts. It is probably impossible to be 100%, but the closer you are, the more you benefit.

Consider the example of a guy who coached youth soccer and had never played. He told the league that he was unqualified but available if they could not find someone else. They called, and he managed a team with the help of two assistants that could teach skills. They worked things out. He managed the team rather than coached, and the kids had fun. This same guy also managed a youth hockey team and could not skate. He committed and got the job done.

One of my jobs was training people new to sales in the business world. A trainee working with me heard the word commitment a lot. If you were the one that got back to the customer and if the customer trusted you would be prompt, you would get the first call and the most orders. Fortunately, most of the competition lacked the passion or desire to be fully committed in sales.

I took liberty with the "do ..." I wanted it to be generic. It goes on to "...sure to do because you made your vow freely to the LORD your God with your mouth." If you read these messages at some time in your life, you committed to God. These messages are an opportunity to review that commitment and recharge your batteries, a way to keep engaged and stay on track in a world of distractions.

Thought for Today: Let's renew our commitment to the Lord and our local church.

Prayer for Today: Dear Lord, we have not always been faithful. We pray for forgiveness and make a new commitment to do your will. Amen

July 3 Pelham Beach
Hastings, East Sussex, UK

Independence Day

It is for freedom that Christ has set us free.
Stand firm, then, and do not let yourselves
be burdened again by a yoke of slavery.
(Galatians 5 vs 1)

Independence makes America great, and our many freedoms make this a great place to live. Our constitution relies on our ability to self-govern. Below is a quote from Abraham Lincoln about our system.

"This country, with its institutions, belongs to the people who inhabit it. Whenever they shall grow weary of the existing government, they can exercise their constitutional right of amending it or exercise their revolutionary right to overthrow it."

Pray for the future of America.

Thought for Today: Today, let's celebrate our independence by obeying the Lord's commandments.

Prayer for Today: Dear Lord and Father, our country celebrates its independence. Our freedoms are based on your laws and our abilities to obey them. Today we pray for spiritual growth, honesty, integrity, and ethics. Amen

Stand Free

> It is for freedom that Christ has set us free.
> Stand firm, then, and do not let yourselves be burdened again
> by a yoke of slavery.
> (Galatians 5 vs 1)

You that know me probably have heard my definition of retirement; having four days a week without a calendar commitment and a long to-do list with the opportunity to choose. That is the definition of freedom and the way Christ would want us to live. Unfortunately, few careers offer that kind of flexibility, and most families today have two jobs working to clutter up their calendars.

The new normal economy and the financial status of the American family do not always allow freedom. It is easy to get caught up in the pursuit of becoming an average family or average Joe. It takes a certain amount of control to take a deep breath and step out of line to seek peace. The "…yoke of slavery..." has become habitual, and many feel uncomfortable when they have free time. We need to evaluate that, each on our terms.

We can experience freedom through meditation and prayer. It takes a few minutes to unwind when we focus on being at peace. My old standard of balance, the YMCA triangle of Spirit, Mind, and Body, is a model we need to keep in our lives. We must stop, look, and listen to Christ, be at peace, and be the best we can be.

Thought for Today: Let's evaluate our "yoke of slavery" to determine what is necessary and what is not. Let's accept the guidance from Christ and take one step closer to being free.

Prayer for Today: Dear Lord and Father, we pray for a light at the end of our tunnel. Amen

Belief

Therefore, I tell you, whatever you ask for in prayer, believe that you have received it, and it will be yours.
(Mark 11 vs 24)

When we pray, we generate a certain amount of doubt in our minds. Often we ask God for something out of reach. We Elders often pray for extended youth or capability to do things we did 20 years ago. Those prayers essentially go unanswered. Our pastor talks about praying for the terminally ill. He prays that they will find peace with the Lord and pray for the family and their future.

Recently, we prayed that a person would receive a liver transplant on our prayer chain. That is a catch-22 because the donor has to die. For a prince to become king, his mother must pass on—what a conundrum. We were not praying for death. We were praying that if someone died, they could make the ultimate gift, the gift of life. That is still something to consider.

It seems that Mark is correct, though, when he says, "believe that you have received it …" A strong belief appears to improve the success rate through prayer.

Thought for Today: For today, let us keep it simple and enjoy the day.

Prayer for Today: Heavenly Father, today we pray a simple prayer. Today is the day you made for us, and today we thank you for that and the opportunity to enjoy it. Amen

Landmarks

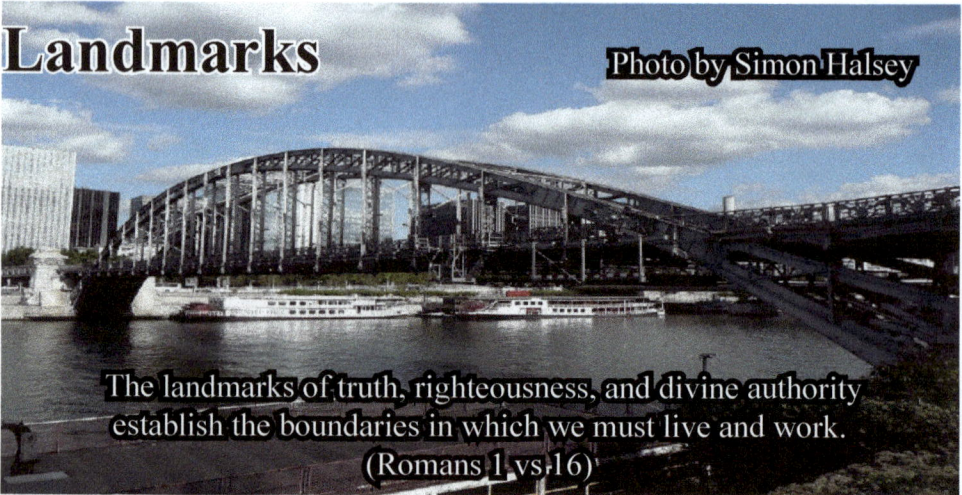

The landmarks of truth, righteousness, and divine authority establish the boundaries in which we must live and work.
(Romans 1 vs 16)

As adults, our lives are full of memories. They are landmarks in our minds. They are what makes us who we are and often determine our self-image. A very early landmark in my mind goes back to the 1940s in Massachusetts at a post-WW2 parade. A color guard led it, a platoon of soldiers in full packs, and a marching band followed closely. Parades are always impressive, and we, a group of five to eight-year-olds, were very excited. The older kids jumped up and marched alongside the big base drum, and I followed.

As Christians, we also have positive memories. The exciting parade memory returns every May and stays through Independence day. It is a positive and patriotic landmark celebrating the end of a World War. Christmas and Easter are positive Christian landmarks relating to Christ. In our lives, there are personal memories that we cherish. We all have personal memories we cherish, landmarks.

Thought for Today: Today, let us think back and remember what brought us to this point in our lives. Focus on "landmark" events that shaped us to be what we are and understand God's role and how he shaped and
developed us.

Prayer for Today: Heavenly Father, as a nation, we celebrated independence, our many privileges, and especially our religious freedoms. We pray that people can learn to appreciate their faith and the love that comes with it around the world. Amen

July 7

Bridge on the Tiber River
Rome, Italy

Follow Your Heart

Above all else, guard your heart,
for everything you do flows from it.
(Proverbs 4 vs 23)

We need to make decisions to get through every day. Sometimes we know we are wrong when we make them. My bad choices involve skipping exercise sessions, eating an extra cookie, and putting off something until tomorrow. During the 1960s, my dark period, my daily decisions were challenging and created a life of darkness. My focus during those years had much to do with "self." I was not listening to my heart and ended up divorced and chemically dependent.

As a young married adult, my focus was education, earning enough money to survive, and my golf game. Family life was a distant fourth priority. I attended Northeastern University two or three evenings a week, worked full time, had a part-time job at the YMCA teaching fitness, and maintained a seven handicap. My focus was all on myself.

Dr. Joyce Meyer says, "You cannot be selfish and happy. The two never go together." My life from the late 1950s through the mid-1960s confirms that. Somehow, there was a conversion through my church, twelve-step programs, and my newfound attention to family. I am blessed.

Today, my message is simple: if you are not as happy as you would like to be (And is any of us?), the solution lies in spiritual growth, both personal and within our family and friends, or being true to your heart.

Thought for the Day: For today, stop when you feel stressed or unhappy. Chances are, it will be a conflict between doing what our heart says rather than what our calendar says.

Prayer for Today: Dear Lord, today we give thanks for the many blessings you have given us. We are incredibly blessed by friends, family, and those around us. Amen

Bridge on the Tiber River
Rome, Italy

Forgive and Love

Praise the LORD, O my soul, and forget not all his benefits who forgives all your sins...
(Psalm 103 vs 2)

Grace means that we are forgiven. We all have had reasons to be forgiven and memories of being forgiven. Growing together spiritually within a family or social structure so that faults are forgiven creates landmarks in our lives. I pray that all readers find the previous statements true and ask that we think about the many times in our lives when we were down and out, possibly guilt-ridden.

Children often misbehave. Fight over toys, sneak a treat before dinner, the simple things. We almost always forgive them after a consequence. That is an excellent example of our love. Some behaviors are more extreme as teens, but we again excuse the behavior and show our love.

Forgiveness and love create a family and social landmarks in our lives. They create memories that make us what we are. It is important to be aware of the many times that God's will has generated forgiveness in our lives and be grateful. We have all experienced His grace through these landmark events.

Thought for Today: God forgives us for our sins. We receive the reward of "good feelings" and a growing relationship by forgiving others. Let us focus on being tolerant and forgiving.

Prayer for Today: Dear Loving God, often we find ourselves offended by the behaviors of others. We have noisy neighbors, careless drivers, inconsiderate fellow employees, and other life factors. It is challenging to be a good Christian when dealing with irritants. We pray that we can behave as Christ when tested by our society we display tolerance and love for all. Amen

Grand Amore Rose

Mile Markers

Teach us to number our days,
that we may gain a heart of wisdom.
(Psalm 90 vs. 12)

Each day of our life is a present and special in some way. Each has a memory, some fade but the great ones stay forever. We often catalog them, and many hide in our subconscious. Numbering our days is an excellent thought.

The major ones do not take rocket science to remember. I am an elder and remember where I was for Pearl Harbor (27 months old), JFK's assassination, the twin tower assault, and Ted William's last at-bat (a home run at age 41).

The unconscious ones are often more fun when brought to the front. Recently, an old friend from 1955 and I reconnected and reviewed our memories together; high school football experiences, school days, former teachers, and cheerleaders. He brought back so many memories that he called me one evening while online. We talked for two hours.

The Lord has been good to us. We are not wealthy but rich in memories, full of love, happiness, and wisdom. The numbering of our days has paid off in a worthy life. It will also work for you.

Thought for Today: Today, we will create a memory. Whether it is a major or minor event remains to be seen. Either way, let us recognize its contribution to our memory.

Prayer for Today: Dear Lord and Father, we thank you for all the great memories and blessings you have given us. Today we pray that we serve your will here on earth as we go through our day. Amen

Real Freedom

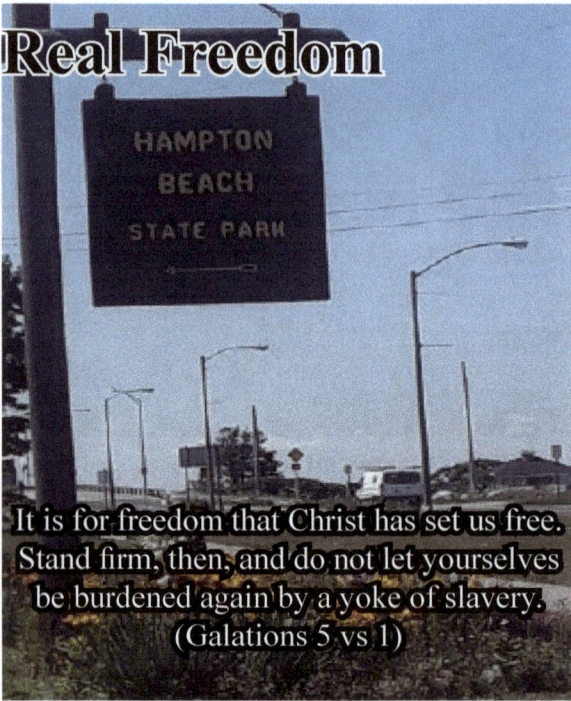

It is for freedom that Christ has set us free. Stand firm, then, and do not let yourselves be burdened again by a yoke of slavery.
(Galations 5 vs 1)

In society today, we find too many ways to become slaves. We take on church projects, youth sports, charity events, etc. Then we become aware that we have little time left for meditation and rest. In today's world, we tend to create our brand of slavery, all in the name of lifestyle.

At some time, we have all tried it and then backed off. Often our pastors ask us to put down the morning paper, turn off the TV news, and pick up the daily meditation book; start the day with meditation and love. That's how my Good News messages began. My willpower kept going back to the news and sports.

Paul said above, *"The only thing that counts is faith expressing itself through love."* We are better people and have a better life when we keep our faith at the forefront and recharge our spiritual batteries. When aware of our faith, problems seem to have less impact, it is easier to show others we care, and tranquility comes to the surface. Take the advice of my favorite philosopher, NIKE, and "Just Do It."

Thought for Today: Keep meditation at the forefront today. Yes, we are too busy and need to get to the lake home mow the lawn; the kids have three games, etc. But no one says we need to be formal in our thoughts regarding our faith. Take a mini-break a day; at a stoplight, in the parking lot- a few minutes of charging the batteries goes a long way.

Prayer for Today: Heavenly Father, we have become calendar slaves. Our lifestyles and fear of losing our lifestyle have dominated our days. Today we pray that we can trust in you and recognize that your grace is what we need. Amen

Let Go and Let God

I will never leave you nor forsake you.
(Hebrews 13 vs 5)

What do you do when a problem seems unsolvable? The solution is to let God show you that there is a solution. Do not be troublvs ed if you are uncertain about the future or have difficulty releasing the past. Let go and let God guide you in this present moment. God is with you now.

Let go of worries or concerns about how you think something should be done, and let God guide you to the best way to do it. Do not become overwhelmed by the number of tasks before you. Let God's spirit lead you step-by-step to a new life of fulfillment.

As you let go and let God take charge of your life, you will realize that seeming obstacles can be opportunities in disguise. God will never fail you.

Thought for Today: Let go of the stress and tasks that seem impossible and out of our control; do what we can and pray about the rest.

Prayer for Today: Dear Lord, today we thank your presence in our lives and our future. We have confidence that by letting go and turning things over to you and living by your laws, grace will be ours. Amen

Ethical Business Wins

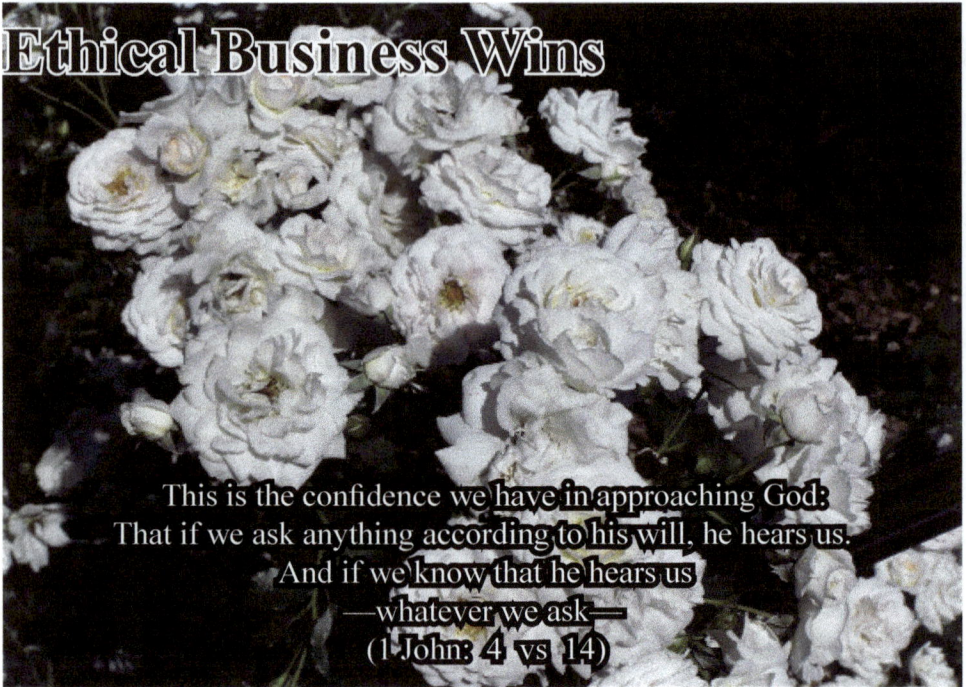

This is the confidence we have in approaching God:
That if we ask anything according to his will, he hears us.
And if we know that he hears us
—whatever we ask—
(1 John: 4 vs 14)

In business and life, aggressive and opportunistic behavior is typical. Our economies are generally cash-driven; sales are often "let the buyer beware." Service has become a lesser part of the equation in our more modern Internet-friendly economy.

In my younger days as a salesman, my youthful enthusiasm, lack of confidence, and immediate financial needs generated behaviors that may not have been as professional as they were later in my career. I used the tools of the opportunistic salesman. Win the negotiation. The term "win-win" should be in the bible, but I couldn't find the right passage. Good ethics and Godly behaviors generate good rewards. In the long term, they do not work. In fact, over the 30 years of sales, my experience has proven, without a doubt, that open and honest sales and people in business outperform the sharks and slippery every time.

Thought for Today: Today, let's focus on being open and honest in our dealings.

Prayer for Today: Father, we thank you for our Christian ethics. Life is good when we do business or play a game using our rules. Amen

Snowdrift Shrub Rose
Minnesota Landscape Arboretum

Doing God's Will

> We know that we have what we asked of him.
> We know that anyone born of God does not continue to sin;
> the one who was born of God keeps him safe,
> and the evil one cannot harm him.
> (1 John 4 vs 16, 17)

We are a society of checks and balances, and our scale seems negative or evil. Keep the faith as we proceed, I believe that God plays a role here, and we will tip the scale back to more Godly behaviors.

An early TV personality, Arthur Godfrey, had Lipton Tea as a sponsor for several years. He touted the great flavor, the best way to make it, and praised it highly. Then he changed sponsors and commented on how glad he was to have a great American cup of coffee. His network did not renew his contract. He lost half of his audience because he admitted his deception. Somehow, actors who never used or checked out a product have become the norm and accepted.

In my mind, faith and values are important in advertising and business. Sales and marketing are services to the customer and reflect a company's integrity. Buying is getting a fair deal; everybody can win, but only when there is confidence and a Godly presence.

Thought for Today: Let us ask a simple question as we go about our day; let us ask where God in all of this is?

Prayer for Today: Heavenly Father, we seem to be in a downward spiral. There is fraud, scandal, anger, and war in abundance. Evil appears to abound, and there appears to be no end. Please help us focus and demonstrate that your ways are the correct ways. Please help us maintain the confidence and maturity to overcome evil around us. Amen

Snowdrift Shrub Rose
Minnesota Landscape Arboretum   **July 14**   Page 205

Safety

Peace I leave with you; my peace I give you.
I do not give to you as the world gives.
Do not let your hearts be troubled, and do not be afraid.
(John 14 vs 27)

Peace is something that all religions teach, and somehow we manage to mess it up. If we could ask, "What would Jesus do?" we would not go to war in our Christian sense. Onward Christian soldiers and The Battle Hymn of the Republic would not have been written in a world of peace. That is the reality of our world.

June and I are considered world travelers. Several years ago, we made a western Mediterranean trip that was wonderful. But, every country and city we visited but one had riots and revolution since we were there; the one exception was Monte Carlo. When traveling, we feel that we need to understand what they are saying on the evening news to feel safe, and in most countries, we did not find English-speaking news.

As believers, we must contribute to the scale's other side. There are three essential contributions we need to make daily. First, we pray for our enemies so that they can find a better way through the Lord. Second, for our safety and happiness. Live confidently and without fear. Third, give thanks for the opportunities provided to us to contribute.

We live in a world of differences. We need to live and set an example for others and ask WWJD!

Thought for Today: Let us exercise our freedom through Christ and not be critical of others. Demonstrate our love as we do our daily activities.

Prayer for Today: Heavenly Father, today we pray for lasting peace. Amen

Letting Go

> So if anyone is in Christ,
> there is a new creation:
> everything old has passed away.
> (2 Corinthians 5 vs 17)

With God's help, we can release the past and live in the now. Accepting God's presence in our lives can release the past rather than reliving it. Holding on to hurtful memories takes us down roads that lead nowhere. With God's help, we can choose new directions and turn from a nowhere destination to live in the here and now.

A piece of all of us seems to need to live in the negative past. Divorced people can hold resentments for years; accident victims often resent the other driver; workers frequently hold grudges against their managers in the workplace, and it goes on. It is easy to do, but in the scope of Christianity, it does not fit. Forgiveness is what leads to peace and happiness.

Today is a new day where we can discard the baggage of old habits that limit us. Start anew with God, take control of our lives, and be receptive to all the goodness God has to offer through divine guidance.

Yes, today is the first day of the rest of our life.

Thought for Today: Today, think about what wears us down. When it is a historical issue, deal with it. If you can adjust to the situation, do it. If you can switch to something positive, do it. If you can not resolve the negativity, pray about it.

Prayer for Today: Dear Lord and Father, we need you in our lives more than ever. There are so many negative issues it is often difficult to focus on your goodness. We thank the blessings you bring to our lives, the friends we need, the world that surrounds us with beauty, and our families that bless our lives. We thank you as our creator for it all. Amen

Why Judge

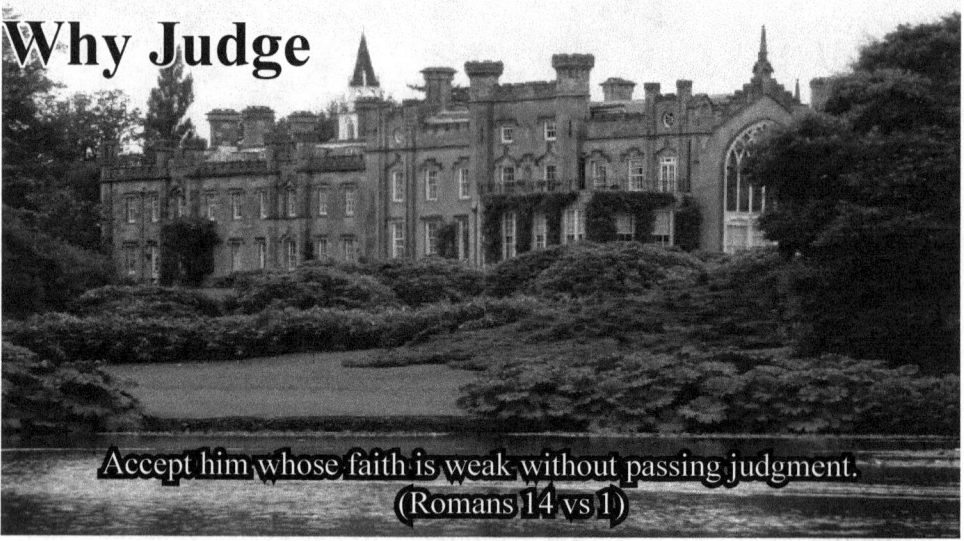

Accept him whose faith is weak without passing judgment.
(Romans 14 vs 1)

Since 1978 I have been involved in twelve-step programs that emphasize spiritual growth. When people walk in the door, they usually have lost touch with their spiritual side. They often never had one. Those who offer help typically have problems getting them to the second step, "Come to believe that a power greater than ourselves can restore us to sanity."

Often referring to God at this point in their lives will scare them away, so the term "higher power" is accepted as a starting point. It always bothers me when I hear that term because God was never an issue in my life. However, when a person is hurting and in need, it is a good start that opens the door to God and generally works.

The active people who sponsor and work with new members in need cannot pass judgment. Paul's message to the Romans is the key and the start of helping people sort out their lives.

Thought for Today: Today, we will interface with people who do not believe the way we do. Let's practice acceptance of our differences without being judgmental.

Prayer for Today: Dear Lord, please help me understand and accept others. Please help me understand those who do not practice the principles taught by Jesus in their daily lives. Please help me welcome them and live my life in a loving and caring way. Amen.

Sheffield Park, House and Gardens

July 17 East Sussex, UK

Differences

..let us stop passing judgment on one another.
Instead, make up our minds not to put an obstacle in our brothers' way.
(Romans 14 vs 13)

Growing up in Boston in the 1940s and 1950s, my family was strict on who was acceptable and not; prejudicial to the max. I believe that the feelings existed from the fear of competition within our society.

The good news is that I was blessed to be a YMCA brat growing up, and they were leaders in treating people as equals. I mixed with all and never saw any difference, so it was hard for me to buy into my family's ideas. My grandmother advised me that my Italian friends were not welcome at her house.

At the YMCA, our director, Jim Goodwin, was a leader in educating us on equality (in the 1950s). Jim was exceptional and well before his time. His daughter tells me he spent time reaching out to the Jewish Community Center and scheduling joint events.

My senior year of high school was at Huntington Prep in downtown Boston. It was my first exposure to a truly mixed nationality and race community. It was confusing because all were great guys, and my family had a true WASPish background. We studied together, trained together, and were fond of each other. We all had a shared goal, get into a good college.

My story has a point. Somehow I was blessed by being exposed to worldly people and was blind to the differences. My friends were varied. The moral is clear, love your neighbor, and do not be afraid to show it.

Thought for Today: We will interact with people of all kinds; recognize them as equals and the blessings of our differences. Love them all unconditionally.

Prayer for Today: Dear Lord and Father, somehow America, home of the free, still harbors prejudices within our society. We pray that we can learn to accept others as St. Paul suggested. Amen

Rain over Park Guell
Barcelona, Spain

July 18

Consequences

*Let us make every effort to do what leads to peace
and mutual edification.
(Romans 14 vs 19)*

Yes, we are beating on the same drum. It is a vital drum to beat, not for those we call "Them" but for us. The term "network" became popular in the 1980s and generally referred to business relationships and started as a business terminology. It has grown.

The internet has created more formal systems of business and social networks. In a social network, people are called friends, and I like that. My grandparents would exclude over half my friends from my Friends list of over 200 people. That is half the opportunities to learn, enjoy, assist, and help. It would be sad.

It is our right to form groups and decide what to say to whom. For example, Christian Friends and God is my Spinach have been viewed in over 170 countries and support people, not just Christians. It is a humble effort for "peace and edification."

My point is that the exclusionary attitudes taught in the 1950s are a deep-rooted problem. When we exclude others, we are the losers. Paul closed with the term "…mutual edification." And we lose that when we exclude.

Thought for Today: Extend our Christian love to everyone we meet and not exclude anyone.

Prayer for Today: Heavenly Father, we give thanks for the Grace of Jesus and the forgiveness of our faith. We have not been perfect in our treatment of others. We pray for the gift of love and that I may accept and love everyone. Amen

At Peace

You will keep in perfect peace
those whose minds are steadfast,
because they trust in you.
(Isaiah 26 vs 30)

Perfect Peace. Is that something we dream of? Many dreams are about troubles, potential troubles, and past experiences. Do you wonder what negative and scary dreams mean? Are they punishment or weak faith? Or was it too darn much sugar in that desert eaten after dinner? It could be all of the above.

It is one thing to master peace while awake. When awake maintaining a positive focus and feelings and having a great day are choices we can make. We can handle a water ball and fourth putt on the golf course. The red lights and traffic jams can be a chance to take a deep breath and relax. Life can be good, darn good.

Recently, there was a cartoon regarding the patience we develop as we grow older. It mentioned how things that bothered us in our youth don't seem as important as they once were. The punch line in the cartoon was, "maybe we just don't dive a darn anymore." I assure you that this is not the case. Seniors generally have matured and put things in perspective.

One of Webster's definitions of "steadfast" is 'extremely steady and loyal." The prophet Isaiah tells us that a strong faith rewards us with peace in our hearts. Reading devotionals helps us be steadfast!

Thought for Today: Today, let's be steadfast and optimistic in our search for peace.

Prayer for Today: Dear Lord, we pray for a positive attitude as we deal with our activities. We pray that we may contribute to the peace of those around us in your name. Amen

Pre Race Sunrise
Lake Phalen, St. Paul, Minnesota   **July 20**   Page 211

Being Humble

Now Moses was a very humble man,
more humble than anyone else on the face of the earth.
(Numbers 12 vs 3).

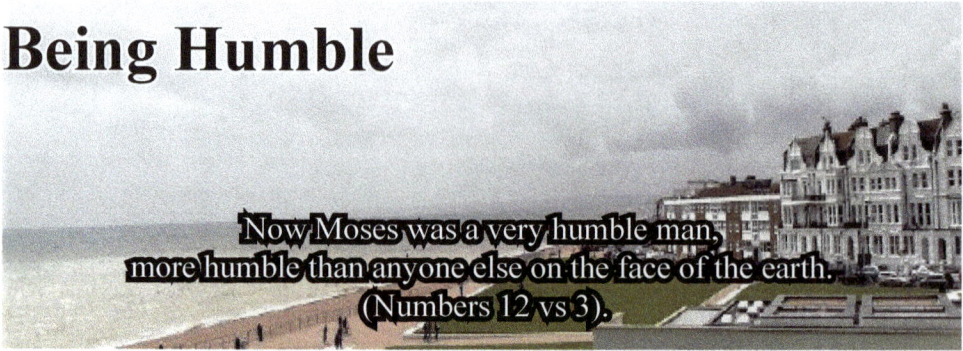

Is there a meek person in your life? What do you think of the meek or humble person at work, in the family, or at church? Would you like to avoid him? We tend to equate humble or meek with being a wimp. In the case of Moses, he was not passive. He took on an Egyptian overseer, stood up to Pharaoh, and hiked the desert for forty years. It is hard to see him as a wimp.

Humble is a choice. It is being humble before God and deliberately harnessing your strength, and tempering it to use in a controlled way. Humble is not weak. It is believing and obeying God when you don't particularly want to when it is not the path of least resistance.

Moses was not always enthusiastic about what God wanted. He did not feel capable when God called him to lead the people out of bondage. He didn't exactly say, "right on." It was more like, "Me, you have got to be kidding. Try someone else." (see Exodus 4 vs 10-13).

God's response "I will be with you."

When you feel hesitant and inferior, God says, "I will be with you."

When you are wondering if you can make it another day with the job stress, he says, "I will be with you."

When you're faced with a tough decision and wondering what to do, he says, "I will be with you."

Like Moses, you may be a bit reluctant. But he obeyed God. Moses believed him and did what he said. We can, too, when we humble ourselves.

Thought for Today: Let's be humble before the Lord today.
Prayer for Today: Dear Lord, we pray that we can do your will in our everyday actions. We pray for the guidance and humility to accomplish that. Amen

July 21 Stormy Sky over
Bexhill on Sea, East Sussex, UK

The Sabbath

Remember the Sabbath day by keeping it holy.
Six days you shall labor and do all your work,
but the seventh day is a Sabbath to the Lord your God.
On it, you shall not do any work.
(Exodus 20:8-10).

Rest. God says that we need to take a break once a week. He is saying there is more to life than work. He is also urging us to follow his pattern: "For in six days the Lord made the heavens and the earth, the sea and all that is in them, but he rested on the seventh day. Therefore the Lord blessed the Sabbath day and made it holy" (Exodus 20 vs 11).

We need to rest physically. There is a rhythm to the seventh day of rest that is a good balance
of work and rest. In the early 1990s, my seven-day-a-week running buddy, Bill, advised me that he would no longer do long runs on Sunday. We both stopped Sunday runs, and our overall running improved. Many people put themselves out trying their plans.

Spiritually we need this time to refocus our lives. God wants us to spend one day looking
to him and thanking him for being liberated. The Sabbath is a great day to recharge our spirit and rest our bodies.

In America, Sunday blue laws requiring stores to close are gone. That enables us to carry on and skip the day of rest. Take a look at how you use the Sabbath. Is it a day to serve, worship, rejoice, and rest?

Thought for Today: Take some time this week to meditate and pray for rest and peace in our lives.

Prayer for Today: Let's pray for those people who can't take time to rest and meditate. May they somehow find joy in the Lord. Amen

Stormy Sky over
Torquay Pier, Devon, UK

The Good Times

Then Jesus told his disciples...
that they should always pray and not give up.
(Luke 18 vs 1)

There are always good and bad times, and they are relative terms. At a recent bible study, we asked if anyone in the room ever had really bad financial times. We all thought the answer was yes. Well, after a brief discussion, we changed our minds.

In one case, a fellow had been divorced and certainly had some cash flow issues, feelings of loneliness, and despair. However, he kept a job and a relationship with his children, remarried, and stayed that way for over 50 years.

Several others were raised on farms, lived in small communities in the mid-west, and experienced the highs and lows of farm life. In two cases, the towns where they grew up are now ghost towns. No town was left after the corporate farms bought out the family tract; communities have gone forever. However, none of us had ever gone a day without food or a family presence.

We were all very blessed.

Sad stories are all too familiar in our new world economy. Many people's dreams have crashed down, and we fear for future generations. In this environment, the Christian church seems to grow. In troubled times the Lord is more visible than in good times. People reach out for His and our support, and we need to be there for everyone who comes. "The Lord said, 'Call to me, and I will come to you.'" (Jeremiah 33:3)

Thought for Today: Today, let's focus on being there for others. Not just those who seek us, let's be approachable to all.

Prayer for Today: Heavenly Father, today we had three square meals, tonight we will have a warm bed today we have your grace. Thank you. Amen

New Beginnings

Give thanks to the LORD, for he is good;
his love endures forever.
(Psalm 118 vs 1)

Often I awaken before sunrise and feel the need to share some good news. Frankly, it has not happened enough this year, but today I am blessed, and the good Lord will bless me with a nap this afternoon.

Times are certainly challenging, as yesterday's Good News "Inventory" pointed out. Several of our good news buddies with challenges or heavy hearts. If you are reading this, you know there is hope and that you will be a winner.

Psalm 118 is one of my favorites because it says it all in my mind. This year the news is sad and often scary or depressing to read the paper or watch the news. My recommendation is don't start the day that way. Start the day with a meditation, coffee with a friend (spouse?), or some exercise. There may be other options, but those are mine. It will change your outlook.

New beginnings are a great experience. My friend George asked, "What if we let Jesus come into our life every morning at our early service Sunday?" Would our life change? Indeed, it would be a new beginning.

Blessings to all of you, for I probably would not be here writing without you.

Thought for Today: "This is the day the Lord has made…" so let's go out and share it with someone. If possible, share it with someone with a heavy heart.

Prayer for Today: Today, we give thanks for our abundant lives. We pray that you will place someone in need in our path so that we may help them. Amen

One God ?

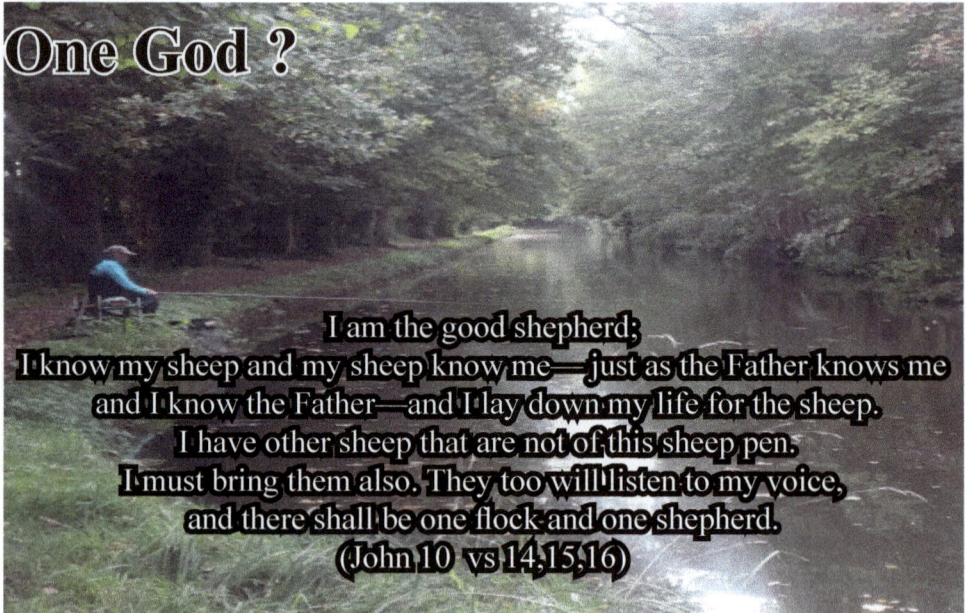

> I am the good shepherd;
> I know my sheep and my sheep know me—just as the Father knows me
> and I know the Father—and I lay down my life for the sheep.
> I have other sheep that are not of this sheep pen.
> I must bring them also. They too will listen to my voice,
> and there shall be one flock and one shepherd.
> (John 10 vs 14,15,16)

At a meeting recently, I expressed my belief that there is one God worshiped worldwide in many different ways. Several people in the conversation jumped on me and advised me on why I was wrong. It was one of those uncomfortable moments because we would never agree.

As many of you know, I am twelve-step programs. In fifty years, the blend of people attending has evolved to reflect our society today. In almost any meeting, Hispanic, East Indian, and Asian were to what used to be a dominant WASP and Afro-American mix. The program works for all.

The real question is how and why? The reason is simple. Although there is a mix of beliefs and worship practices, everyone recognizes that they need a "higher power." They always start with that "higher power" terminology because it works. In today's world of un-churched and varied beliefs, AA and other twelve-step programs have not lost their effectiveness. They still serve individuals by creating recovery through spiritual growth.

Thought for Today: For today, let's set two goals: First, let us find a personal way to have some spiritual growth; increase our faith. Second, let us contribute to another person's spirit and faith; be ecumenical.

Prayer for Today: Dear Lord and Father, we need your help and support. We are weak, tired, and too busy. Today we ask for a vision of tour will and the ability to help through prayer. Amen

July 25 River Wey Navagation
West Byfleet, Surrey, UK

Our Grace

May our Lord Jesus Christ himself and God our Father,
who loved us and by his grace gave us eternal
encouragement and good hope, encourage your hearts and
strengthen you in every good deed and word.
(2 Thessalonians vs 16, 17)

My friend Michael is the master of simplification and understatement. His style is simple; he has accepted the grace given to us through Jesus. He has a great life, donates to more causes than I even know of, and is one that is always joyful.

He often makes me a bit jealous because when I am confused by the facts of life, he will often ask where grace fits in. Recently I was bemoaning all the lost jobs in America, the state of business, and the markets, none of which I have significant control over. Michael pointed that out and asked, "Bob, you are so blessed. Why wreck your day on that stuff? Do what you can, but the best thing you could probably do is be happy.",

He was correct. My light was not shining at that moment, so my contributions would be negative that day. However, life will always be good with the oversimplification of accepting grace. Grace powers the lamp inside us to help light the world.

Thought for Today: This is the day the Lord has made; rejoice and be glad in it. Accept our God-given grace, and enjoy.

Prayer for Today: Dear Heavenly Father, We are blessed with your grace. We pray to keep that thought in perspective as we work through our society's confusion. Amen

Always Be Joyful

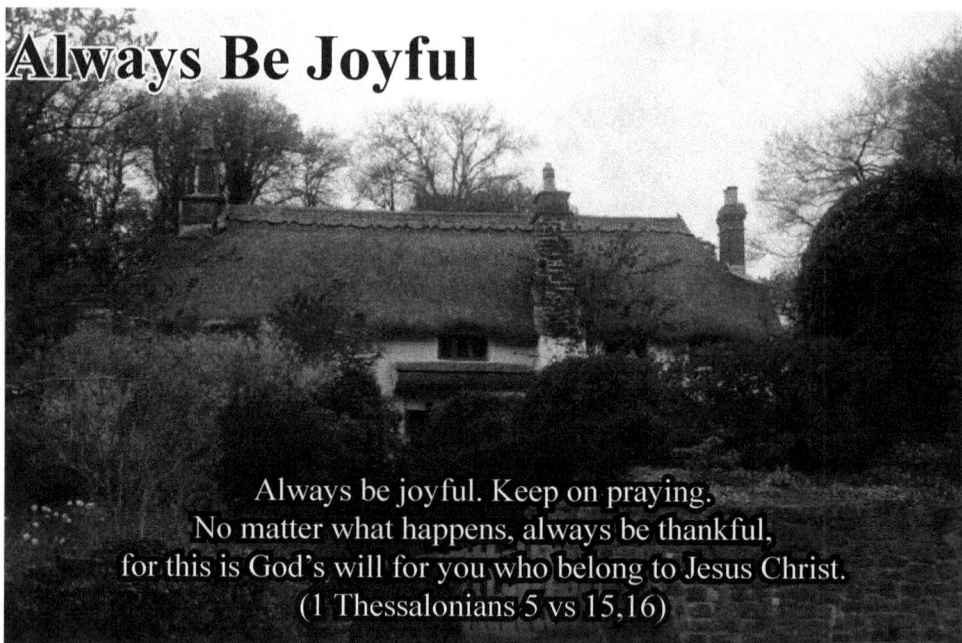

Always be joyful. Keep on praying.
No matter what happens, always be thankful,
for this is God's will for you who belong to Jesus Christ.
(1 Thessalonians 5 vs 15,16)

Writing during a summer sunrise is cool and clear, and the view from our balcony is beautiful and serene. There is no difficulty being joyful and praying. It is a great moment, but.

This month has been a challenge in our world- Racial and financial inequities are troublesome, the pandemic and its variants seem to be accelerating, and severe weather was rampant last evening. But, today is the first day of the rest of our lives, and we need to rejoice in it.

Out of adversity comes greatness. Today, hundreds of beautiful people volunteer to help in the cities that lost buildings in riots; more are collecting and distributing food for the unemployed due to the pandemic; many are simply praying for love to prevail and bring joy.

In summary, life is not always great, and it is sometimes difficult to "Always be joyful," but we can always "Keep on praying."

Bless you, all.

Thought for Today: Let's find a way to enjoy life despite the challenges and recognize the challenges that will strengthen us. The Lord will see us through.

Prayer for Today: Dear Lord, today we thank you for the joy in our lives and the ability to sustain it in hard times through prayer. Amen

July 27 Cockington Village
Devon, Uk

Marriage 50th

A wife of noble character who can find?
She is worth far more than rubies.
Her husband has full confidence in her
and lacks nothing of value.
(Proverbs 31 vs 10,11)

On July 28th, 2018, June and I celebrated our 50th wedding anniversary. We were married on her 30th birthday. She has been a blessing to me, and I often refer to her as the light at the end of my tunnel. She helped escort me from my dark period of the 1960s into something better- that seems to be still growing. Fifty years is a long time, and it was not all romance and happy times. There was alcohol treatment, recovery, career moves, stress, the challenges of raising four children, and just living with Bob, who does not always make sense.

I often discuss the many benefits of a good marriage: the great mutual support, the care when illness arrives, and the joint celebrations of the many events that occur. Yes, marriage is truly an extraordinary institution when things are well and blessed by God.

Thought for Today: Let's keep it simple and enjoy our significant other and those others around us.

Prayer for Today: Heavenly Father, today we give thanks for the people that you have placed close to us in our lives. We pray that as this week progresses, we can share our love with friends, family, and others we meet. Amen

Lechlade on Thames
Gloucesteshire, UK

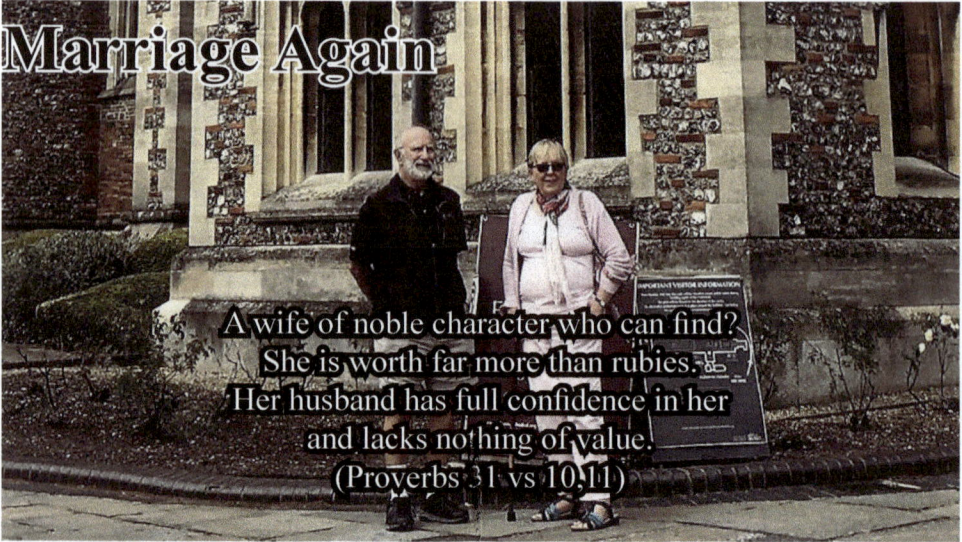

Marriage Again

A wife of noble character who can find?
She is worth far more than rubies.
Her husband has full confidence in her
and lacks nothing of value.
(Proverbs 31 vs 10,11)

Marriage is one of the world's most challenging jobs. Let me quote from The Mystery of Marriage by Mike Mason.

"Marriage, even under the best of circumstances, is a crisis; one of the major crises of life. It is a dangerous thing not to be aware of this. Whether it turns out to be a healthy, challenging, and constructive crisis or a disastrous nightmare depends largely upon how willing the partners are to be changed, how malleable they are."

"Crises" seems a bit extreme to me. Still, undoubtedly, marriage is an excellent opportunity for the fulfillment of life, and it certainly is not without its opportunities for either success or failure. A marriage blessed by God, where the partners have allowed God's love to grow in their relationship, is one of the world's greatest experiences.

Thought for Today: We face many distractions in our daily lives; work, busy schedules, pandemics, war, and financial issues are some. This week let us look at our primary relationships and focus introspectively, up close. Let us understand that when things are fine in our relationships, the outside problems seem less intense; focus on our loves.

Prayer for Today: Heavenly Father, today we thank the people you have placed close to us in our lives. We pray that we can share our love with friends, family, and others we meet as this week progresses. men Amen

July 29

St. Albans Cathedral
St. Albans. Hertfordshire

Who's Macro

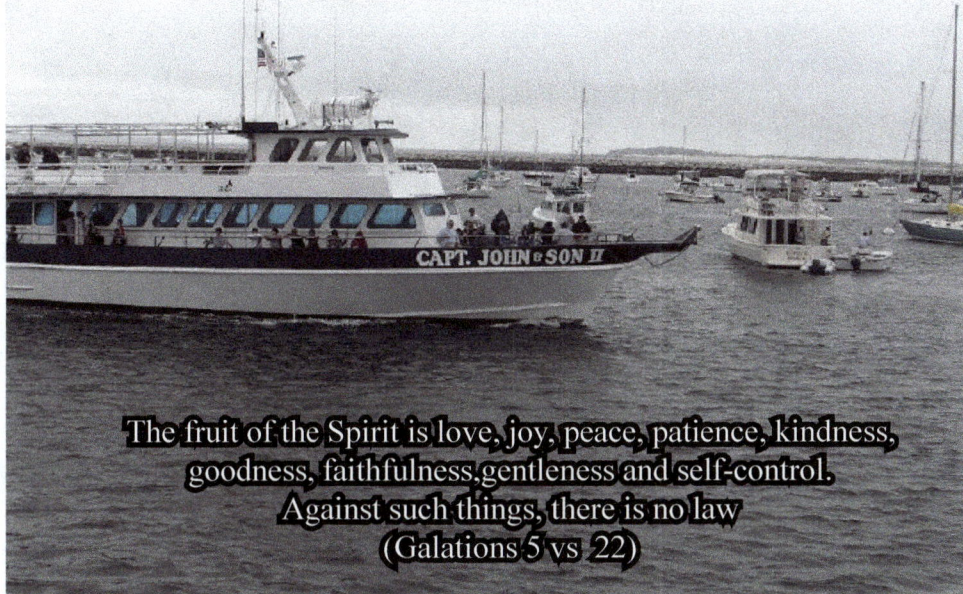

The fruit of the Spirit is love, joy, peace, patience, kindness, goodness, faithfulness, gentleness and self-control. Against such things, there is no law
(Galations 5 vs 22)

Please do not take this as a political piece, but my life is out of control. Not the daily issues, but in computer terms, it seems my Macro needs resetting. Where is the land of milk and honey, the golden years, or to live happily ever after? We are trained to look for that in all those books our mom read when we were growing up.

Well, another old-time expression is "life begins at 40". It may not seem like that as you approach that milestone, but looking back at over eighty, it seems that way. Believe it or not, the period age fifty through seventy are most often the best years of our lives; enjoy them. It is all a matter of perspective.

Thought for Today: We need to focus on our daily lives for survival. With that said, today, let's do what we need to do to survive but keep Paul's letters and the word of our Lord in our daily lives. It will fit in if we let it.

Prayer for Today: Dear Lord, today we pray for our world and country. We pray we can find a way back to Jesus's word and Paul's Macro. Amen

Plymouth Harbor
Plymouth, Massachusetts   **July 30**   **Page 221**

Macro Issues

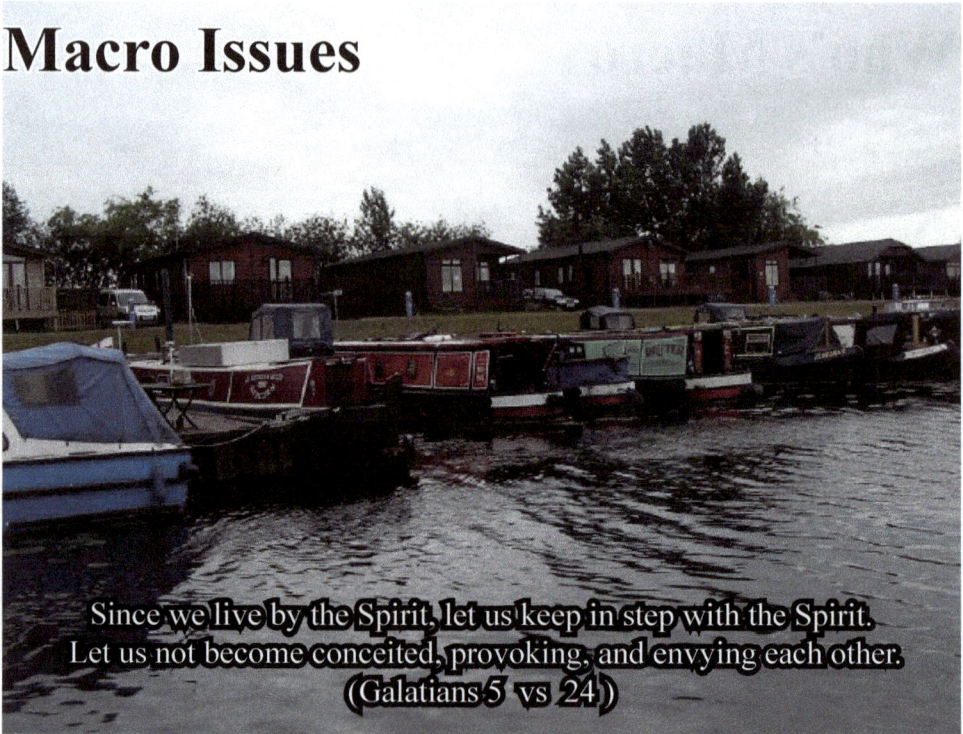

Since we live by the Spirit, let us keep in step with the Spirit.
Let us not become conceited, provoking, and envying each other.
(Galatians 5 vs 24)

My macro issues are with the new world economy and what is happening worldwide. It is like "we the people" do not get our say in the issues. We all want to have income, end war, reduce taxes, and live happily ever after. That is the challenge.

Over the years, politics around the world changed things. The new world economy seems more autocratic and has less supply and demand. The new normal created by illness and war has altered lifestyles. The words of the Lord have not changed. The solution is to focus on the correct Macro, the spirit of our Christian Faith, as opposed to the Government macro. Saint Paul wrote the real Macro.

Thought for Today: Let's focus on the message and do what we knowhow.
Prayer for Today: Dear Lord, we pray for our world and country; that we can find a way back to Jesus's word and Paul's Macro.
Amen

July 31 Boat Camp, River Nene
Peterborough, Cambridgeshire, UK

August

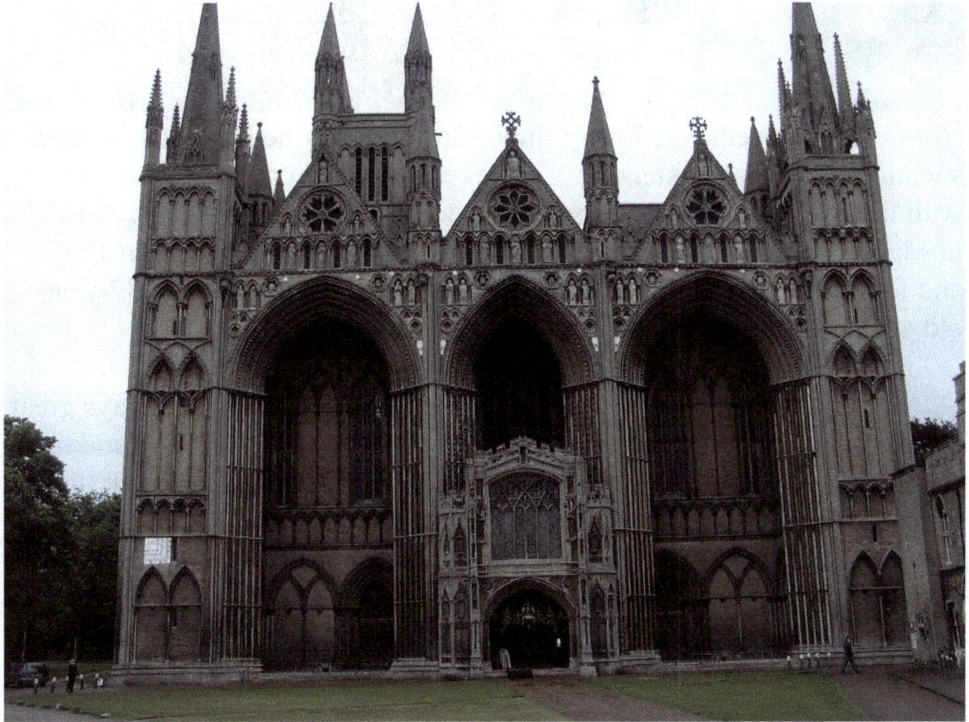

Peterborough Cathedral

Peterborough Cathedral is one of the finest Norman cathedrals in England. Founded as a monastic community in 654 AD, it became one of the most significant medieval abbeys in the country It is the burial place of Catherine of Aragone and Mary Queen of Scots. (Moved to Westminster Abby in 1612)

Vacation Time

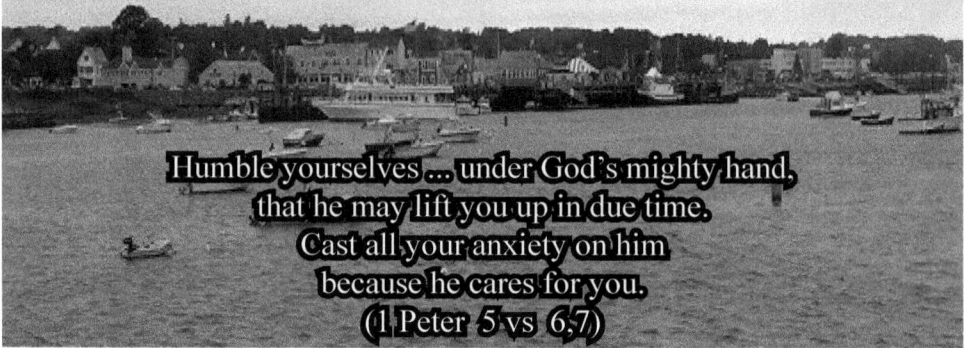

> Humble yourselves ... under God's mighty hand,
> that he may lift you up in due time.
> Cast all your anxiety on him
> because he cares for you.
> (1 Peter 5 vs 6,7)

Grand events are lovely. June and I just returned from a two-week vacation that was an extended grand event. We spent the first weekend with family in New Hampshire; we visited friends from the class of 1957 in Maine, then on to lunch with a whole group of classmates from 1957, and followed that up with a visit with my 94-year-old mom and 87-year-old aunt.

We enjoyed hearing their memories and laughter. It is always great to listen to them and share the good times. Indeed, all of us had good times and bad to talk about, but the focus was on the joys and pleasure of the past, and there were smiles all around. Good times were the focus. I am sure that there was anxiety amongst us. Some had experienced cancer scares, some lost loved ones, and certainly, we are battling the aging process with the age group from 70 to 94. We cast our anxieties aside and let joy and love abound.

Moments like this are a gift from God, and we need to focus on them.

Thought for Today: Let us focus on casting away our angst and turning our lives over to the Lord while focusing on the older generation. Reach out to them with love and share the good times.

Prayer for Today: Heavenly Father, we pray for ourselves, friends, and loved ones. Many are ill and experiencing fear, uncertainty, loneliness, or hurt. We pray that we may help be the conduit that strengthens their faith and eases their anxieties. We pray for a way to do your will in this way. Amen

The Harbor (cropped)

Forever

Enter his gates with thanksgiving
and his courts with praise;
give thanks to him and praise his name.
For the LORD is good, and his love endures forever;
his faithfulness continues through all generations.
(Psalm 100 vs. 4, 5)

In Saugus, Massachusetts, in the forties and fifties, each school day started with saluting the flag, reading the 100th Psalm, followed by the Lord's Prayer. It was a great reminder of who we were and what America was and represented. I believe that hearing them repeated so often was the best training for a life they could have passed on to us.

Many events, dinners, award ceremonies, and high school sports started with a prayer, to name a few. The prayer leaders rotated by faith, but the message was always clear, we are one people.

The overall theme of Psalm 100 is Joy through faith. Try making a simple comparison in your mind. Think about those who are angry, having trouble with stress, etc. Identify and pray for them.

Thought for Today: Today, let us stay focused on being joyful Christians.

Prayer for Today: Dear Lord, today we give thanks for the grace guaranteed us by Jesus when he died on the cross. We give thanks for his grace and the joyous lives that we lead. Amen

The Harbor
Plymouth, Mass   **August 2**   **Page 225**

Giving Back

Treat others as you want them to treat you...
Never criticize or condemn, or it will all come back to you.
(Luke 6 vs 31)

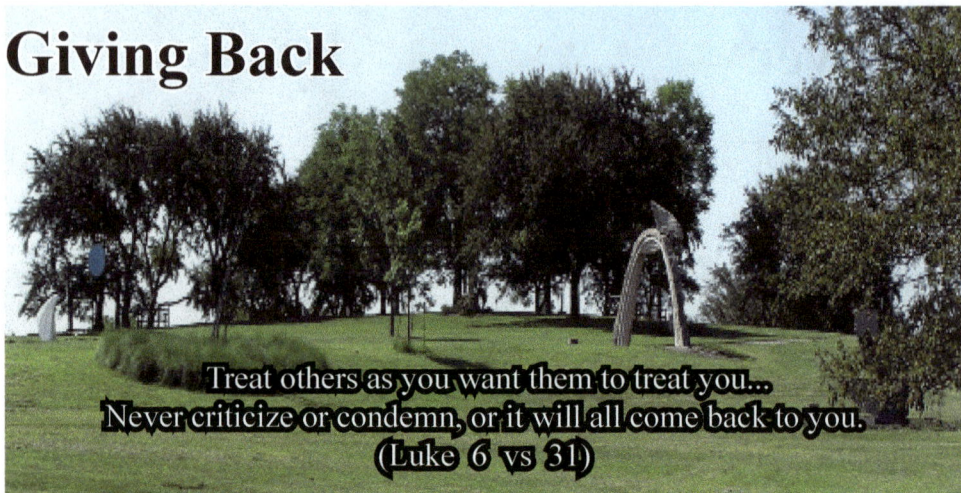

Every day as people and Christians, we are giving. In the workplace, in family, or driving alone, we participate and give to those around us. What we give overwhelmingly affects our lives, society, and environment.

Let's look at where being positive is the easiest; love is the strongest in the family. Indeed, we have always been positive, loving, and "really cool" within our families. Most of us do not meet that standard. You better take a reality check and ensure your other family members see it the same if you think that.

Sometimes we are tired, and our career is not working well; we anger when we should stop and meditate. Perfection is our goal, perhaps not our reality. When we are down, it is essential to remember that we are the children of God, and we have His support in both the good and testing times. He wants us to work with Him to bring peace and good while sharing His love with others. Sharing His love instead of "our frustrations" with others is a lofty goal.

Thought for Today: When we feel stressed out today, let us focus on not bringing it home. It is OK to ask the family for support during stressful times, but unfair and destructive to pass our stresses on to them.

Prayer for Today: Heavenly Father, we are truly blessed through your love. We pray we can reach out to you during tough times and feel and share that love. Amen.

Sculpture Garden

August 3 Minnesota Landscape Arboretum

Priorities

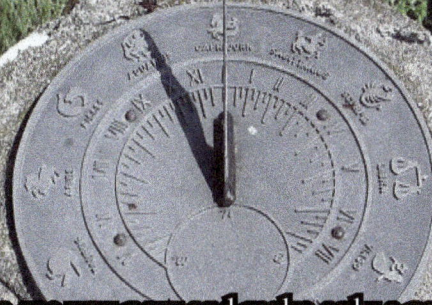

"I do not want to see you now and make only a passing visit;
I hope to spend some time with you if the Lord permits."
(1 Corinthians 16 vs 7)

His accomplishments seem incredible when reading about Paul's work for the Lord. It is hard to understand how it all happened. Today's letter hints that his life had similarities to ours. He was not without stress, and he had to set priorities. He could have said, "I am too busy right now to …, I will get to you later." We hear that a lot today. Here are some questions for us that are over fifty:

Did you carry a calendar when you were twelve?

Were there sports, scouts, or other activities on Wednesday or Sunday evening?

Did anyone bring a phone to the dinner table or a meeting?

Once upon a time, Wednesday and Sunday nights were reserved for Church, and the kids did not carry calendars. Things have changed. Today is the era of cell phones functioning as personal assistants. High school kids take college classes, and college students help in high school. They are excellent training for the future, teaching them to make choices and set priorities.

When reading bible stories, it is essential to recognize that the issues are different from now but are also very similar. Disciples were expected to support the Church and spread the word. Paul recognized his responsibilities and set his priorities for the Lord. We have similar responsibilities and need to keep our discipleship high on our priority list.

Thought for Today: Let's think about where we can work for God. He will present opportunities if we are willing and alert.

Prayer for Today: Dear Lord and Father, thank you for your many gifts and the opportunity help others in your name. Amen

Sun Dial

Minnesota Landscape Arboretum **August 4** Page 227

We

Two are better than one,
because they have a good return for their work:
If one falls, his friend can help him up.
But pity the man who falls and has no one to help him up.
(Ecclesiastis 4 vs 10)

When I write, I try to avoid using the same words repeatedly. The term "we" is used 14 times for the next two days. It is a good word.

Those who have known me a while have heard me say, "Two people working together can do four times as much as the best of two could do alone." It seemed that way, and I always had a partner or best friend. It is something that I learned from experience- back in my teens.

In my early years, it was a cousin who lived next door. We were inseparable; we fished, canoed, played ball, and had our first jobs together. When we fished, they would seem to follow my lure and bite on his. I always got to take the photo. Playing ball, he pitched, and I caught. We played every day and became very good at it. It would be hard to do that alone.

We took a job at Howard Johnson's as counter-men, walked to work together, and dealt with the public side by side. We started on July 4th,1955- the busiest night of the year. Walking home at 2 am, the police stopped and gave us a ride. They picked us up a lot and used to look for us. That was the only reason we were ever in a squad car.

We were a team, accomplished, and learned more together than we could have.

Thought for the Day: Today, let's remember our partners when we were young and learning; think about that special relationship.

Prayer for Today: Heavenly Father, we thank our life partners you sent us, who have helped us grow and become who we are. Amen

August 5

Parkers Lake
Plymouth, Minnesota

We Again

If one falls, his friend can help him up.
But pity the man who falls and has no one to help him up.
(Ecclesiastis 4 vs 10)

A great example of teamwork can be a married or significant other relationship. June married me when I was a single parent- that took courage. June saw something that she wanted, which may have been the challenge. She married a single parent with two small girls on her thirtieth birthday. She went from carefree and single to a mother of four in three short years. We worked hard together to figure out how to survive. We still do work as a team and are proud of our successes. Things did not always work well, but we are proud of our efforts even when they failed. It has been a good ride.

Returning to my cousin from yesterday, we went separate ways for fifty years, and in 2009, we reacquainted ourselves at several family functions. He is married to a fine lady whose name is June. We have established a new relationship and recently visited him at his cottage in New Hampshire. Guess what? He needed to move 6 yards of sand, and we are still a good team.

Thought for Today: Let's think about our life partners and thank the Lord for them. There are times in our lives when we do not have a partner and other times when it is hard to identify one. We must remember our ultimate partner, who is with us always and will never let us down. That partner is God.

Prayer for Today: Dear Lord, we thank all who have helped us in our lives; those we know and those we do not know. We also recognize your contribution to our lives and thank you for that. We pray that we can do your will by helping others as others have helped me. Amen

Cedar Lake
Minneapolis, Minnesota

Winning

Praise be to the God and Father of our Lord Jesus Christ,
the Father of compassion and the God of all comfort,
who comforts us in all our troubles, so
that we can comfort those in any trouble
with the comfort we have received from God.
(2 Corinthians) 1 vs 3,4)

Who in our lives are the winners? Some say the one with the most toys wins. That is a materialistic one-liner that gives me goosebumps. However, in our society today, we pursue "things" instead of happiness and peace. So who are the real winners, and how do they win?

God placed us here to be his stewards, with our priority to be sharing the gifts we received from Him with others. That seems to be a very tall order. However, we always feel great when we have reached out and helped a friend or stranger.

God gives us resources in many different forms. We have money that we earn and the knowledge that we have learned. We graciously share these things with our families and children, making us feel good. Many people also reach out beyond their family units and share. There are ways to share and sow the seeds God has given us to plant, and we are real winners when we share our gifts.

Thought for Today: Let us look for an opportunity to help someone, perhaps someone who is sick, hurting, or lonely. If we fail in finding someone, let's share some extra with our Church. Sharing a bit will make us feel better.

Prayer for Today: Heavenly Father, we live in a troubled world. Civil unrest, road rage, families in strife, and other tragic incidences. Today we pray for an opportunity to help and share with someone and demonstrate your Grace through our actions. Amen.

Importance

I saw that there is nothing better than that all should enjoy their work, for that is their lot; who can bring them to see what will be after them?
(Ecclesiastes 3 vs 22)

A job can provide great satisfaction. As Christians, we must guard against the temptation to live for our careers instead of God. Our rlationship with the Lord and the people around us will outlast our jobs.

Luke 12 vs 15 speaks to us about greed and our attitude toward possessions: "Take care! Be on guard against all kinds of greed, for one's life does not consist in the abundance of possessions." Christ tells us to remember what is crucial as we approach our work and the people we encounter daily.

We will no longer have a job at some point in our lives. That does not mean we will not have a career. There will be service to humanity, family, friends, and the Lord. It is not that lifestyle is not important because it is. However, a lifestyle can be empty and unrewarding without good health and strong faith.

Thought for Today: Today, let us make every part of our lives an arena for deepening our faithfulness to God. and our fellow man.

Prayer for Today: Dear Lord and Father, please help me have a healthy attitude toward my daily activities and relationships. Please show me how to put money and possessions aside and people upfront. Amen

Joy and Peace

May the God of hope fill you with all joy and peace
as you trust in him,
so that you may overflow with hope
by the power of the Holy Spirit.
(Romans 15 vs 13)

We Christians often seem celebration conscious. Birthdays, anniversaries, and holidays trigger family gatherings and create great memories in our private lives. Easter, Christmas, Pentecost, rally day, etc., are grand celebrations holding our church families together.

The memorial service celebrating one's life is one of joy, hope, and the power of the holy spirit, a time when the faults, idiosyncrasies, and character defects are forgotten. The end-of-life experience brings grief and sadness and is often a time of depression for close loved ones.

We often encounter people experiencing or expecting end-of-life events in their families. We need to pray for them, pray that the Lord will help them celebrate the lives of their loved ones, and they find joy and peace as they move forward in their grief.

Thought for Today: This is the day that the Lord has made. Let us rejoice. We will experience ups and downs, but with the hope of God in our hearts, the downs can be short, the ups can be high, and a day of joy. It is our choice.

Prayer for Today: Dear Lord and Father, we live amongst the wonders of your creation. We have four seasons, mountains, oceans, and the grandeur of creation. Today we thank you for everything and the beautiful lives we live through you.
Amen

August 9 Great Grebe, River Nene
Cambridgeshire, UK

Values

I saw that there is nothing better
then that all should enjoy their work,
for that is their lot;
who can bring them to see what will be after them?
(Ecclesiastes 3 vs 22)

Several years ago, we attended the birthday party of a businessman and mentor of mine. There was a roast, and nearly every speaker's underlying theme had little to do with money. The recipient was undoubtedly focused on money during business hours but was gracious and generous with his outside activities.

Outside of business, he demonstrated tireless generosity. The general discussions involved how many young people he helped along with their careers. Among the guests were former interns, people from help organizations specializing in helping people who had lost their jobs, and representatives from schools where he had helped out with programs and placements.

There is room in business for solid Christian values. We need to be profitable to survive, which requires good financial practices. However, we owe it to ourselves to keep Christian values in all areas of our lives and make every attempt to create win-win situations. Jesus' words in Luke 12 vs.15 speak to us about greed. "Take care! Be on guard against all kinds of greed, for one's life does not consist in the abundance of possessions." Christ tells us to remember what is important as we approach our work and the people we encounter each day. We need to share and demonstrate our values every day.

Thought for Today: As Christians, we need to keep our principles in focus. We need to keep our positive attitudes and demonstrate them daily.

Prayer for Today: Dear Lord, we thank you for the principles and ethics we have learned at Jesus's knee. Today we pray that we may keep them in focus and apply them in all situations. Amen

Nesting Swan, River Nene
Cambridgeshire, UK

Helping Others

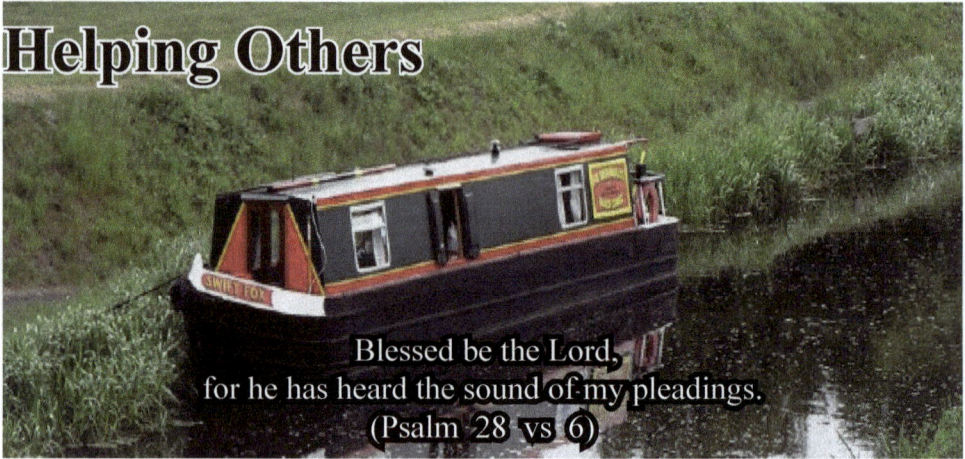

Blessed be the Lord,
for he has heard the sound of my pleadings.
(Psalm 28 vs 6)

Last year a friend called after a twenty-year lapse. June would say he was "down on his uppers." (I think that is English for on the rocks.). He was broke, getting divorced, and having a "nobody likes me, everybody hates me, I'm going to eat some worms..." kind of day. He was suicidal.

These kinds of calls are never convenient. They often trigger the question in my mind, "Why me, Lord?". The first conversation lasted around an hour and finished with my refusal to visit him (a good rule to follow) but to call him back. I also committed to praying for him if he would pray with me.

We have been talking regularly since, and he is doing better.

We often need another set of ears to hear our problems. Sometimes the listener can be a friend, but we also have another wiser, more faithful listener- God.

In Psalm 28, David cries out for help. Like David, when we express our feelings to God, we always find a patient and willing listener. At the end of the Psalm, David demonstrates trust and confidence in God.

Thought for Today: Let's take that call, pray that someone asks for our help and that we may contribute to their success or recovery.

Prayer for Today: Dear Lord, we ask you to hear our prayers and pleadings. We pray for the faith to let go of our stresses and have confidence in your solutions rather than our own.
Amen

August 11

Narrow Boat, River Nene
Cambridgeshire, UK

Rewards of Faith

"You reward everyone according to what they have done."
(Psalm 62 vs. 12)

We live a long time, and often, the road is bumpy. The statistics on our world economy indicate some long-term economic decline. Economic difficulties always hurt the lower third of the income range first and hardest. Globally, decisions and priorities are changing. We need to deal with changes.

My thoughts are not about policy, elections, or the economy. They are about prayer and priorities. First, we must pray for the lower third of our global socio-economic world. Food in the US is expensive but is scarce and unaffordable in many nations. More people will be starving around the world next year than this year. We need to pray for those that are suffering from hunger.

When times get tough, we need to stick with our faith and beliefs as followers of Christ. Pray for our neighbors and those less fortunate and give more of ourselves. Follow the basic principles of our faith. The Psalmist states that we will not be disappointed- we need to believe. It is now that we all need to gather our resources to help. We need to believe that the Lord will be there for us, and we need to be there for Him.

"
I am the LORD your God,who brought you up out of Egypt.
Open wide your mouth, and I will fill it.
(Psalm 71 vs 14)

Thought for Today: Let's think about trusting the Lord to be there when we need Him. Some on this email list need help, and some can help. Let us all do what we can in the name of the Lord.

Prayer for Today: Father, we pray for the resources to relieve hunger where we live and worldwide. Amen

Railroad Bridge, River Nene
Cambridgeshire, UK

August 12

The Lord's Will

Photo by
Jackie Collins

Be very careful, then, how you live—
not as unwise but as wise,
making the most of every opportunity, because the days are evil.
Therefore do not be foolish, but understand what the Lord's will is.
(Ephesians 5 vs 14)

In life, there are temptations. Opportunities to take more than we know we deserve, the relentless pursuit of things or money. Most of the World thinks that is the American way of life. After all, that is what makes our economy run.

A classic example is the negotiations between young athletes and the drafted team. Often, these people grapple over extra millions, and the relationship and respect between those involved are permanently damaged.

One of my favorite people, Harvey McKay, wrote about this subject in his weekly article. He pointed out that good negotiations were not opportunistic but "win-win." The temptation to go for it all leads to ultimate failure because the team spirit is damaged.

Harvey is a businessman, tennis player, marathon runner, and author. He is a winner in all his endeavors and has that burning desire for excellence. Harvey built his life around playing by the rules and constructing a win-win lifestyle. I do not know Harvey well enough to know his spirituality, but he does God's work very well from my casual observation.

Thought for today: Let's search out the temptations in our lives. Let us recognize them for what they are and follow good Christian ethics in our decisions. Everyone can win.

Prayer for today: Heavenly Father, our World seems full of ungodly events. Kidnappings, suicide bombers, illness, and many others cause us to focus on the negative. This week, please help us maintain our focus on the good things in our lives and give us the will to spread goodness. Amen

Straight to Our Heart

In the wilderness prepare the way for the LORD,
make straight in the desert a highway for our God.
(Isaiah 40 vs 3)

When driving in the UK, where the roads are windy and twisty, occasionally we come to a long straight road that goes on for miles. My wife, a Brit, explained that those are ancient Roman roads laid out 2000 years ago. I found that impressive.

In ancient times leaders built roads for their armies to move. They are long and straight and efficient so that they can move quickly. The valleys are filled by pushing the tops of the hills. They facilitated the need. There are very few straight roads in New England where I grew up. They paved the cow paths and horse trails that tended to follow the river beds. It is challenging for strangers to find their way.

Today's message is that we need to be sure of our road to the lord; it needs to be straight. There needs to be a straight connection between God and our hearts. We need to allow the simplest two-way travel possible in our complex world, straight to our hearts.

Thought for Today: Today, let's think about where our road takes us; where are we going. Perhaps we can take a few bends out and travel straight.

Prayer for the Day: Heavenly Father, we live in a complex world, are surrounded by too much activity, and are overcommitted. Today we thank you for being with us and pray that we may keep our hearts open to you and stay on a straight and holy path. Amen

Lieutenant Island
Wellfleet, Massachusetts

August 14

Acceptance and Happiness

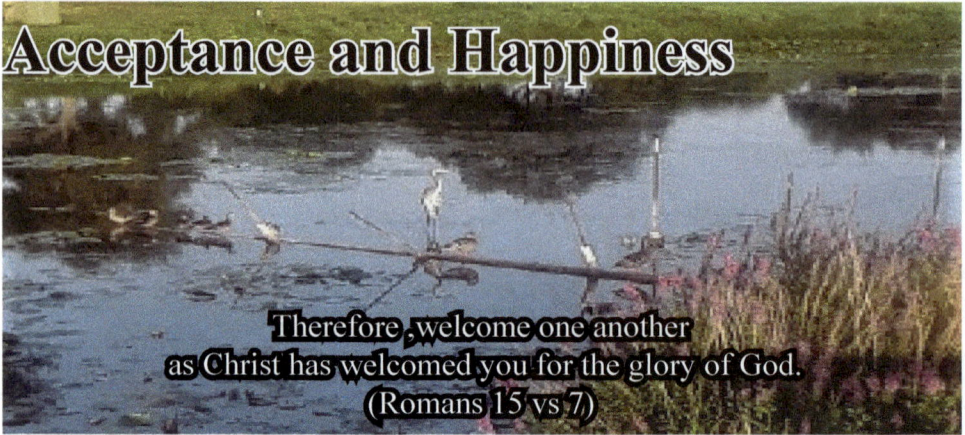

Therefore, welcome one another
as Christ has welcomed you for the glory of God.
(Romans 15 vs 7)

We are often happiest when surrounded by family and people we love and demonstrate that love in demonstrative ways. On a recent vacation, we attended a family reunion of around thirty people aged two to ninety. It was a wonderful experience, full of hugs and compliments. Grace and love were everywhere.

At other times we were in crowded tourist areas and were uptight, not as openly caring. We made ourselves uncomfortable. The situation became somewhat competitive; service lines competing for the best view of the fireworks, the best seat on the beach, etc. During these times, I suggest the difference is a choice that we made; a choice to feel different.

It is socially acceptable to be more cautious when in public. However, being reserved in our behavior does not mean we need to feel uncomfortable. We do not need to lose sight of ourselves and our caring nature. We can be loving, considerate, and demonstrate God's will in a crowd. We will have a better time and be happier and less stressed when we do.

Thought for Today: We all will make choices this week. We will choose to be angry, stressed, or frustrated by other people's actions and social situations. As Christians, we can select prayer and meditation to turn the stressful issues over to God and be happier. This week let us focus on being a happier person through prayer.

Prayer for Today: Heavenly Father, we have often failed to use your tools. We know better, but in our daily lives, we forget your lessons. Today we pray that we may use meditation and prayer when we become stressed, fearful, or angry. We pray that we can use your tool kit to improve our lives and the lives of those surrounding us. Amen

August 15 Brookview Golf Course
Golden Valley. Minnesota

God's Code Of Ethics

May integrity and uprightness protect me,
because my hope, LORD, is in you.
(Psalm 25 vs 21)

A classic error of human ways is that we tend to hear what we want, which defines miscommunication. Thus, expectations will not be met, and disappointment will occur. Often there is a disagreement after the fact. This even happens with written contracts in business because people do not read the same meaning into the words. Lawyers get wealthy on this.

In a profit-driven economy, the focus often becomes dollars and return on investment. Thus a win-lose mentality can develop. That is not how God planned the world. Experience shows that the consideration of others always creates a win-win in our society and works best.

In our own lives, we need to have a clear conscience. ".... My (our) steps have held to your paths; my (our) feet have not slipped." We must meet God's code of ethics in all dealings to sleep at night. We must keep that in mind and God in our operating style. People that follow the Lord's principles are the real winners in life.

Thought for Today: Tomorrow will be a great day. We will be cooperative rather than competitive and seek win-win situations in our dealings with others.

Prayer for the Today: Heavenly Father, we pray for a good life and that we may contribute to the goodness in the lives of others. We are often confused by the negativity and violence in our society and feel incapable of helping. Today, we pray that we can see a way to contribute more of ourselves and share your love with others. Amen

Pleasant Temptations

> Blessed is the man that endures temptation, for when he is tried, he shall receive the crown of life, which the Lord has promised to those that love Him.
> (James 1 vs 12)

In the words of Dr. Norman Vincent Peale," Temptation is the urge to do or say something wrong, something contrary to the will of God and the law of Christ. Temptation often comes in pleasant and seductive form, and the mind always attempts to rationalize it to make it seem right." We face it every day.

We can choose the right or wrong path throughout our lives, the opportunistic or the Godly way. None of us has always chosen the right path that follows the law of Christ. We have all crossed that line and felt remorse, guilt, or doubt. Yes, admit it; you are not quite perfect.

It is common for us to hold on to the memories of when we slipped and took temptation. Often this sorrowful thinking leads to a low self-image or guilt that affects our lives. Working with others for the last 25 years, June and I have seen people turn their lives around by accepting the concept of "spiritual growth" and making amends to those they have harmed.

We are not perfect, but when we grow spiritually, we feel good about ourselves and turn down the temptations that confront us daily. The secret of success is spiritual growth through prayer and daily meditation.

Thought for Today: In our personal lives, there are temptations; ways to cheat, subtle dishonesty, procrastination, lust, etc. We can choose to follow the Lord's commandments. Let us note our wise decisions and thank the spirituality and maturity that gets us through the week.

Prayer for Today: Heavenly Father, wars and terrorism are a problem. We have many opportunities to help and pray we may bring peace and love to replace the fear and hate in our world. Amen.

August 17

Minneapolis Sky Line
from Lake Harriet

Speak The Word

In the same way, let your light shine before men, that they may see your good deeds and praise your Father in heaven.
(Matthew 5 vs 16)

Few of us flaunt our Christian beliefs in business and life in general. Few of us are willing to stand on a corner or go to a podium and speak the word. Rarely do we speak out that our goals are to follow Jesus's Laws. In business today, the human resources rules generally state that religion is a taboo subject in the office. We certainly would not want to make a person of a different faith "uncomfortable in their workplace."

Several years ago, I started wearing a gold lapel pin that is two feet. They represent Christ's feet from "Footprints in the Sand" and lead to a discussion of faith. I have made many fine acquaintances this way. We do not stand on a soapbox, but we want to share our faith and need to open the door to the discussion.

The feet in my lapel are my light for everyone to see. Yes, even as a salesman, I am reluctant to stand on the corner and speak the word until I have screened the audience. We Christians are an interesting group.

Thought for Today: Today, let us all know that we are the light. Yes, people see what we do and copy our example. We can choose to have a positive or negative influence on our surroundings. Let all of us recognize our position and be a positive force following the laws of Christ.

Prayer for Today: Dear Lord. Today we pray for the opportunity to share our faith someone who needs to hear the story. Amen

St. Anthony Falls on The Mississippi
Minneapolis, Minnesota   **August 18**   Page 241

Do It

Photo buy
Stephanie Symmes

MOUNT WASHINGTON STATE PARK
CRAWFORD PATH
AT THIS POINT THE GEOGRAPHICAL SUMMIT
OF MOUNT WASHINGTON, ELEVATION 6288'
THE CRAWFORD PATH TERMINATES. THIS PATH,
THE OLDEST MOUNTAIN HIKING TRAIL IN

Never tire of doing what is right.
(1 Thessalonians 3 vs 13)

One of my Pickeringisms is that there are two types of people: givers and takers. That is undoubtedly a gross oversimplification used to describe humanity originating from sales and business training and has overflowed into my teachings on living.

Many want to win at any cost; they think they are climbing the corporate ladder rather than building a support pyramid. In the pyramid, you build a base, wide and tall, as you move forward and up. You step on the rungs as you climb, and often the ladder breaks.

In Christian life, there are also givers and takers. We are all people in need, and that need level is relative. Our requirements vary from year to year, decade to decade. When June and I raised four children, we were active in our Christian family. However, we often needed love and support from our peers. There were times when we took a bit more than we gave, emotionally and financially.

Today, we are in the elder mode; we have more time and cash; we give more than we take. That gives us a much warmer and more rewarding feeling. Both being a taker and a giver in the Christian sense is OK. If there were no people in need, there would not be anyone to give to, which would be a conundrum.

Paul's message never says tire of doing what is right. When you are doing what is right, you will not get tired. OOPS- is that a Pickeringism?

Bless you, all, for being my friends.

Thought for Today: Let us live as good Christians. Recognize that we have made the giver feel good if we need support. If we are givers, let us freely give where needed and graciously accept support.

Prayer for Today: Dear Lord, we pray for those in need. Whether the need is great or small, physical or emotional, we pray that we recognize it and give them support in your name. Amen

One Loving God

Photo buy Stephanie Symmes

In this way, love is made complete among us so that we will have confidence on the day of judgment, because in this world, we are like him.
(1 John 4 vs 16, 17)

Our world changed in 2020 and on 9/11/2001. Both impacted our society and affected church attendance. The nine-eleven attacks changed how American citizens viewed the world; they had increased doubts and fears. Church service attendance increased, but not for long. Per Quora, "Unequivocally, yes. (Attendance increased). However, this attendance change was short-lived."

In 2020, the pandemic emptied Church buildings, and the church moved elsewhere; to Zoom, the street, but many turned to their faith at home. Church online became a norm, along with casual attire and coffee. Progressive churches left the broadcasts in place, and home services are still common today and probable will be forever. That said, declining attendance returned, and we are back on the curve (slide).

We, the USA, had embarrassing COVID 19 numbers. Something like four percent of the world's population and twenty percent of the world's cases. Our callous and make our own rules population created an embarrassing situation. We must pray about that and attempt to demonstrate a more Godly lifestyle.

Gospel 1 John 4 vs 16 states, "Whoever lives in love lives in God, and God in him." It does not specify any qualification other than a Love of God.

Thought for Today: Let's think about what happened in 2020 and focus on the golden rule.

Prayer for Today: Heavenly Father, we are trying to live our lives showing love and compassion by following Jesus's laws. We get confused about hate in the world and neighborhoods around us. We pray for the ability to effect negative forces in loving and caring ways. Amen

Birthday Special

Each year on my birthday, I give thanks for something learned as a YMCA brat in my youth. The symbol for the Y is a triangle, and each side has a meaning, "spirit, mind, and body." Each year I give thanks for my role as a father, son, and place in society. But let's talk a bit about what it takes to be in a good place with ourselves. It is being selfish, yes, being selfish in pursuit of a healthy self: mentally, physically, and spiritually. In each of our lives, we must fit into niches in society; a family, a workplace, and a social setting. We fit best when the three sides of our triangle are in a healthy balance.

In all areas of our lives, it is essential to demonstrate the forgiveness and love that comes from spirituality. We need to be physically fit enough to deal with the long days without being fatigued and run down. Also, we need to be mentally sharp when making life decisions. That is a lot to ask of mortals and not an easy task. So be a bit selfish. Take care of yourself so that you may be all that

God wants you to be and be capable of doing His work when the opportunity presents itself to you. Take care of yourself to be all that your family needs you to be. Remember the logo of the YMCA, spirit, mind, and body. Keep fit and enjoy life.

Birthday Thought: Today is the day the Lord has made, a day for me to enjoy. Friends will recognize it, the family will celebrate it, and I will enjoy it. It is a blessing that we all have and a great day to give thanks to the Lord for all of our many blessings.

Birthday Prayer: Heavenly Father, today is a special day, the day that you brought me into your service. Throughout this day, I thank you for all the opportunities you have provided me and the chance to have a healthy relationship with family and friends. Today I will often hear the words "happy birthday." To those words, I say, "Thanks be to God.". Amen

Birthday Party

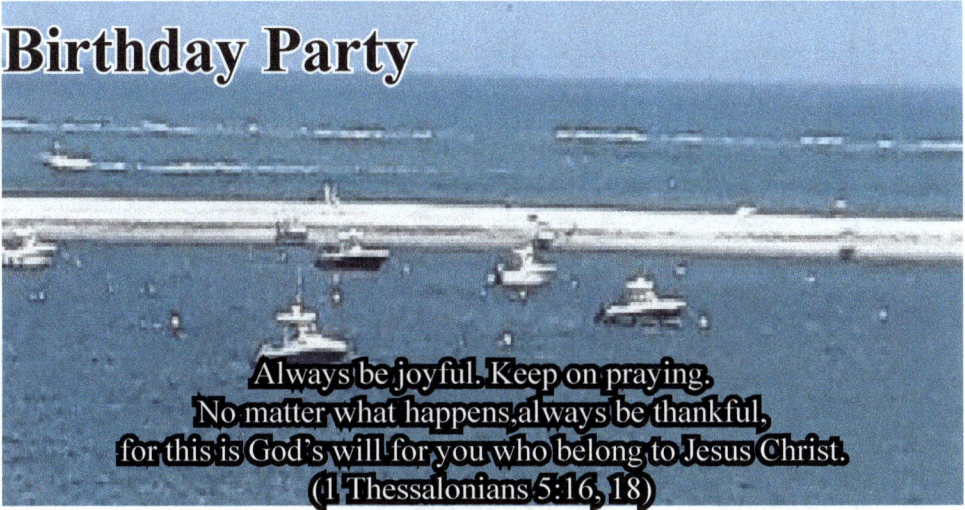

Always be joyful. Keep on praying.
No matter what happens, always be thankful,
for this is God's will for you who belong to Jesus Christ.
(1 Thessalonians 5:16, 18)

As leaders and teachers, we must recognize that those around us often need encouragement. Romans 12 lists one of God's gifts as "encouraging." In the 1950s, parenting seemed critical. Slogans included: walk softly and carry a big stick; I'm taking you out behind the woodshed; switches and wooden spoons were commonplace.

I had two coaches to compare. My football coach was a very successful negative motivator. I left football in my senior year and went to a private school to swim for a great coach. The newspaper published an article quoting the coach saying thet my leaving left a big hole in the program. That was the first positive thing I had ever heard from him.

The swim coach was a positive motivator and sent several swimmers to national championships and Olympics. Our small prep school defeated high-ranking first-year college teams with several future 1960 Olympians. When one of us lost, we were surprised- Coach Al was a positive motivator and teacher that had us believing in ourselves.

Today's teachers use positive reinforcement, and most parents also do. Future generations will benefit significantly from enlightened parenting and teaching. People with the gift of encouragement are blessed, and I pray all of you have it.

Thought for Today: We will all have an opportunity to "encourage" someone. It will be a natural "gift" to some, but it will be a chore to many. Let's recognize where we fit and utilize God's gifts in our lives to make God's world a better place.

Prayer for Today: We pray that we may use ou God given skills and knowledge to encourage as we lead our families and others. Amen.

Helping Hands 1

Praise be to the God and Father of our Lord Jesus Christ, the Father of compassion and the God of all comfort, who comforts us in all our troubles, so that we can comfort those in any trouble with the comfort we have received from God.
(2 Corinthians 1 vs 3-7)

It is an early Saturday morning, and I am guilt-ridden because the world events over the last few years have not affected me as much as they have several of my close friends. That does not make sense, but that is where my feelings are. We need prayers for the people of the world.

Here is my list: Several friends are financially stressed and are losing their homes; three recent widows are adjusting their lives; two elderly couples have given up their homes and moved to assisted living; friends have lost their businesses; our children and grandchildren's future. The list is only partial because everyone's problems and fears would be too much! But what does Paul ask the Corinthians? "…who comforts us in all our troubles?"

All days are not created equal, nor are months or years. However, the constant in our lives is God. He is always with us to assist in new beginnings.

Thought for Today: We choose to look forward or look back each day. Today let us recognize the new opportunities presented to us and be thankful as we work through them.

Prayer for Today: Dear Lord, today is a new beginning. We thank you for all you have let us have and welcome your help as we face the new challenges before us. Amen

Helping Hands 2

*For just as the sufferings of Christ flow over into our lives,
so also through Christ our comfort overflows.
If we are distressed, it is for your comfort and salvation;
if we are comforted, it is for your comfort,
which produces in you patient endurance
of the same sufferings we suffer.
(2 Corinthians 1 vs 5,6)*

Following yesterday, one of the widows, who I do not know very well, is closing on the sale of her house. On the one hand, she is sad about selling the home she and her husband shared; she is excited about a new home closer to her children and grandchildren. As a new beginning, how positive is that!

Another widow had difficulty finding the spiritual support that fit her needs when her husband died three years ago. She shared that she focuses on helping others work through their grief and feeling good about herself. God is with her as she helps others.

In another, a friend went through the loss of a family home and bankruptcy. She is regrouping and building her life. They have put together a new beginning and a life plan that will work. They have their eye on the sky and welcome God as their helper.

These Christian friends are experiencing opportunities for new beginnings, and the Lord is with them to help. We all are in that mode each day when the sun rises. Every day we will be challenged, and we have a helper. That helper is God.

Thought for Today: Today is the first day of the rest of our lives. Let's move forward and enjoy it.

Prayer for Today: Dear Lord, today we thank you for your support; for being with us during good and bad times. Today we look forward to our new beginnings. Amen

Garden for Wildlife
Minnesota Landscape Arboretum

Peace

Who is God besides the Lord?
And who is the Rock except for our God?
(2 Samuel 22 vs 32)

In late August, Christian church ministry teams make many phone calls and home visits. Our pastor calls everyone in the church directory and invites them to the fall programs. With the help of his team, there will be home meetings, coffee shop visits around the city, and often just messages on answering machines saying that we care. It is a time of invitation to lead people back to the Rock of stability and Peace.

For families, school is about to start. The fall activities are about to begin, the summer slowdown, and the vacations are over. Empty nesters are looking at the leaves turning and thinking about winter, warm weather travels, and the holidays. For the most part, the human race is kicking into high gear- back to being too busy. In many cases, it means not being at Peace.

In the next few months, we may find ourselves in complicated situations and need to be reminded not to leave the Rock, our Lord, behind as we move forward into these exciting times. It is time to accept the invitations from our ministry teams and keep the Lord in our everyday lives. We need to keep Him in our lives to maintain our tranquility and keep us on an even keel.

Thought for Today: Let's look at our calendars and schedule a few minutes with our Lord, a few minutes for meditation, and a few minutes to give thanks. And a few minutes for ourselves. Let's do this so that we will be at Peace and be better able to help others.

Prayer for Today: Dear Lord, let's be calm and relaxed, patient and observing, caring and loving as we deal with others. Let us shine your light, so others will recognize we are at Peace. Amen

August 25

Country Path
Cockington Devon, UK

Hitch Hiking

You cannot serve both God and money.
(Matthew 6 vs 24)

In the 1950s, hitchhiking was a primary means of transportation for teenagers. We hitched to the ball field, the next town, the beach; we hitched wherever busses did not go. We have fond memories of the people we met and the rides shared. When mom would give me a nickel for the bus, I would stand there with my thumb out, hoping to save the nickel to buy candy.

H. Norman Wright, in his book All My Strength, writes about hitchhikers. Below are his thoughts:
"But consider the hitchhiker for a moment. He wants a free ride. He has no responsibility at all for the vehicle. He doesn't have to buy a car, pay insurance, upkeep or gas. Have you ever had a hitchhiker who volunteered to pay for gas? Not likely. He wants a free ride, a comfortable ride, a safe ride, and sometimes imposes upon you to take him out of your way. It's as though he expects you to do this for him.

There are a lot of spiritual hitchhikers today. They know the Lord, but they want a free ride. They want all the benefits of being a Christian but none of the responsibilities or the costs. They bail out without accountability, commitment, willingness to serve, and if it begins to cost.

The decision to serve God or serve ONES self is a big one. We can't do both. We can hitchhike in our faith, or we can serve our God. The ride is better with Him.

Thought for Today: Let's think about the hitchhiker and the driver. The hitchhiker has a need and thus is a taker. The driver is a willing giver. That describes Christians well, and it is OK to be a taker. We must decide who we are and who we will be rather than what we want to be. This season let us take a step forward and up. Let us pursue a better ride.

Prayer for the Day: Dear Lord, today we offer prayers of thanks for the opportunity to serve and contribute to peace on earth. Amen

Country Path
Cockington Devon, UK

August 26

Page 249

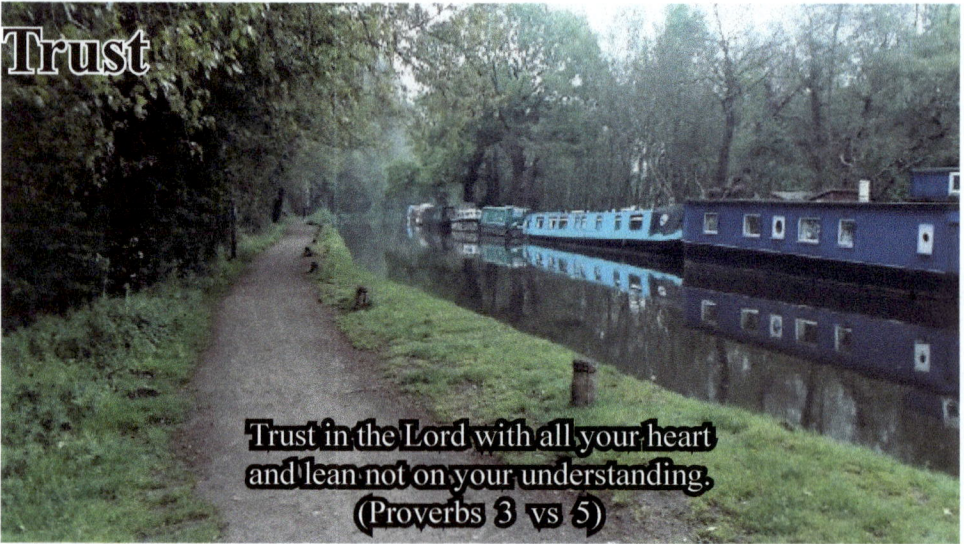

Trust

Trust in the Lord with all your heart
and lean not on your understanding.
(Proverbs 3 vs 5)

We often try to make things happen in our lives, driving toward human goals while conforming to modern society's standards. It is easy to get diverted from a solid spiritual track functioning our way rather than the Lord's way.

Am I ready and willing to do God's will? If so, how do I know God's will? The ten commandments are a good place to start. What the Lord has in mind for you may take you by surprise. Perhaps it is best expressed by Isaiah 55 vs 8,9.

"For my thoughts are not your thoughts,
neither are your ways my ways, declares the Lord.
'As the heavens are higher than the earth,
so are my ways higher than your ways
and my thoughts higher than your thoughts."

Knowing God's will cannot be a power struggle; he wants our will to be submissive to him. The more we value control and power, the more significant battle we will have. To be at peace, He needs to be in charge.

Thought for Today: Today, let's try to do God's will through our daily activities. He can and will resolve our problems.

Prayer for Today: Heavenly Father, we search for clues to help do your will. We pray that we can contribute to making your world a better place. Amen

River Wey Canal,
Surrey, Woking, UK

August 27

First Commandment

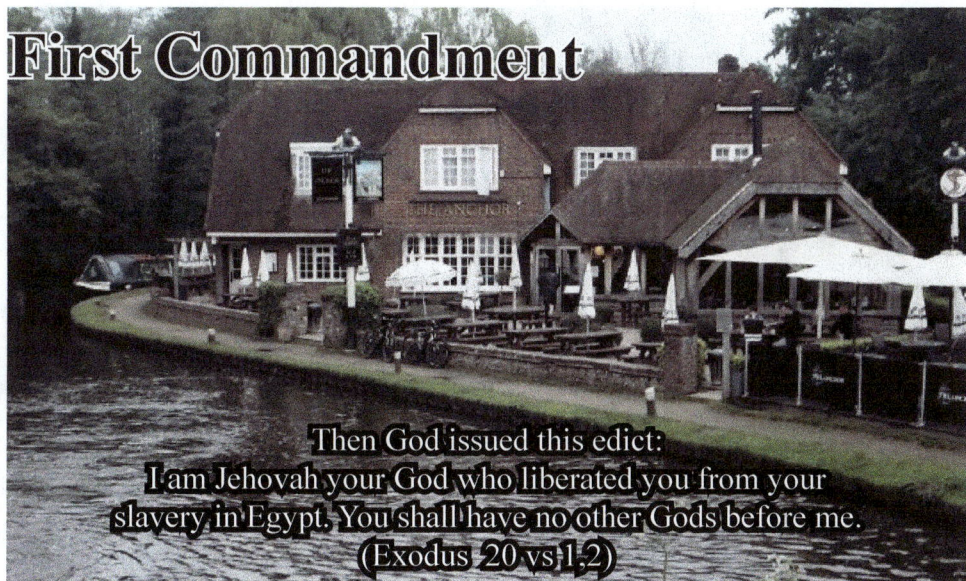

Then God issued this edict:
I am Jehovah your God who liberated you from your slavery in Egypt. You shall have no other Gods before me.
(Exodus 20 vs 1,2)

Kent Hughes has written an excellent book on the ten commandments titled "Disciplines of Grace." He gives a provocative summary of the first four commandments. He calls each one a word of Grace. Let's look at the first commandment.

The First word of Grace- the primacy of God: "You shall have no other God before me." That is, you shall have Me. I must be in the first place." If God is first, if there is nothing before Him, you will love Him more and more. Is He truly first in your life?

Frankly, there have been times in my life when there was not a conscious space for God. That was terrible news for me and those around me. All of us have had those times, and they are not pleasant. If you are reading this, I suspect you have gotten through that period and placed God first. You are blessed.

Thought for Today: How may we keep God first in our complex lives? What a question, there is an answer.

Prayer for Today: Heavenly Father, help me find a way to keep you first in my life at all times. When the going gets tough, lead me to creativity and solutions; When anger overtakes me, lead me to forgiveness; When things are going great, let me be thankful. Amen

The Anchor Pub
Surrey, Woking, UK

August 28

Page 251

Second Commandment

So then, men ought to regard us as servants of Christ and as those entrusted with the secret things of God.
(1Corinthians 4 vs 1)

In his book titled The Discipline of Grace, Kent Hughes gives this summary of the second commandment.

The Second Word of Grace- The person of God: "You shall not make for yourself an idol in the form of anything..." That is, you shall not make a material image or dream up a mental picture of God according to your design. God wants you to see Himself in His word and His Son because if you do, you will love him more. The clearer your vision, the greater your love. How is your vision?

Often when I arise early in the morning to write, nothing happens; nothing transfers from my fingertips to the keyboard. Is it a temporary lack of vision or not enough caffeine and sugar? I will never know the answer to that, but it is dastardly inconvenient.

None of us seem to have perfect vision to see the way. We seem to lose it, and often it is cloudy or blurred. Frankly, that is the mystery of our faith and something we can always correct.

Thought for Today: Let us place our vision on our calendar so that we stop and try to clear our image of God and improve our lives through Him.

Prayer for Today: Dear Lord, there are many days that my vision is cloudy. Calendar items block my view, family activity does not give me time to stop and look, and my agenda comes before you. I pray for guidance to take the time each day to clearly understand your presence in my life. Amen

RHS Kew Gardens

August 29 Richmond on Thames, London, UK

Third Commandment

Then God issued this edict: "I am Jehovah your God who liberated you from your slavery in Egypt."
(Exodus 20 vs 1,2).

In his book The Disciplines of Grace, Kent Hughes summarizes the third and fourth commandments.

"The Third Word of Grace- the person of God: "You shall not misuse the name of the Lord your God." That is, "You shall reverence God's name." Reverently loving Him in your mind and with your mouth will elevate and substantiate your love."

I was once golfing with my pastor, and he committed golfings biggest error. He missed his third putt. I commented that I always wanted to hear what comments he would make while lining up his fourth putt. He stated that he thought everything I would say, but I would never hear it. I wonder if he took the name of our Lord in vain.

The Fourth Word of Grace- the time for God. "Remember the Sabbath day by keeping it holy." This tells us to keep the Lord's day holy. Are you week by week offering it up in love to Him?

When we moved to Minneapolis, I was shocked to find stores open on Sunday. We had come from Massachusetts, which still honored the "blue laws." Frankly, not having them has led to kid's sports on Sunday and Wednesday evenings; this change has contributed to the wearing down of the family. Few people today honor the Sabbath.

Thought for Today: Let us remember in our thoughts and prayers the families of the children, youth, and young adults struggling with their faith.

Prayer for Today: Dear Lord, we need to slow down and keep you in our sites today. We pray for the focus and patience to make it happen. Amen

RHS Kew Gardens
Richmond on Thames, London, UK **August 30**   Page 253

Time Out

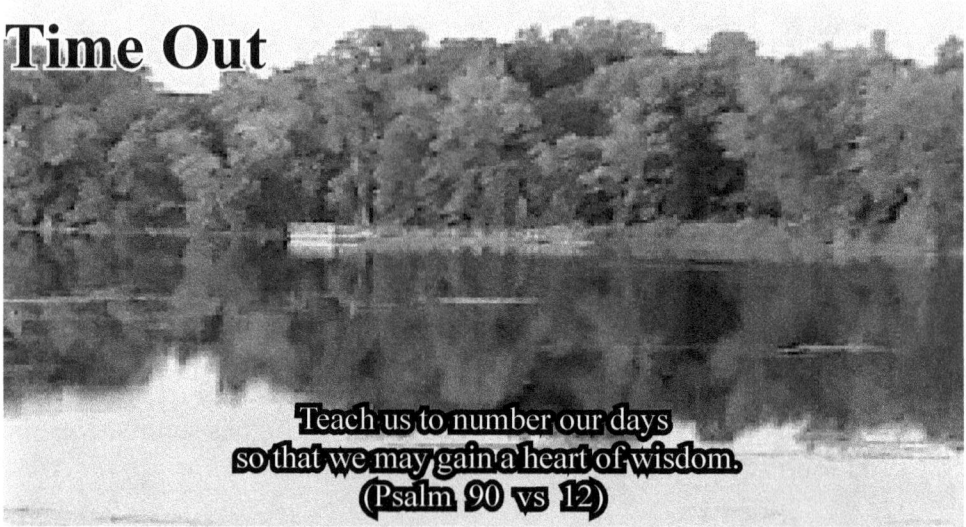

Teach us to number our days
so that we may gain a heart of wisdom.
(Psalm 90 vs 12)

Citizens of the World and America are dealing with pandemic issues, environmental challenges, and a world war. We just finished a long summer; youth sports, yard work, vacation trips, and ball games took our time away. Yes, we relaxed through our activities. Many people are still uptight.

Attendance in Christian churches goes down in the summer, and people go the entire period without recharging their batteries. They get to the end of August tired and feeling empty. There is a better way and a way to a better peace. My message is that what we do is fine, but if we feel a bit empty, that is the message to bring the Lord's holiness into our day. Lincoln put it like this:

"All we want is time, patience, and a reliance on a God who has never forsaken his people."

I say that when we are feeling empty, we need to recharge our spirituality.

Thought for Today: Today, let's reach out and show the world our Christ-like side.
Prayer for Today: Dear Lord, it has been a long busy summer. We are renewing our fall and winter activities. Thank you for the rest and recreation of vacation times as we move forward into the school year and the fall season. Amen

September

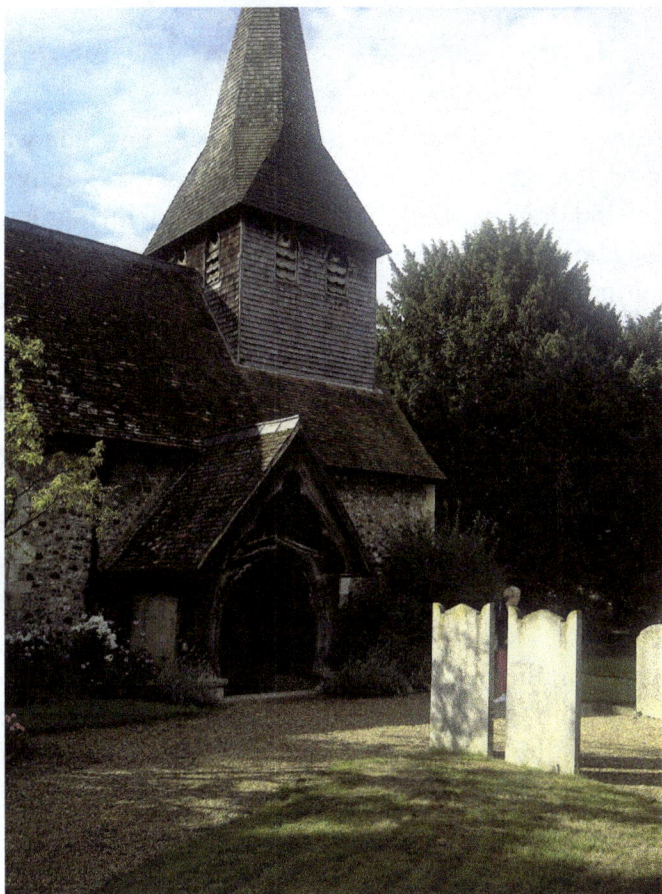

Saint Mary's, Byfleet, UK

The Church of England's vocation is and always has been to proclaim the good news of Jesus Christ afresh in each generation to the people of England.

Rally Day

If I was trying to please men,
I would not be a servant of Christ.
(Galatians 1 vs 10)

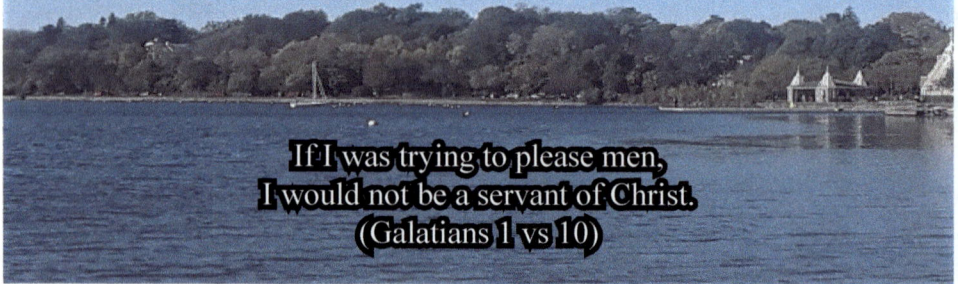

We learn that life is easier and more rewarding when we please those around us at a very young age. Grandchildren work diligently trying to please nana and gramps. They help in the kitchen, the garden, and other non-child-like chores. They love to help and love the approval they receive in return.

In the context of Paul's message to the Galatians, what are we teaching children? To please others gives good feelings. That is what I learned growing up and was in my thirties before realizing that being a "people pleaser" was not always in everyone's best interest. When pleasing people, honesty is sacrificed, and everyone involved misses a chance to grow closer to God.

What is the best way to get this message to the next generation?

Christian education, Sunday school as we used to call it, is probably the best answer. Through Christian education, the children learn what is important and meaningful. As they grow, they will choose to follow Christ and please God rather than people.

Soon it will be Rally Day at most Christian churches. There will be thousands of children returning and thousands not coming. It is a time of coming together for the Lord after a long summer.

Thought for Today: As leaders in our community and family, let us focus on visibly doing God's work in our lives.

Prayer for Today: Heavenly Father, we thank the Christian educators who work with children and youth. Those who teach the belief and faith will guide them throughout their lives. Amen

September 1 Lake Harriet
Minneapolis, Minesota

Courageous

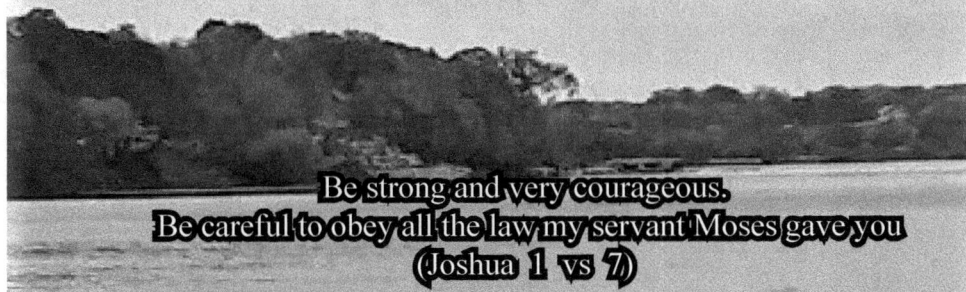

Be strong and very courageous.
Be careful to obey all the law my servant Moses gave you
(Joshua 1 vs 7)

We need to apply the passage above in our daily lives. We have overcomplicated our lives in developing our post-pandemic lifestyle. Our society is a distraction and getting through each day without drifting from our Christian standards seems more challenging than ever.

Our Friday Bible study group has several guys who grew up on farms in the midwest. They talk about caring for the livestock in the morning, attending school for the day (often a long mile walk), and the prize was getting home to help on the farm before doing the homework. That was not my life in New England, my children's lifestyle, and is undoubtedly not my grandchildren's today.

The easy path is not always the Godly path. Even as a retiree with reasonable calendar control, we get waylaid and off-target. It takes a certain amount of courage to say no to a distraction and do God's work. It is essential to recognize when our control is slipping away. Then we need to slow down, meditate and pray for guidance. The correct path will always be clear, and the courage to take it is available. God is with us, but we must let Him into our day.

Thought for Today: Let us slow down, smell the roses, and exhibit our good side. Let this be a relaxing and productive day.

Prayer for Today: Heavenly Father, as COVID changes our world, we pray for peace, love, and enjoyment. We pray that we can contribute to each of those things by doing your will. Amen

Medicine Lake
Plymouth, Minnesota

September 2

Page 257

Daily Diligence

> Whatever you do, work at it with all your heart,
> as working for the Lord, not for human masters,
> since you know that you will receive an inheritance from the
> Lord as a reward.
> It is the Lord Christ you are serving.
> (Ephesians 6 vs 8)

My first real job was as a drafting trainee at Bell Labs in Andover, Massachusetts. It may have been the lowest of the lows and the least significant position in the company. However, it was a great experience working with experienced, caring professionals who wanted everyone to grow and succeed.

My mentor talked a lot about teamwork and told me something I never forgot. He came over with an AT&T annual report and opened it to the pie chart showing their revenue breakdown. He had placed a dot of ink with a quill pen and explained that I was smaller in the big company picture than that dot. There were over 50,000 employees during that era. His message was that my dot could only grow when the whole pie grew and that I should always "…work at it with all my heart." He encouraged me to be a company man and a team player.

In our Lord's world, we are one of the billions, smaller even than my dot on that pie chart; but in no way are we insignificant. Every day and in every activity, each of us has the opportunity to affect those around us positively. We need to be diligent in pursuing happiness, love, and peace in God's world.

Thought for Today: Let's remember who our real boss is, our Lord. Let us make every effort to represent him well as we move through the day by having a positive influence on those around us.

Prayer for Today: Dear Lord, we give thanks for the opportunities we will have to help others. We pray that we will have a positive impact on those around us and the world with your guidance. Amen

Hosta, The Hosta Glade

Minnesota Landscape Arboretum

September 3

More Grace

Because of the service by which you have proved yourselves, others will praise God for the obedience that accompanies your confession of the gospel of Christ, and for your generosity in sharing with them and with everyone else. And in their prayers for you, their hearts will go out to you, because of the surpassing Grace God has given you. Thanks be to God for his indescribable gift!
(2 Corinthians 9 vs. 13-15)

We are supposed to be the light of the world, born to give, receive graciously, and accept Grace. This simple paraphrase can oversimplify aul's message: "Through service to others we will find grace and peace."

We positively impact our world when we give, help, and demonstrate Grace. That needs to be our mission, charge, and way of life as Christians: "Thanks be to God for his indescribable gift!"

Thought for Today: OK, I understand Paul's message for today- Now let us use it.

Prayer for Today: Dear Lord, today we desire to serve. We pray that we recognize the chance to help when you place it before us. Amen

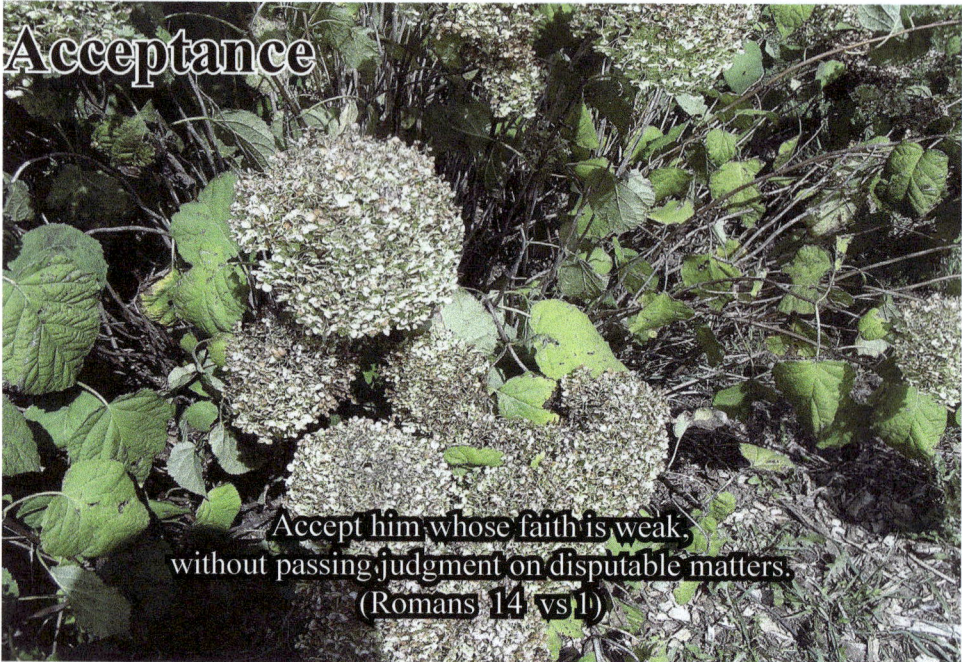

Acceptance

Accept him whose faith is weak,
without passing judgment on disputable matters.
(Romans 14 vs 1)

So how do you deal with antisocial, aggressive, opportunistic, and un-Christian behavior? We encounter it daily, and sometimes we act Christ-like and other times not. Wouldn't it be great if we always forgave with prayers and did not cross the line between hurt and anger?

Condemnation. Hmm, is it usually associated with a prison term? As practicing Christians, we think about forgiveness. In life, my one-word answer is prayerful.

My 37-year sales career was during the win-win industrial era. Most businesses, suppliers, and customers negotiated fairly and honored the contracts. It was always time-consuming work but enjoyable. Of course, there were always a few sharks and unethical individuals.

Paul's message is always about acceptance.

Thought for Today: Let's all be more accepting of others and their decisions.

Prayer for Today: Heavenly Father, let me accept those things that I do not understand; allow me to trust other people's decisions. Amen

Judging

Trust in the Lord With all your heart
and lean not on your own understanding.
(Proverbs 3 vs 5)

As an octogenarian, I constantly wonder about the direction society is going. Remember the good old days? It seems that whatever age you are, they exist. Two of my mom's favorite expressions were "Live and Learn." and "The more you know, the more you don't know." By now, we "Octos" know it all. Hah.

In the 50s, TV was going to ruin us. We spent more time watching it than reading, but we still read books. Then years later, we bought an Apple IIE computer, and a new age began. In our ever-evolving society, the only constant in the human race is "change."

What has not changed? Nature. We still have four seasons; the sun rises and sets; tides ebb and flow. It is September, and here in the northland, the evenings are cool, school has started, and a few leaves are turning.

Man's technology changes the way we operate. Our constant is our God-given world. We will read on our phones and tablets and send emails through cyberspace. All the while, God's world will continue to evolve. We are blessed.

Thought for Today: Let's give thanks for the many fall activities; school begins, kids are excited, and the formal learning process starts. To some, the start of the fall sports season is meaningful. To others, the fall means hunting and being outdoors. It would be easy amongst all the activities to forget God. Remember that all this is God's work, and give thanks for it all.

Prayer for Today: Dear Lord, we thank you for your patient love. We hope and pray that we may use that love to understand this complex world and apply it to everyone's benefit. Amen

Hydrangea Garden
Minnesota Landscape Arboretum   **September 6**   **Page 261**

Assertiveness

For God did not give us a spirit of timidity,
but a spirit of power, of love and of self-discipline.
(2 Timothy 1 vs 7)

Kenneth Haugk's book, "Speaking the Truth in Love: How to Be an Assertive Christian, did not promote standing on the corner rattling beads and waving the bible. It asked us to be unafraid to tell people who and what we are through our words and behavior. The simple act of a blessing at the lunch counter, a quiet time during a coffee break, and having a daily meditation on our desk are all subtle but assertive statements.

In the workplace today, the human resource departments have declared that religious issues may make someone uncomfortable and therefore are inappropriate. Many companies' email screens quarantine religious terms and other words with language scans. Being an assertive Christian in the workplace is not a good idea. However, behaving in an ethical Christ-like manner will improve the chance for success.

Here are three examples of semi-assertive Christian behavior in the workplace. A small business owner begins each week with a voluntary prayer breakfast; a second has a daily meditation calendar on his desk and says a blessing at all lunches; the third wears a lapel pin feet from footprints in the sand. All three inevitably lead to discussions with other Christians and improve the work environment.

We are given power, love, and self-discipline through our faith. It is important to remember to display and practice it every day.

Thought for Today: This week let's freely discuss our Christian ethics and beliefs with others so that they may better understand why we are who we are.

Prayer for Today: Dear Lord and Savior, we are approaching the time of year when all faiths have a special recognition of their beginnings. We pray that we may focus on similarities rather than differences . Amen

Peace Together

Remain in me, as I also remain in you.
(John 15 vs 4)

Often people say they are no longer interested in organized religion. The ritual, rules, money, and hard work did not do it for them; shame on them and shame on their church. Others change churches, often searching for something they never quite find. (It may be in their hearts.) we need to pray that they locate it.

In general, those described above are less than happy in their lives.

Jesus' message is clear; He is with us always. When we are searching and restless, the ball is in our court; we are the problem. These are the times we are out of touch with the Holy Spirit, not taking the time to open our hearts. When spiritually down and out, we need to look at ourselves first.

In 1954, Stuart Hamblen published the song "Open up your Heart" (and let the sunshine in.). Google shows that it was a big hit by the Maguire Sisters that year. It has been used hundreds of times in cartoons, children's messages, and TV shows. Jesus is our Lord and sunshine; we, the people, need to allow the sunshine in so that we may find peace together.

Thought for Today: Let's open our hearts to the Lord and find peace with Him.

Prayer for Today: Dear Lord, today we thank you for being with us; on our walks, at work, in our cars, and all phases of our day. Today we pray that we may stay in touch with you under all conditions. Amen

Plymouth Harbor
Plymouth Massachusetts

September 8

Page 263

Our Shield

Days are not equal as we go through life. There are highs and lows, and we have to deal with them.

One day in July 1998, it was too hot for golf. I did not want to walk the course at 95 degrees, but I was the league captain and begrudgingly went to the course. It was hot and steamy. At the start, my practice swings made my hands sweat, so the club was slipping, but I had an extra towel to keep them dry. My confidence was low, and being out there seemed like a bad idea.

By the third hole, my extra hand towel was already soaked from keeping my hands dry, and my shirt was sticking to my body, but I had parred the first two holes. It was on this par three that my negative attitude changed. I dried my hands, did my setup, and put the ball in the cup, my first hole in one! My two partners kidded me because I had been complaining. That is a good way for an 11 handicap to start.

As I said, things change; that day went from miserable to great.

In our ever-changing life, there is one constant force available, and if you are reading this, you more than likely understand; that constant force is our faith. We read that God is always with us. Paul advised the Ephesians to take up the shield of faith. We must remember him when things are not perfect and give thank him when things are going well.

Thought for Today: It may rain or the sun may be hot on our foreheads. Either way, let us keep our faith strong and have a great day.

Prayer for Today: Dear God, some days are good, others not so good. Today will be good because we are thinking about you and know we have you with us. Amen

Stormy Sky
Rome, Italy

September 9

Everlasting Faith

I do not hide your righteousness in my heart;
I speak of your faithfulness and salvation.
I do not conceal your love and your truth
from the great assembly.
(Psalm 40 vs 10,11)

We all remember where we were on nine-eleven. The physical world changed that day. For several months after that, Christian churches experienced a measurable increase in attendance. The best news regarding that is the very high increase in "un-churched guests" and the percentage that has kept coming.

Most of us will remember that day forever. I want to share a few memories of my own with you. On November 22, 1963, while donating blood in Salem, Massachusetts, the nurse told me that she had heard that the president had been shot. I told her that she should not even joke about stuff like that. Many people remember that day.

Solidly burned in my memory is sitting in a darkened room listening to the radio on Haverford Street in Hamden, Ct. We were listening to reports of the attack on Pearl Harbor. December 7, 1941. I was only 27 months old. (My mom confirmed that is all true; we think it is my first memory.) Both events changed the physical world in which we live. They changed society's operations, but not our hearts.

Worldly events cannot harm our spirit. Remember significant events and accept changes while keeping Lord in your heart. He will be with us.

Thought for Today: Let us find a friend and share the story about how September 11, 2001, has not changed our faith or how our faith is helping us through society's changes.

Prayer for Today: Dear Lord and father, today we give thanks for the joyous summer we experienced and look forward to the fall colors as they arrive. We are thankful for the opportunity to do your work here on earth and the pleasure we receive.   Amen

Storm over the Tiber River
Rome, Italy

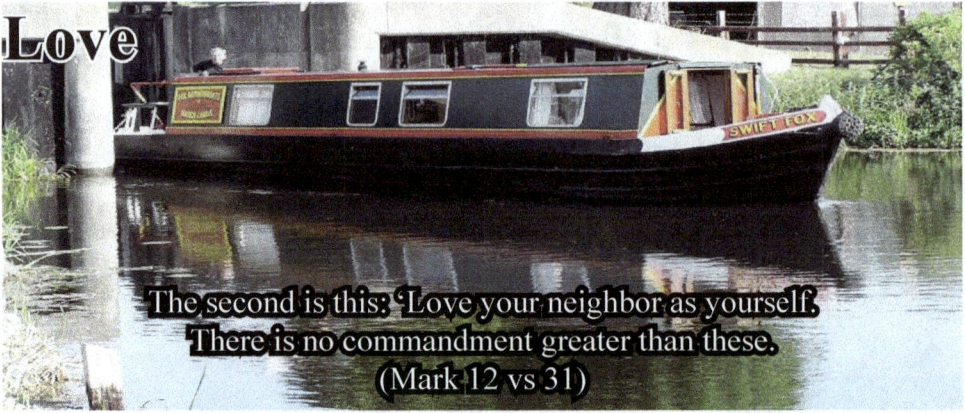

Love

The second is this: 'Love your neighbor as yourself.'
There is no commandment greater than these.
(Mark 12 vs 31)

September 11, 2001. We all remember this day twenty years ago. It negatively affected all. If President Roosevelt had been alive, he would have called it "A Day of infamy." Yes, that is a quote from December 7, 1941, after the attack on pearl harbor.

My wife, June, was born in London in 1938. Her life was permanently affected by six years of bombing during the war years. Twenty years ago, a discomforting awareness took over the American people when the twin towers were attacked. In many cases, the awareness quickly became fear, hate, or both. Children growing up in that era learned more about hate than love.

Our Christian faith, through Jesus, has the answer, written above by the disciple Mark. With that said, I fear that not enough people go to church or read the bible anymore, so below are some other places it is said that we may remember.

1955, the song and movie Love is a Many Splendid Thing,
1967, All You Need is Love by the Beatles.
1987, Forever and Ever, Amen by Randy Travis

Thought for Today: Let us think about our contact base with lov in our hearts.

Prayer for Today: Heavenly Father, often stress builds up in our lives. It is a combination of hurts, anger, and resentments kept hidden inside ourselves. When this occurs, I pray that I find a way to let you help and accept the guidance, protection, and support promised through our Christian faith. Amen

Share Your Spirit

And you show that you are a letter from Christ delivered by us, written not with ink but with the Spirit of the living God, not on tablets of stone but tablets of human hearts.
(2 Corinthians 3 vs 3)

In the early 1990s, the pastor at our small church introduced the concept that we were all the ministers and his function was facilitator or spiritual leader. He encouraged us to speak our faith, demonstrate our spirituality daily, and reach out to people. He used to say that the average Methodist invited a guest to church every 22 years.

In our wildest dreams, we may someday achieve world peace, resolve world hunger, and become an ethnically and racially blended society. When that happens, it will not happen through our politics today. It will be a Godly event that we cannot perceive.

We are all ministers and have the opportunity to work every day towards an improved society. Language and color divide us into nations and social groups. However, there is a common language,".., not on tablets of stone, but tablets of human hearts." We all have a job to do.

Thought for Today: We can find it easy to get caught up in our activities. Families have sports programs, school issues, and business issues, while singles have their way of filling the week. Yes, most of the world's people keep busy. Today let us seek the opportunity to demonstrate and share our spirit with someone.

Prayer for the Day: Heavenly Father, today we thank you for the people you placed in our lives that have supported and led us to grace. Today we pray for the opportunity to contribute to your will here on earth. Amen

Lock and Dam, River Nene
Cambridgeshire, UK

Somebody

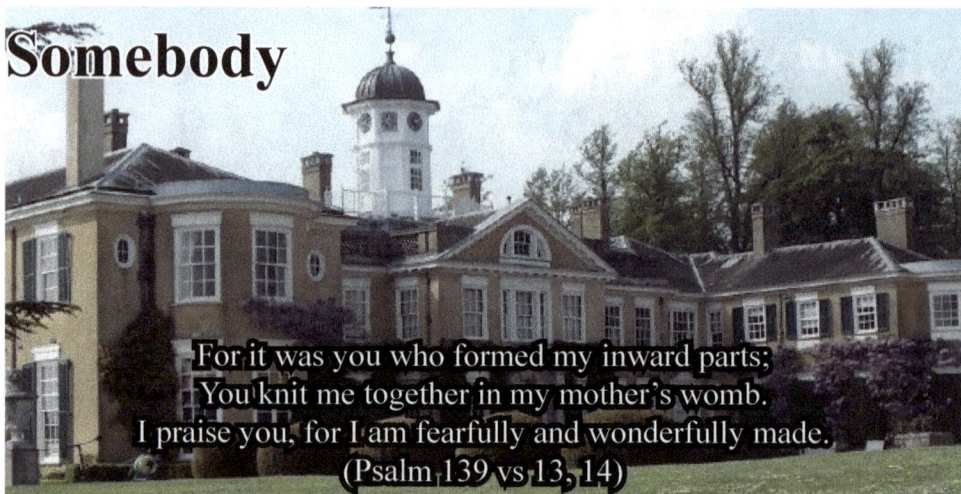

> For it was you who formed my inward parts;
> You knit me together in my mother's womb.
> I praise you, for I am fearfully and wonderfully made.
> (Psalm 139 vs 13, 14)

The Lord works in strange ways. When I write these devotions, I do not know what the results will be. Sometimes it is from an outside source placed before me during the week. This is one of those occasions, and it is close to plagiarism.

A pastor, good friend, and retired minister wrote, "Everybody is Somebody-including you and me." We all know that we are winners because the Lord is with us. Pastor Mike said it in a similar way that reinforces the thought. Below is a crucial paragraph from Mike:

"…My theology and values are centered on the conviction that because we are created in the image of God, each of us is valued and has deep within us the potential to reflect the goodness and beauty of our Creator. Therefore, being of Norwegian or German descent, African or Korean, tall or short, gay or straight, rich or poor is not a determining factor in our worth as human beings. We are valued because we are created in the image of God."

My thanks to Pastor Mike Miller.

Thought for Today: Today, we will have battles we do not expect. Let us be winners with God's help, no matter how the battle turns out. Plus: We have the parts and the image to be of value. Enjoy.

Prayer for Today: Dear Lord, we give thanks for who and what we are; your image here on earth. Amen

Start The Day

The path of the righteous is like the first gleam of dawn,
shining ever brighter till the full light of day.
But the way of the wicked is like deep darkness;
they do not know what makes them stumble.
(Proverbs 4 vs 18, 19)

Those who have known me long know I have always been a morning person. I think there is no better time of day than early morning, even sunrise. There is no prettier sight than the sun coming up out of the sea off of Boston, the early light on the first tee waiting for enough daylight to see the ball's flight, or the sun coming up over a mountain when viewed from a canoe while fishing. I am blessed because the first light is a spiritual event to me.

Each sunrise starts a new beginning, a new opportunity to do better, and a new opportunity to do God's work. Yesterday is gone and can not be changed, and our future is today and beyond.

The devotionals started as something to do during the early hours. The newscasts on TV were (and still are) depressing. The newspapers are full of bad news. It seems that bad news sells.

Tomorrow you will see a "first light." It may be mid-morning if you are a late sleeper or a sunrise. Either way, it is a new beginning, a new opportunity. It will be the first day of the rest of your life. Spend it with hope and joy.

Thought for Today: There will be seven days this week. Each is a fresh start. Let us feel the spirit in the first light, the blessing of a new day. Let us live the first day of the rest of our lives with faith and the joy of the Lord.

Prayer for Today: Dear Lord, we thank you for the sunrise, the new beginning, new opportunity. We pray we may use this opportunity to do your will here on earth. Amen

Wisteria at Polesden Lacey,
Dorking, Surrey, UK,

September 14   Page 269

Temptations

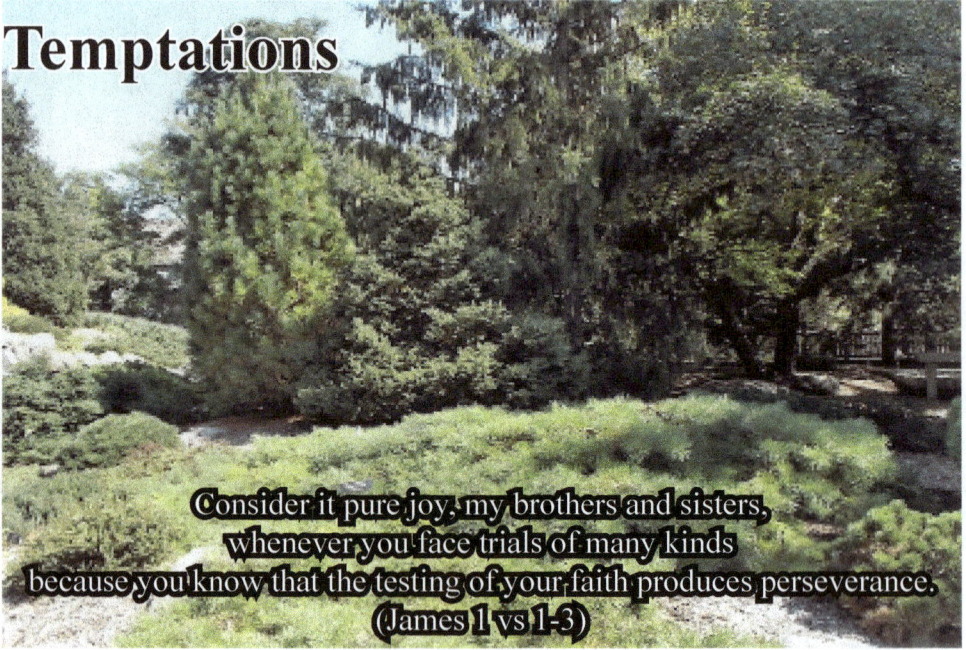

Consider it pure joy, my brothers and sisters,
whenever you face trials of many kinds
because you know that the testing of your faith produces perseverance.
(James 1 vs 1-3)

We will face trials in our lives. Some are simple, some are complex, and all help us become better people when we deal with them correctly. James is correct; tests of our faith develop character and perseverance.

Remember the story about the tortoise and the hare? The hare is overconfident and loses the race. My favorite poster was on my office wall for 30 years. It was of a very long windy road, miles long, and showed a lone runner. The distance to the horizon appeared to be out to infinity. The caption read, "The race is not always to the swift but to those who keep running." The title was persistence. The hare was the fastest, had all the advantages but lacked commitment and persistence.

James and Jesus knew it; we hear and understand it; we must persevere in our faith to improve the world.

Thought for the Day: Today, this week, month, and year let us remember our faith. Each day let us spread our love and joy to make our presence a positive force.

Prayer for Today: Dear God, we give thanks for your presence in our lives and the ability to resist temptations. Amen

Dwarf Conifers

September 15   Minnesota Landscape Arboretum

Whoever Has Ears

Whoever has ears, let them hear what the
Spirit says to the churches.
(Revelations 2 vs 7)

Today is my first try at using a passage from Revelations. Today's quote also appears in Revelations 2, a message from the Angels to several church congregations. It is used three times in Rev 3 and summarizes a newspaper article, "No religion, too? A recipe for trouble…" by Katherine Kersten. She discusses a strong connection between virtue (as taught by religious organizations) and successful self-government (democracy).

In her article, she points out that the intellectual or "psychological" man replaces the Christian model of man. Otherwise stated, the soul is being replaced by the "self." Since the Christian model places very high demands on virtue, she fears that our ability to self-govern is being sacrificed. I think this describes many issues bothering America and the free world.

A famous quote often credited to James Madison, our fourth President, said it this way: "We have staked the whole of all our political institutions upon the capacity of mankind for Self-Government, the capacity of each and all of us to govern ourselves, control ourselves, and sustain ourselves according to the Ten Commandments of God."

Christians have a personal obligation to demonstrate their faith, invite others to join, and somehow keep open to inspection. When others learn what we have in terms of happiness and satisfaction, they will join in.

Thought for the Day: Let us radiate our happiness and wear our faith on our sleeves. Demonstrate our Faith.

Prayer for Today: Lord, today we pray that we may hear the Spirit in our daily activities and can do your will here on earth. Amen

Overachievers

> Dear friends, let us love one another, for love comes from God. Everyone who loves has been born of God and knows God. Whoever does not love does not know God, because God is love.
> (1 John 4 vs 7, 8)

Many of you have known me for years and have heard me comment on over-achieving salespersons. My comments are that no one would deal with the frustrations of sales and dealing with the public unless the reward was internal. Somehow, all overachievers feel they are helping others.

In a sales career, the more interested you are in helping others, the more successful you become. In thirty years of sales, I saw people enter the field "for the big bucks." These people do not become long-term overachievers, and most seem to underachieve and disappear.

Many of my mentors were of this type, and I thought of them as boy scouts. I had not made the connection between them, love, and God. My weekly devotional mail list includes them today. Also on this list are clergy from many faiths and business people from receptionists to CEOs- all successful, primarily through a love of serving.

Love, caring, and sharing God with others will lead to success and happiness in business and daily life. Let us follow Nike's lead and "Just Do It."

Thought for Today: Let's search out and focus on the many things we do to serve. Not just the big things, but the little. The times we allow someone into traffic, open or hold a door, a phone call to say hello, etc. These are all acts of caring. Let us enjoy it when someone does these things for us. Let us share our caring spirit and enjoy the week.

Prayer for Today: Heavenly Father, we must understand your "love." The world is full of hate, distrust, and doubt of others. Personally, each of us shares these at some level. We pray that we learn to "love" the way Jesus did and apply that love in our daily lives as an example. Amen

Rejoyce Always

Do not be anxious about anything, but in everything, by prayer and petition, with thanksgiving, present your requests to God.
(Phillipians 4 vs 6)

Our active overcrowded lives can be stressful. Often conversations start with how busy we are; adding things to a calendar seems the norm. Even retirees often say they do not know how they ever had time to work. Then they go home and take their blood pressure medication.

Several years ago, a friend had severe back problems and high blood pressure. She had tried too many chemicals to work on the issues and was addicted to the pain killers. The addiction upset her tranquility and affected her blood pressure—a widespread and vicious cycle for many.

In desperation, she and her physician reduced the chemicals and substituted hypnosis and meditation. The meditation evolved into prayer. Well, I can't say that all her problems were solved. She had a diseased spine and a family history of high blood pressure. This story is not about healing.

However, most of her problems went away. The meditation and prayer brought her peace and relaxed her back muscles, and her blood pressure went down. The disease did not leave, but the symptoms were relieved. She found peace and a better life.

The effect of slowing down and taking time out for prayer will make God's peace be yours.

Thought for Today: Slow down, pray for peace, the tranquility, and serenity God has for you when you are willing to let it in.

Prayer for Today: Heavenly Father, with these words, we pray for the ability to live quiet and peaceful lives doing your work:

"God grant me the serenity,
to accept the things we can not change
The courage to change the things we can
and the wisdom to know the difference."

Japanese Garden
Minnesota Landscape Arboretum

September 18

Always Joyful

I have told you this so that my joy may be in you
and that your joy may be complete.
(John 15 vs 11)

Joy is in the heart, and our heads seem to want to control it. Does that make sense? The Holy Spirit is always with us; sometimes, we do not recognize its presence. I am writing in the seaside village of Torquay in Devon, and the rain is pelting down for the eighth or ninth day of this visit. We just had breakfast with 50-60 other hotel guests, some joyful and others sorrowful.

One fellow was looking forward to his round of golf wearing his wellington boots and slicker. He loves his golf and was very optimistic about the day. Another was going to catch up on his reading and walk to a restaurant for lunch. I am writing and then walking in the expected rain. We are a positive force in the room. The spirit of joy and peace is with us.

Several others have long faces and are complaining about the rain. Their heads have taken control and are missing out on their joy. The reality is we are in a beautiful place with great people. The views are magnificent, the food excellent and there is always tomorrow. Yes, there will not be any sunning on the beach; sitting under the palms and the umbrellas will keep us dry rather than protect us from the sun.

.   Today is the day the Lord has made; let us rejoice and be glad.

Thought for Today: Let's recognize that we can be full of joy or worry. Let's choose to be joyful.

Prayer for Today: Dear Lord and Father, today we give thanks for people, the individuals that makeup humanity. They come in all sizes and shapes and worship you in many different ways but are overwhelmingly great to know. You created them all differently but somehow in your image. Amen

Mint and Thyme

Peace

> Nevertheless, I will bring health and healing to it;
> I will heal my people and will let them enjoy abundant peace and security.
> ...they will be in awe and will tremble at the abundant prosperity and
> peace I provide....
> (Jeremiah 33 vs. 6, 9)

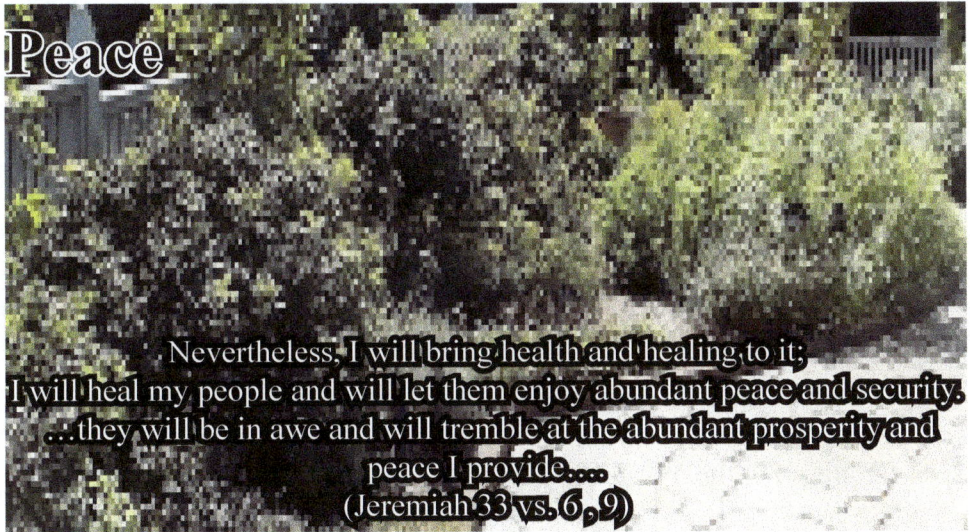

Today is a great day here in Minnesota. The sky is blue, the temperature is in the mid-seventies (That's the twenties for my Euro-friends), and I have had a swim, a jog, and nine holes of golf. I am tired and at peace as I write this. I hope that world peace (which includes family, city, county, national, and any other peace!) is like good weather. It will come someday.

After World War II there was the famous picture of the soldier kissing the nurse in Times Square. After all, that was the war to end all wars. In the fifties, a friend from New Hampshire received the Silver Star for his contributions to "keeping the peace" in Korea. At my fiftieth high school reunion, the list of deceased was overwhelmingly male. It had a lot to do with Vietnam and agent orange. These people contributed to peace and protected our country, and I greatly appreciate their efforts.

The prophet Jeremiah talked about peace 2600 years ago. We are hopeful and pray for it to come, and most of us are willing to help it along. For all of us reading this today, let us contribute a bit of love to the situation. Let us enjoy our peace and hope that it spreads.

Thought for Today: Think about how peaceful life is and appreciate it.

Prayer for Today: Dear Lord, we pray for world peace and peace in our families, communities, cities, and nations. Please show us how we can apply your will toward this lofty goal. We pray for the safety of the world's soldiers through the end of hatred and war. Amen

Herb Garden
Minnesota Landscape Arboretum

Consideration

On my 72nd birthday, we had a grand celebration of fitness, friendship, and family. Oh, for some reason, I could not resist doing a sprint triathlon in the morning with my brother, granddaughter, and daughter.   When several hundred people are swimming and racing across a lake, consideration of others is often not visible, tenderness does not come to mind, and selfish ambition is everywhere. Most people were racing for themselves, and most did not share their space with you if you were in the way.

The good news is that "most" is not everyone- the Lord was with me, and he sent me plenty of Christ-like people to support me in crises. I had an asthma attack about five minutes the swim. Rather than being one of the strongest swimmers, I was trying to figure a way to survive,

Several swimmers heard my rather loud wheezing exhales and offered assistance- macho me advised them that I would be OK. Lifeguards in kayaks asked if I needed help. My answer was not yet; finishing was important to me. In the last 200 yards, a lifeguard wanted to pull me from the race. I told him I was a good swimmer and couldn't breathe right now. He looked concerned and kept close by in his kayak. By the Grace of God, things worked out well in all my bad judgment.

The summary was the great support and encouragement other swimmers had for me. One fellow swam alongside me for several hundred yards, the officials in the kayaks were concerned but gracious, and when in the transition area, a spectator offered me her inhaler.

Thought for Today: Let's look out for others- let's lend a helping hand in Christ's name.

Prayer for Today: Dear Lord and Father, we thank your followers, those Christ-like people who are there every day when people need them. We give thanks to all who are blessed by their beliefs. Amen

Rye Harbor Nature Preserve
Rye Harbor, East Sussex, UK

Success

I saw that wisdom is better than folly,
Just as light is better than darkness.
(Ecclesiastes 2 vs 13)

Our democratic society is a competitive marketplace for goods and services. That is supposed to be what makes America great. Success is often a matter of having more "stuff." We are building five, six, and seven thousand square foot houses, owning bigger boats, luxury cars abound, etc. All this is very good for the economy, but is it good for our souls?

Aristotle Onassis's definition of success was to "... keep climbing higher and higher-just for the thrill." Barbra Streisand said, "success for me is having ten honeydew melons and eating only the best part of each."

Because you are reading this Good News today, I pray that your definition is more closely better represented by Dr. Gary Rossberg's perspective:

"Success is not just a matter of money, power, and ego, but also issues of heart-like compassion, bravery, generosity, and love. It is an issue of character, not performance of being the person God wanted you to be, not how much salary you can pull down. ...".

If we sit in our homes surrounded by our "stuff" and still feel underachieved, If we sit on the couch next to our spouse and still feel lonely, we need to go back to the simple things we learned growing up and search our faith for the definition of success. We will find that Rossberg is very close to the answer.

Thought for Today: Let's look at our calendars and evaluate where our efforts are taking us. Let us fit our lives into Rossberg's perspective rather than the more material views of success.

Prayer for Today: Dear heavenly Father, our world has changed. Terror seems to be taking over well beyond faith and love. Somehow we pray for an answer to how it all fits Your plan. Amen

Rye Harbor Nature Preserve
Rye Harbor, East Sussex, UK

September 22

Page 277

Trust

I rejoiced greatly in the Lord that at last, you renewed your concern for me. Indeed, you were concerned, but you had no opportunity to show it. I am not saying this because I am in need, for I have learned to be content whatever the circumstances. (Philippians 4 vs 10-13)

It always amazes me and reinforces my faith when something Paul said 2000 years ago applies directly to today's world. For several years our free world economy has been flaky. Trust in government has faded as the leaders of America and the world have become polarized. The advent of Ponzi schemes and fraud by high-powered executives have hurt the trust we need in our financial markets for them to be strong. Even at low levels of government, doubts about their ability to perform are stronger than ever. Frankly, it is scary because our country relies on trust. Look at your money, "In God We Trust."

I promise to turn this around. I try not to be political, but that seems to be the case today. Paul is pointing out a simple truth, and we must pay attention. In a recent telecast, televangelist Joel Osteen said, "We do not know what the future holds, but we do know who holds our future." Hmmm, there is something to think about.

Thought for Today: Each day take time to focus on our savior. Take a few minutes to appreciate and welcome Him into our life.

Prayer for Today: Dear Lord and Father, today we give thanks for Paul's words and encouragement. We pray that we may accept his advice graciously and lean on you to get through our daily stresses. Amen

Positive Christian 1

Photo By Jackie Collins

He gives strength to the weary
and increases the power of the weak.
(Isaiah 40 vs 29)

It is another early morning. I am thinking about the summer of 2018 when June and I moved into our eighties and fifty years of marriage. It is great to celebrate and reminisce about the victories and challenges we have worked through over the years. We are truly blessed.

The story is not all that positive; however, we are getting older, and my mom used to say, "Growing old is not for sissies." It comes with its challenges; getting tired easier, recovering slower, and requiring fewer calories (eat less). Several years ago, June and I set the goal of not becoming grumpy senior citizens. We decided to pray and always try to be positive Christians. It is not always easy.

Thought for Today: Today will be a milestone; things will happen we do not expect. Let's recognize the blessings we will have, even if they seem like challenges.

Prayer for Today: Heavenly Father, today we thank you for our many fond memories. As we face today's challenges, we pray that we accomplish your will, deal with issues Jesus way, and generate more fond memories for tomorrow. Amen

Ossipee River
Effingham Falls, New Hampshire   **September 24**   Page 279

Positive Christian 2

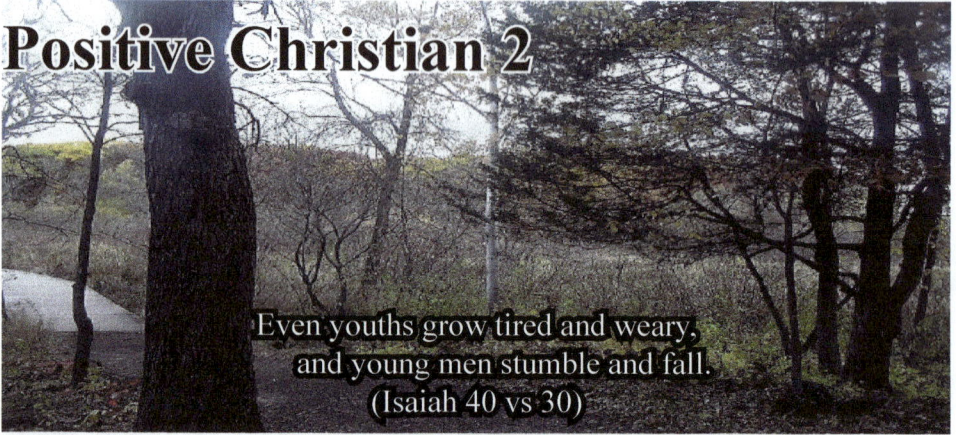

> Even youths grow tired and weary,
> and young men stumble and fall.
> (Isaiah 40 vs 30)

I have exercised with an older retired physician, Phil, for over ten years. He has completed over 25 marathons and 20 ultra-marathons, and most of you know my triathlon history. Phil and I talk about those youthful days. We walk/jog/waddle 15-20 miles a week, and we have a lot of time to talk. We have determined that we do not recover as fast as we used to.

Phil and I have several friends who lost their spouse, They are dealing wuth a challenge that half od us will face. We will respond in different ways.

All of the above sounds a negative but is just data. The reality is that it is great to be a Christian. We have a great perspective on life and a lot to share with future generations. In our later years, we have the support of our Lord and have time to help others. We need to be positive Christians and set an example on how to live happily. Remember this:

> "but those who hope in the LORD
> will renew their strength.
> They will soar on wings like eagles;
> they will run and not grow weary,
> they will walk and not be faint."
> (Isaiah 40 vs. 31,32)

Thought for Today: Be happy and positive and share our enthusiasm with others.

Prayer for Today: Dear Lord, we thank you for our blessings and the ability to focus on positive feelings through your love. Today we pray that we may be positive and radiate joy to those around us. Amen

Busyness

I have fought the good fight
I have finished the race, I have kept the faith.
(2 Timothy 4 vs 7)

Over the years, I came to relate closely with the race analogies used by Paul in his letters. They are meaningful today because the events around the world have thrown us into a high state of BUSYness. (Spell-check hates that word, but I like it!). Paul's message above is not about a marathon, a workweek, or getting to the children's activities; it has nothing to do with our BUSYness. It has to do with keeping our faith peaked during the process of life.

BUSYness! I wrote this today because retired old Bob is too busy with retirement stuff; writing, blogging, helping others in need, increasing my exercise program, and generally being Bob. For the second day in a row, my morning meditation did not fit. In the early 1990s, my daughter gave me a devotional, "With All My Strength" by H. Norman Wright." Before that, I skimmed the newspaper while watching the morning TV news and drinking my coffee. That would increase my stress and negativity. Reading the devotional improved my attitude, and life improved through spiritual growth

Today, I read Paul's message to Timothy before tackling the day's tasks. You see, life is excellent but longer than a marathon! Sometimes called the daily grind. Life is good when the good fight is supported by spiritual growth. Finish your race by keeping the faith.

Thought for Today: In a counter to Paul's message about the race, I read the following from the 23rd Psalm: "He makes me lie down in green pastures, he leads me beside quiet waters, he restores my soul." Take a prayer break today and every day.

Prayer for Today: Dear father, we pray for personal peace. Amen

Brotherly Love

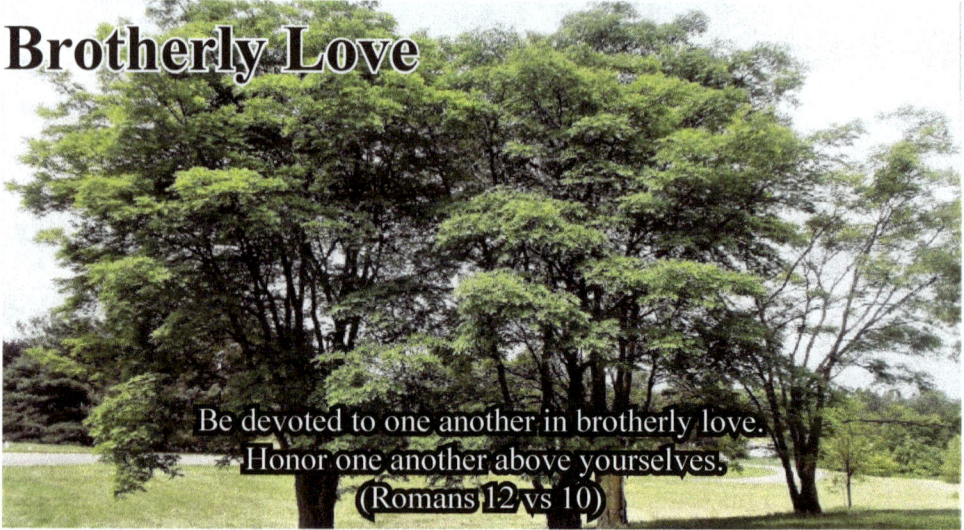

Be devoted to one another in brotherly love.
Honor one another above yourselves.
(Romans 12 vs 10)

Paul says that the person closest to or standing next to you deserves dignity and honor at any moment. In many cases, that is not how it works. We are an overloaded society and rarely give the person near us enough of our thoughts. We are about thinking too far ahead rather than the present. We need to slow down.

Christ served everyone; He made time for lepers, prostitutes, tax collectors, the "unclean" and needy, and his disciples. We should not forget to consider or care for everyone, even when we do not have time. We are often called or approached by a friend or acquaintance for advice or help at an inconvenient time. When that happens, we often look at our watch while they talk, space out and not listen, and then brush them off as quickly as possible- Wow, WWJD on that one.

The above is a real problem faced by all of us almost daily. We have deadlines in our lives and people that matter long term; our families and career colleagues. With that in mind, how do we deal with others who come for help when we do not have time. We need to pray about how we can be considerate and tolerant.

Thought for Today: Let's focus on being caring when we are interrupted by a friend. Let us ask how Jesus would deal with the telemarketer. We always need to find ways to share our Christian love.

Prayer for Today: Heavenly Father, I will meet someone in need and won't have time to listen. Today when that happens, I pray and hear in your name, as Jesus would. Amen

Amur Maackii

The Prisoner 1

"Set me free from my prison,
that I may praise your name."
(Psalm 142 vs 7)

We are often too busy to stop and pray. That is why I write at five am there are few interruptions and distractions. It is quiet; still, the coffee is hot, and the sugar is sweet. How great can it get?

By 8 o'clock, my calendar kicks in, and prayer and spiritual thoughts will have to fit in between my daily activities. On many days, they do not quite get on the agenda. In a sense, we are victims of our busy schedules trying to meet the needs of family, friends, and business associates. That leads to a good life, and nothing is wrong with that.

In the late 70s, I had an evangelical tennis partner, Ken, who would not shut up in his attempts to recruit me into his congregation. One day he advised me that I was not saving enough time for the Lord, and he was praying for me. That bothered me a lot.

I had a company with a reasonably high cash flow, worked sixty-hour weeks, ran marathons, and played tennis three times a week. He was not very successful in business and had to do everything on a shoestring. My calendar was so full that June and I met at the tennis club on Saturdays after my tennis and her workout to visit each other. It was a full life and very gratifying. There was no room for spiritual growth.

We were happy as clams and did not realize that we were prisoners of our calendars.

Thought for Today: Try to notice how our schedules entrap us.

Prayer for Today: Dear Lord, today we give thanks for our family, our friends, and loved ones. We are blessed by them through you. Amen

The Prisoner 2

I thank God, whom I serve, as my forefathers did,
with a clear conscience,
like night and day, I constantly remember you in my prayers.
(2 Timothy 2 vs 3)

That family schedule mentioned yesterday led us to counsel and a new set of family rules and priorities. It took outside help for us to get out of our self-imposed prison. Yes, we were still busy because four kids had to go to college, and we had obligations to meet. We established new rules and spiritual growth became part of our family equation.

Our prison walls were our calendar items and obligations. When Paul wrote to Timothy, he was in a real prison with actual walls. That allowed him a lot of time to write and pray. He was blessed with the Lord inside him to do that. In our self-induced prison of activity, the opposite happened. We did not take enough time for the Lord.

Over the years, June and I have learned not to judge others. But today, I will ask you to look at yourself and your lifestyle. Is your calendar getting in the way of your spiritual growth? If so, think about altering your long-range plan.

Spiritual growth comes with a "get out of jail free card."

Thought for Today: Let us react to pressure positively and take a prayer break. Cool it, count to ten, take a deep breath, and take control when the going gets tough. Give thanks for having the ability to slow down.

Prayer for Today: Dear Lord, we have woven a web of activity into our daily lives. Often we leave you out and seem to be in a prison of our design. Today we pray that we can keep you with us and that you will guide us and be our get-out-of-jail-free card. Amen

Lake Phalen
St. Paul, Minnesota

Help

In 1912, C. Austin Miles was asked to write a hymn that would "…bring hope to the hopeless, rest for the weary and downy pillows to dying beds". The above reminds us that we are never alone and walk with the Lord at our side.

It is easy to try to be independent when things get tough. After all, we are humans in control of our world. June and I both wanted to fix concerns while celebrating the joy. We needed to listen; "…he walks with me, and he talks with me," We need to let go and let God take control, and sometimes we, especially me, forget who is in control. Yes, all of us tend to take control.

Thought for Today: Let's remember that we do not walk alone. When we are confronted with stress, loneliness, and the everyday events that distract us, let us not forget that God is with us.

Prayer for Today: Dear Lord, this week, many of us rejected your help. We were sometimes angry, often controlling, and occasionally selfish. We succumbed to the pressures that surrounded us. We thank you for being there and pray that we may take the time to allow you to walk at our side and accept your help. Amen.

Lake Phalen
St. Paul, Minnesota

September 30

October

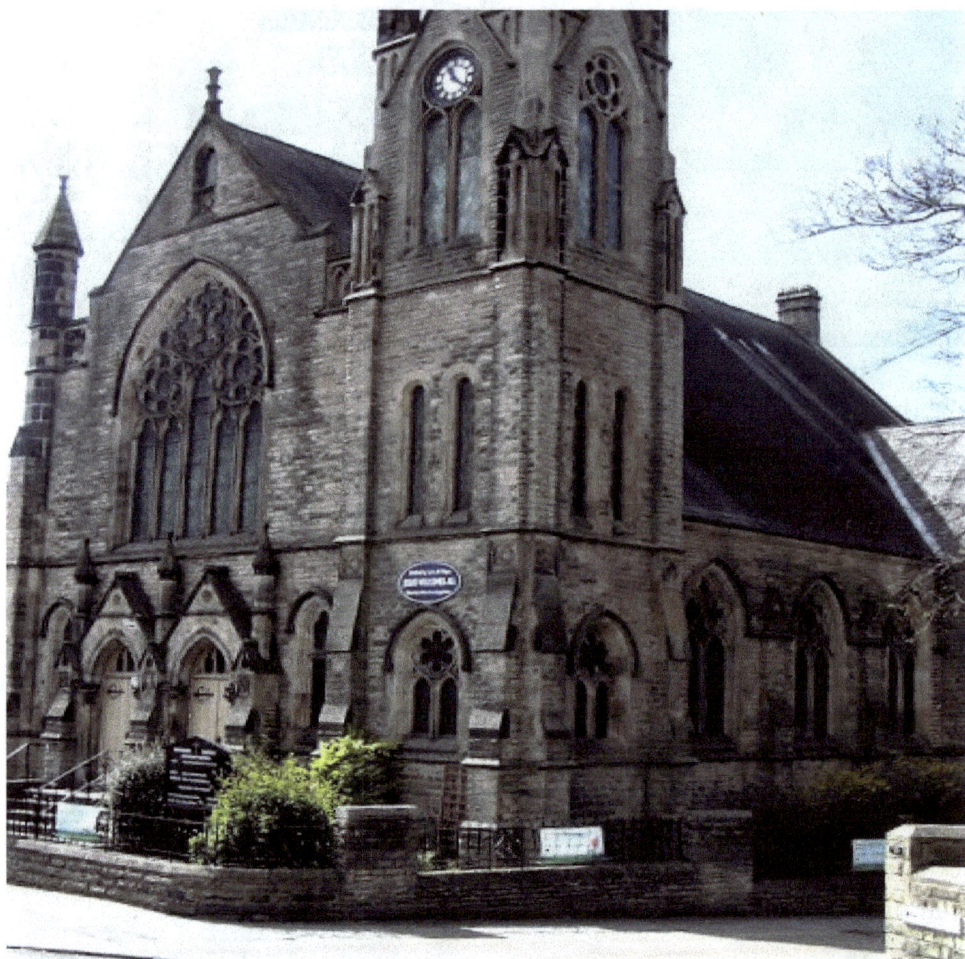

Barnard Castle Methodist Church

The current Methodist church in Barnard Castle was opened on March 30, 1894, so the members are currently celebrating 125 years of service.

'Make desciples of Jesus Christ for the transformation of the world"

Barnard Castle, Durham, UK

Special Days

There are 365 days every year. Our goal and challenge are to enjoy every day. We can not allow our finances, a boss, or other outside influences to steal pleasure from any day. God put us here to be happy, and we need to do that for Him.

OK, let's get real. Some days are just a drag, and things go wrong. God rains on our parade, our back goes out again, etc. When negative things get in the way, we have a hard choice. We can choose to have a bad day or trust our faith and give thanks for what went right. Some days it seems that the only thing to give thanks for its end. Well, that's enough to make it a good day.

We all have problems and challenges that will take longer than one day to resolve. We need to remember two important things. When we live one day at a time, we simplify our solutions. We can work on it tomorrow if we do not get it today. When we believe an issue is unsolvable, we need to remember that the Lord is with us, and He can change the rules. We need to pray and turn unsolvable matters over to the Lord.

Allowing God to be with us daily guarantees that we will have a good day.

Thought for the Day: This will be a wonderful week for all of us. We will walk through the challenges and bless the Lord for the experiences and lessons that we learn one day at a time.

Prayer for Today: Dear Lord and father, we are often confused by our world. There are problems that we want to fix now and can not. We thank you for the many things that go well and pray that we may cheerfully contribute to your plan. Amen

Coco Beach, Playa del Carmen,
Quintana Roo, Mexico

October 1

Don't Fake It

Woe to you ...you hypocrites!
... on the outside, you appear to people as righteous,
but on the inside, you are full of hypocrisy and wickedness.
(Matthew 23 vs 27)

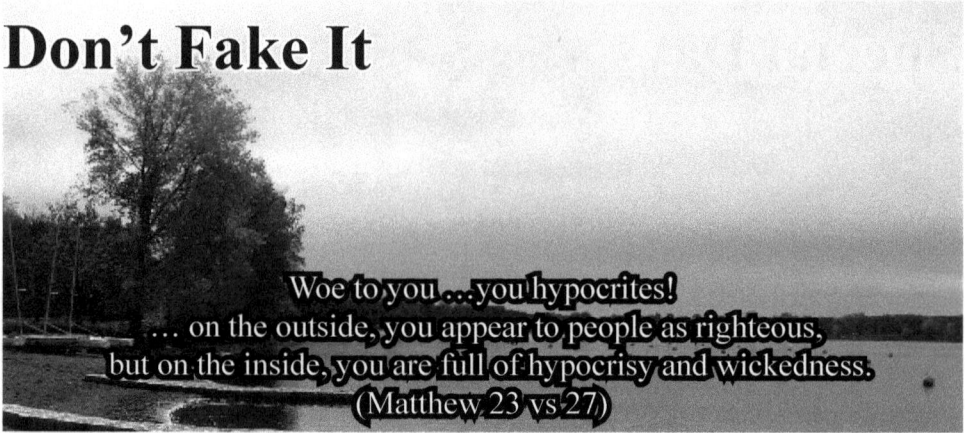

One of my favorite themes is being true to our faith by being open and honest. Too many people in the world have a different reality than Christians. Openness comes with some social consequences.

As Christians, we are taught that the world has an abundance supplied by God, and I believe that is true; but there is a significant distribution problem. It is as if the resources are limited. In America and throughout most of the world, life is competitive.

Dealing with the wealth of Western civilization and how it relates to Christianity is scary. Recently, when discussing a stewardship campaign at our church, it was mentioned that we would not need the government to run social programs if all Christians would tithe. That would be great.

Each of us needs to be as good as we can be to contribute to the positive factor in society. We need to take social risks to reach our real rewards.

"He who has clean hands and a pure heart,
who does not lift his soul to an idol
or swear by what is false.
He will receive blessing from the LORD
and vindication from God his Savior."
(Psalm 24 vs 4,5)

Thought for Today: We must choose today to be straight and true or hold back a bit. We must make tough choices and keep a pure heart to improve the world around us.

Prayer for Today: We pray for the chance to demonstrate our faith to others, to help. We pray to be able to do your will here on earth. Amen

Family 1

Treat others as you want them to treat you... Never criticize or condemn or it will all come back to you. ...If you give, you will get. Your gift will return to you in full and overflowing measure, pressed down, shaken together to make room for more, and running over. Whatever measure you use to give, large or small, will be used to measure what is given back to you.
(Luke 6 vs 31, 37, 38)

In the 1960s, the expression was "giving off vibes" (That probably came from the Beach Boy's "Cool Vibrations"). What we give has an overwhelming effect on our lives, our social environment, and those around us. Every day we are giving. Whether in the workplace, the family arena, or driving alone down the street, we participate and give to those around us.

The place where being positive is easiest and most important is in the family, where love is the strongest. Indeed, within each of our families, we have lways been positive, loving and "really cool." If you think that, you better take a reality check and ensure your other family members see it the same. Most of us do not meet that standard.

Sometimes we are tired. Sometimes the career is not working well. We can be angry when we should stop and meditate. Perfection is our goal, perhaps not our reality. When we are down, it is essential to remember that we are the children of God, and we have His support in both the good and testing times. He wants us to work with Him to bring peace and good while sharing His love with others. Sharing His love instead of "our frustrations" with others is a lofty goal.

Thought for The Day: When we feel stressed out, let us focus on not bringing it home. It is OK to ask the family for support during stressful times, but unfair and destructive to pass stresses on to them.

Prayer for Today: Heavenly Father, we are truly blessed. We stand before you, covered with your love. We pray that during tough times, we can reach out to you, feel, and share that love. Amen

Treat others as you want them to treat you... Never criticize or condemn or it will all come back to you. ...If you give, you will get. Your gift will return to you in full and overflowing measure, pressed down, shaken together to make room for more, and running over. Whatever measure you use to give, large or small, will be used to measure what is given back to you.
(Luke 6 vs 31,37-38)

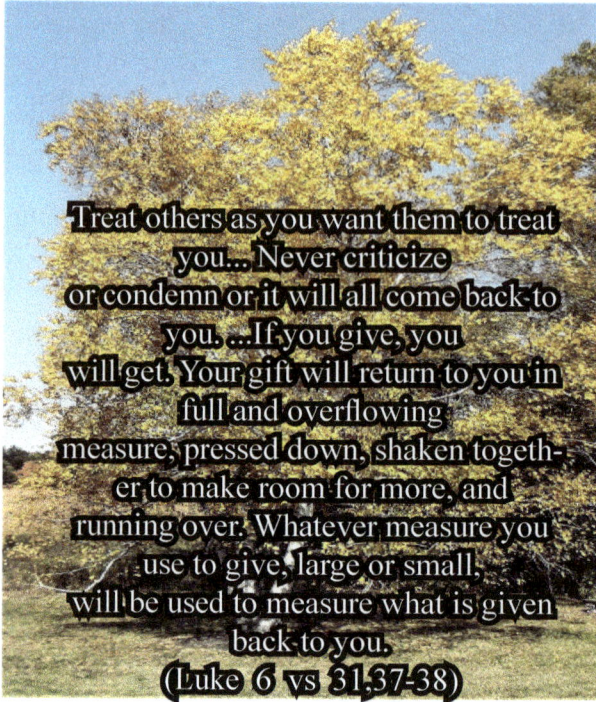

Within the workplace, there can be many stresses that hurt the overall environment. We have deadlines to meet, underfunded projects, professional jealousies that developed, and many issues that are passed on that we cannot control. It is easy to be negative and act differently than a child of God.

Early in my career, a mentor advised me that as an employee, I would always receive a percentage of what I was worth, never 100 percent. His explanation was that difference was required to have a profitable company. After 40 years of working, that seems to have been very accurate advice. His equation appears to work when thinking dollars and cents in the business environment.

A challenge to me is the people who are sharks in the business environment and Christians on Sunday. I mean those that are opportunistic, somewhat misleading (I won't say dishonest), and practice ways that are not part of good Christian ethics. The most successful business people seem to live only by good Christian ethics. My question has always been, "Can you function outside Christian guidelines Monday through Friday and then consider yourself a Christian?"

In the real world, giving is rewarded many times over. I believe that the business world is part of the real world and that we are to act and follow God's guidelines if we live to our full potential.

Thought for Today: Let us be positive and contribute to solving problems rather than spreading them.

Prayer for Today: Dear Lord, we are often tempted to forget our ways and work out problems in a human rather than a Godly manner. I pray for the strength to let you work through me when trying to help, both at home and in the workplace. Amen

Birch Trees
Minnesota Landscape Arboretum

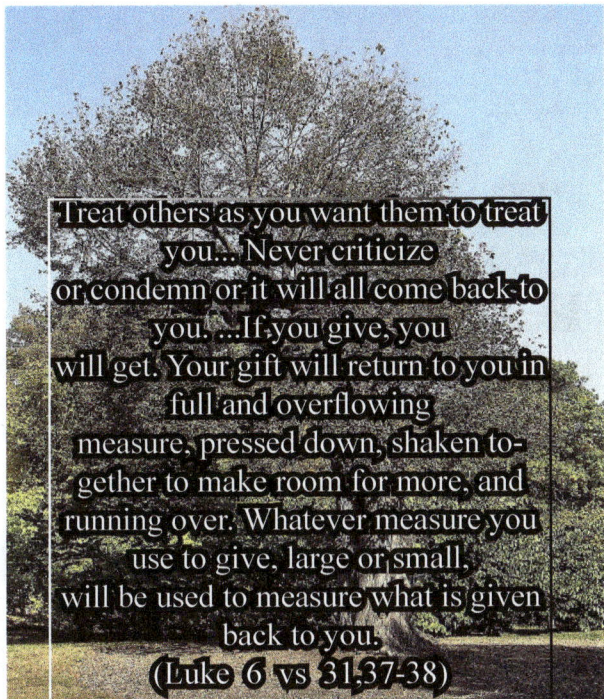

Every day we read of some manifestation of a person's anger against those around them, against society. How do we as Christians avoid getting so far down that we can not control our emotions? We have the tools. Then it must be as simple as using them in our lives. That is how these devotions started. Several years ago, June and I gave up the news for morning meditation and decided to share some of them with you.

Treat others as you want them to treat you... Never criticize or condemn or it will all come back to you. ...If you give, you will get. Your gift will return to you in full and overflowing measure, pressed down, shaken together to make room for more, and running over. Whatever measure you use to give, large or small, will be used to measure what is given back to you.
(Luke 6 vs 31,37-38)

We hope that our messages contribute to your lives.

When we think of our life plans and goals, we think of peace, tranquility, and wealth. In Luke, we learn that when we share our peace, we will receive more back then we gave. Then when we are down and out, we can cuss, strike out, seek a mentor to discuss things with, or pray. As Christians, we have the tools and an obligation to use them. As NIKE (my favorite philosopher) says in its slogan Just Do It.

Thought for the Day: This week, we will all have high and low times, peaks and valleys, frustrations, and celebrations. Let us recognize the "lows" and repeat this week's prayer. Let us be peacemakers rather than facilitating the stresses of our society.

Prayer rfor Today: We recommend the serenity prayer and suggest that we all use it when stressed.

God grant me the serenity
to accept the things that I can not change.
The courage to change the things I can.
And the wisdom to know the difference.
Amen.

American Aspen
Minnesota Landscape Arboretum

Encouragement

> Let us consider how we may spur one another on toward love and good deeds.
> ... Let us encourage one another.
> (Hebrews 10 vs 23-25)

Every day, we may encounter negativity, anger, and difficult situations. When facing this negative force, we choose how we will respond. In our society, we often stand up to be counted rather than perceived as weak, wimpy, or undecided. We can meet the challenge head-on or take the Godly course and work out the problem through love and our hearts. We can demonstrate our love of God through our responses.

When we encounter anger, what happens when we show love? Caring? Calm logic? Prayer? A few years ago, I dealt with a furious neighbor. She was upset with the world and wanted my advice. She had cut herself off from several friends to the point that it affected her family and her overall lifestyle. I was part of her anger equation and saw no real need for what seemed to be misplaced or secondary anger and could not figure out the issue. She was irrational.

I told her she was loved, and we understood she was angry and would pray for her in two ways. First, God would lead me to a better understanding of her will. Second, God helps her find a way of dealing with her resentments without choosing to be angry and lashing out at others. The room filled with silence. We hugged, and I left.

Thought For Today: Let us deal at our level to encourage others to be positive through prayer.

Prayer for Today: Let us pray for the homeless unfortunates, starving and trapped in a place without shelter. Pray for the refugees from society, not just the civilians trapped in a war zone or the poor in remote locations, but for the homeless in our towns. Amen

October 6

Egret on Brookview Golf Course
Golden Valley, Minnesota

Ethics

The entire law is summed up in a single command: "Love your neighbor as yourself." (Galatians 5 vs 14)

We hear of issues where people have chosen to be vengeful, upset, or angry daily. Often property line disputes over a few inches of dirt, changes in the workplace, and noisy fun in the neighborhood cause issues. This week a local woman was assaulted by another because she had too many items in an express checkout line. It is interesting what causes anger and stress in our society.

We live in a complex society that seems to have changed over the last several decades. Is it too much to "Love your neighbor" and show respect and tolerance? Is it too hard to turn the other cheek? Or are people getting so opportunistic we have no choice other than to retaliate?

June and I took a course in behavior where it talked about different feelings. We learned that if we look at anger as a secondary feeling created by a hurt, secondary meaning that we choose to be angry rather than hurt. In the Christian sense, that would mean we chose anger over love. Hmm, that is interesting.

Yes, we all seek freedom, and our country's constitution guarantees it. We need to show love and consideration for all every time. Paul's letter tells us how to use this freedom so that we may all enjoy life to its fullest.

Thought for Today: Today, let us focus on our freedoms. When we drive past a church, note its affiliation. When we notice a different person, make a note of their nationality. Notice all the makes of cars and different shaped houses, and note that we are diverse in all ways. Give a thought to the diversity that demonstrates our freedom and enjoy it all.

Prayer for Today: Heavenly Father, we pray that we may focus on the parts of our lives that practice love, patience, and caring. We pray that in our small piece of the world, we may show your love through our behavior. Amen.

Eighth Hole, Brookview Ececutive
Golden Valley, Minnesota.

Be The Best You Can Be

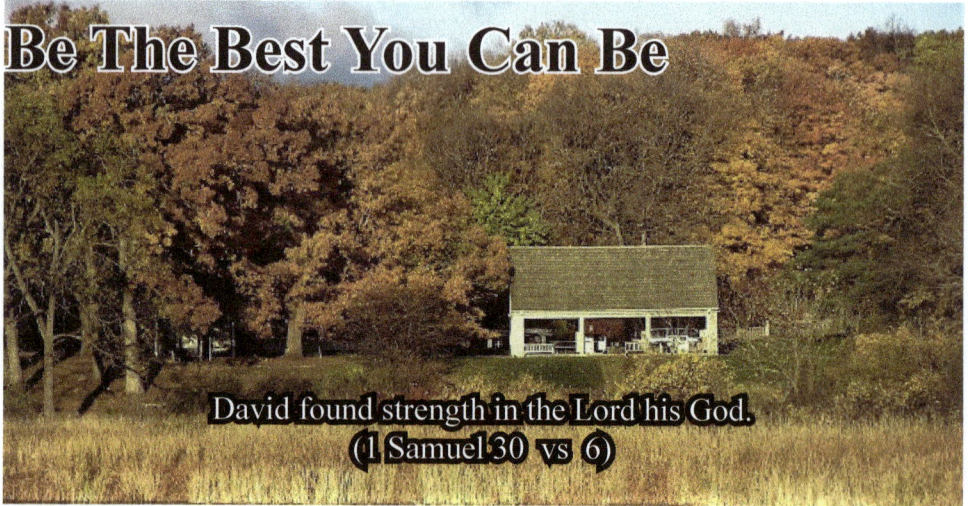

David found strength in the Lord his God.
(1 Samuel 30 vs 6)

Recently I sat alone with Patsy, who was in the middle stages of MS, the part where the disease is starting to take hold, beginning to win. The discussion was not about having an end-of-life experience or about being disabled. It was about doing things differently but doing them. It was about being more tired than before, taking longer to recover, and being OK. It was about waking up sore and using massage, heat, or cold to feel good enough to function for a while. This lady has a heart.

June and I are in our eighties now and considered healthy. Yes, we go to the gym, walk, swim, and do more than most. With that said, there are no more bicycles, skis, or tennis racquets in the shed. We are often out of balance and maybe a bit bent. We are not in our fifties; we were not twenty when we were in our fifties. Our kids were.

As we live life, there will be changes; changes by era and age. Accepting change means accepting diet, pain, vision, balance, and however the good Lord challenges you. We must always be as good as possible in spirit, mind, and body. David found strength in the Lord his God. Pray that you may also.

Thought for Today: We will all have a chance to observe aging or ill people. Let us take a few seconds to pray for them and contribute to their quality of life through our God.

Prayer for Today: Dear Lord, today we pray for those approaching their end-of-life experience. We pray that they recognize your love and that you are with them and work through you to be the best they can be. Amen

October 8 Ordway Picnic Shelter
Minnesota Landscape Arboretum

I Yam What I Yam

I can do all things through Christ who strengthens me.
(Phillipians 4-13)

Was Popeye a philosopher? Cartoonists often are. When Popeye was confronted with difficult situations, he would say, "I yam what I yam?" gulp down his spinach and defend right.

We are not all Popeyes, and we are expected to conform, often to standards below our Christian faith standards, and may face difficulties if we do not. It is necessary to understand who we are, what we are, and keep the Lord in our daily lives. We need our "spinach.".

In many ways, we are continually fighting an image syndrome. Quite often, we get flack because we don't fit. Conformity is the word, and clones are the result.

How did some prophets or John the Baptist fit in with the rest of their society? Probably not too well at times, and they were special. The truth is you are you. You are who God created you to be, and he wants you to know who you are and understand your individual characteristics. No one else is exactly like you. God created you and then broke the mold.

You are unique, and it is all right to be you. Don't let others shape you. That is God's task. He started with you, will finish with you, and will be with you. He is our spinach.
He does want you to be you.

Thought for Today: Let us search for the person that God wants us to be so that we may serve him better.

Prayer for Today: Heavenly Father, as we travel through our weekly chores, we need to see a way to help You. We often lose track of your plan, and sometimes we are too busy and do not understand it. This week we pray that we may find a better way to serve You and make life better for everyone. Amen

Green Heron Pond
Minnesota Landscape Arboretum

Living Lean 1

*I rejoice greatly in the Lord that at last,
you have renewed your concern for me.
Indeed, you have been concerned, but you had no opportunity to show it.
I am not saying this because I am in need,
for I have learned to be content whatever the circumstances
(Philippians 4 vs 10,11)*

Life is exciting, and as we age, we can always look back at our good times and the not-so-good times. Senior citizens will have both in their lives. The interesting piece is that the good times happen when faith is at the forefront of our lives, and the not-so-good tends to be when materialism has taken over. Life is not about things; it's about love and caring. Let me share some stories with you.

We have a friend that is a successful entrepreneur. He owns a plane, three homes, a political career, and an exceptional collection of things. His constant pursuit of things has been of epic proportions. My involvement with his family has let me see the other side. His family does not speak to each other. It is brother versus sister, dad versus mom in a near dysfunctional way. As individuals, each is a friend, and all are beautiful people. However, they are a great example that the love of things does not bring peace of mind or a strong family.

Thought for Today: Let us focus on our spiritual needs rather than our material needs.

Prayer for Today: Dear Lord and father, we live in a glorious world with great opportunities. There are opportunities to serve, opportunities to help others, and opportunities to demonstrate your love through our actions. We ask for the chance to do your will here and support others with our love. Many here forget to do that and chose material and a whimsical lifestyle. We pray for them and ourselves. Amen

October 10

West Waushacum Pond
Sterling, Massachusetts

Living Lean 2

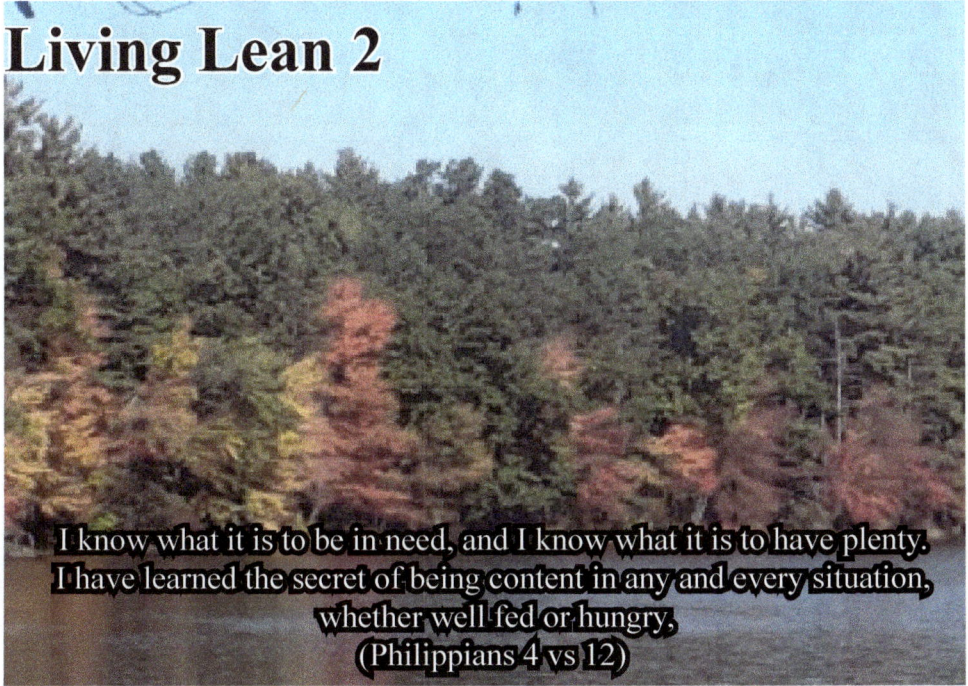

I know what it is to be in need, and I know what it is to have plenty. I have learned the secret of being content in any and every situation, whether well fed or hungry.
(Philippians 4 vs 12)

Following up on yesterday, we know several families with five to fifteen children. They all have good jobs but do not generate millions. They are loving and caring and live life as a family team. Yes, they face the problems of everyday life as we all do. However, when crises are met with caring and love at the forefront and a belief system that allows help from the Lord, the difficult times seem to pass and happiness always prevails. God did not give us a perfect world or a fair world.

My first running buddy here in Minnesota is 83 as I write this. He had six sons and lost his wife several years ago. The dad and two sons live in the family home; one son is disabled, and the other struggles to get a business off the ground. They have worked out a cooperative sharing of talents to be a team. The Lord is with them.

Paul's message to the Philippians was clear. You can be happy when you recognize the spirit of the Lord that is always available to you.

Thought for Today: Let's recognize that we are never alone.
Prayer for Today: Dear Lord, we thank your presence in our lives. Knowing that you are with us is wonderful and satisfying. Amen

Living Lean 3

Whether living in plenty or want,
I can do everything through him who gives me strength.
(Philippians 4 vs 13)

COVID and war changed the world, and large segments of our economy have fallen on hard financial times. The airline and automotive workers are the most obvious. Many of the financially stressed decide to save face by increasing debt. They chose not to live lean and keep all of their things. Others make adjustments to survive and pull together as a team.

The stories of wealth without happiness are many. Mickey Rooney and Liz Taylor had multiple marriages (six or eight?) and everything money could buy, but perhaps not happiness. Are Donald Trump, Brittany Spears, and others happy? We cannot answer that question and must focus on our own needs.

We are often required to live within our means when we feel we deserve more. There is always a temptation to put on a false front. We must remember, "…I can do everything through him who gives me strength."

Thought for Today: Let's use our true strength to help get through the day.

Prayer for Today: Some prayers are worth repeating: Dear lord and father, we live in a glorious world with great opportunities. There are opportunities to serve, opportunities to help others, and opportunities to demonstrate your love through our actions. We ask for the chance to do your will here and support others with our love. Many here forget to do that and choose a material and whimsical lifestyle. We pray for them and ourselves. Amen

Testimony

> For God did not give us a spirit of timidity,
> but a spirit of power, love, and self-discipline.
> So do not be ashamed to testify about our Lord.
> (2 Timothy 1 vs 7, 8)

Paul traveled the world in a constant testimony for God through Christ. He did an easy time in prison once he followed what could only be stated as a hard time. The message above was written while on a kind of death row. Paul knew the end was near; even then, he was testifying and true to his faith.

We had a pastor who used to say that the average Methodist invited a guest to church every 12 years. He was being critical of our ability to testify and invite. He wanted to start including an occasional personal testimony in the Sunday service, so he extended an open invitation to the congregation. No one responded. OOPS! That was a hint as to why we were a declining church. We are very nice but private people.

One of my character defects is that I love to talk (often way too much!). However, that's in my world of family, business, and especially sales. I was way too quiet regarding my faith journey and had a spirit of timidity in that area. Pastor Rick changed that. Thus, now there is this book and weekly messages.

In our world today, we are often in places where testimony regarding our faith is a challenge. We are hushed by rules; at school, scouts, sports, and just about everywhere we go; talking trash is in; talking faith is out. There is hope; we need love and self-discipline to testify and invite people to join us.

Thought for Today: Let us look for an opportunity to discuss our faith. If we are uncomfortable with that, let's find an opening to invite someone to join us this week.

Prayer for Today: Heavenly Father, we pray for the strength to represent you, your ideals, and your will here on earth. We thank you for the opportunity to be at peace and do your work. Amen

Green Mountain
From Freedom, New Hampshire

Eisenhower

He has made us competent as ministers of a new covenant —not of the letter but the Spirit; for the letter kills, but the Spirit gives life.
(2 Corinthians 3 vs 6)

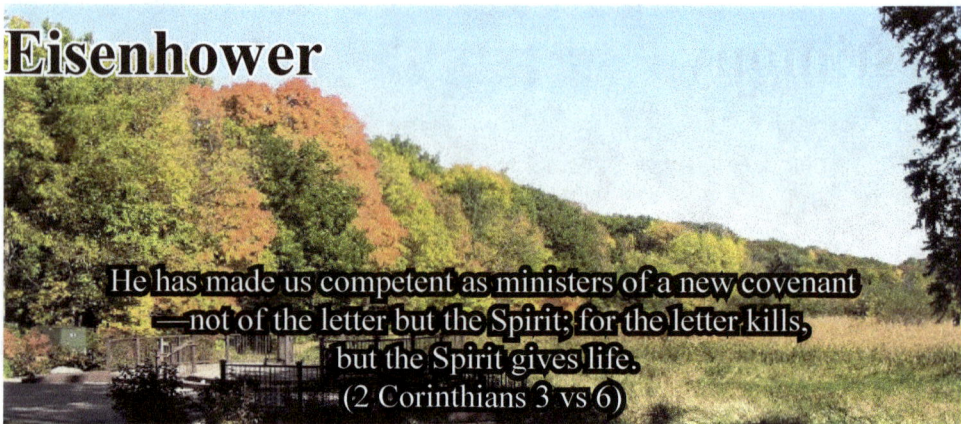

We are in some way the light, ministers of the gospel, or promoters of the Holy Spirit. That is a part of the covenant we make when we join the Christian church. That is a tremendous responsibility, and I certainly don't feel like a "spirit" promoter every day.

I have always had a propensity for relaxing through exercise. Workouts are a daily piece of my life, and pursuing it shows my selfish streak. I made a covenant with myself in my late twenties to be as good as possible. I wanted to be a good dad and husband and believed that fitness was a piece of the equation.

Later in life, June and I decided that fitness was more than physical; i.e., it was spirit, mind, and body. We agreed that we would work on the spirit and mind together, but she was not interested in joining me on my swims, bike rides, and runs. (She was always a bit smarter.) OOPS- that decision meant three times as much work.

Our 34th President, Dwight David Eisenhower, firmly believed in this. He did his morning exercises, and he kept his calendar open for an after-lunch nap. When at the Whitehouse. His colleagues considered him eccentric and selfish, and he felt he needed a scheduled break to be the best he could be for himself and his country.

We all need to be the best we can be for ourselves and our families and serve the Lord. Be a bit selfish so that you can help.

Thought for Today: Today, let's do something for ourselves to help our spirit, mind, and body.

Prayer for Today: Dear Lord, we pray to keep our covenant made to you today, that we are shining your light brightly.. We pray that we are the light of the world so others may find you through us. Amen

Trust In The Lord

But blessed is the man who trusts in the LORD,
whose confidence is in him.
(Jeremiah 17 vs 7)

In the 1990s, June and I enjoyed four weeks of vacation. It was not easy when surrounded by world events. While staying in Pyrford, south of London, there were concerns regarding a serial rapist that had just struck for the ninth time. A sniper started shooting in Washington, DC. There was a bomb in Bali and then a plane crash. It is easy to ask, "Where is God in all of this?" It is logical, by human standards, to feel concerned and helpless. We felt guilty while enjoying a vacation amongst the tragedies.

We need to keep our faith in the Lord through prayer and understanding. He does not expect us to understand everything, love, and trust Him to put it together. Together we need to demonstrate this trust and love to others through times of stress and tragedy. We need to be like a tree with roots planted by the stream. We need to be fresh and always bear the fruit of the Lord; to have this fruit available when others need it.

Thought for Today: Today, let us focus on our fruit and understand what our faith can do for others with less understanding. Let us pray and keep our spiritual fruits fresh to share them with those in need.

Prayer for Today: Heavenly Father, we come to you confused by world events. We are concerned about our issues; unemployment, depleted retirement funds, sickness, and many other problems. Throughout all of this, we pray that we may recognize our role as servants and that we make our spiritual fruits available to those in need. Amen

Exit Maples
Minnesota Landscape Arboretum   **October 15**   **Page 301**

My Body

Praise be to the God and Father of our Lord Jesus Christ, the Father of
compassion and the God of all comfort,
who comforts us in all our troubles, so
that we can comfort those in any trouble with the comfort,
we have received from God.
(2 Corinthians 1 vs 3,4).

Yes, we own our temple, and it needs constant maintenance. Those who know me are expecting a dialog regarding diet and exercise. As an octogenarian, those are important. But being a happy elder is all about the Spirit.

Many octogenarians are angry, and I do not mean unhappy. Life is not perfect, and how we deal with negativity makes the difference. Yes, in aging, we lose capabilities and hopefully taper into our "end of life experience." As Christians, I plead with you to be elderly and happy. Let your family remember your smile and your laugh.

Thought for Today: Let's do what we need to be happy.

Prayer For Today: We Pray that as we approach our end on earth, people will remember us as grateful and happy stewards of our Christian faith. Amen

Who's Law

No one is justified before God by the law,
because the righteous will live by faith.
The law is not based on faith.
(Galatians 3 vs 11, 12)

In Civics class, we learn that we follow a version of the English common law in America. The constitution mixes things up by declaring, "In God, we trust, " then separating Church and State. What a conundrum. We have to deal with the duplicity.

Somehow, each state legislature and congress write thousands of laws, which seem to change yearly. We spend a lot of time adjusting, ignoring, or being unaware of the changes. Governments seem to want to legislate what we know as good Christian ethics; caring about each other, helping others, and developing community. There is no allowance in law for unconditional love and caring for our fellow man.

There is a connection between faith and success. The most successful people follow God's and man's laws. Fortunately, as Christians, when we follow God's law, we align with most government laws and coexist well.

Thought for Today: Let us practice God's law, demonstrate our caring and love of humanity in our actions. Let's show unconditional love in our daily activities.

Prayer for Today: Dear Lord, we pray that we may be strong and follow your law in our toughest moment and most challenging time. Amen

Indian Summer

This is the day
that the Lord has made,
Let us rejoice and be glad in it.
(Psalm 118 vs 24)

In Minnesota, we are experiencing a wonderful Autumn. An "Indian Summer." A freeze followed our first heavy frost; now, we have warm temperatures. A day like this is a gift to us by God that we all appreciate.

During this time, the crabgrass has died; there is color in the leaves; the lawn does not need mowing; the evenings are cool; the garden does not need weeding.

There are many blessings about "Indian Summer," They are easily recognized. Our daily lives have many blessings, but we often do not see and acknowledge them. We try to control our lives and often do not turn enough to God. The more we allow Him to take over, the more blessed our lives become.

The Psalmist says, "...But may all who seek you, rejoice and be glad in you..." As we give thanks for good weather, we also need to give thanks and recognize God's role in our daily lives.

Thought for Today: The fall season is upon us. The busy holidays are approaching us all too swiftly. This week, we can relax and enjoy the dwell-in activities between the end of Summer and the holidays. Let Go and Let God and appreciate the things he will do for us. Let us enjoy by allowing God's will into our daily lives.

Prayer for Today: Father, we pray specifically for those in the world that need food, shelter, and quality of life. For many, the Holy season approaches desperate people. We pray that the prosperous peoples of the world can find a way to do your will. We pray that we may find a way to contribute. Amen

October 18   Lake Harriet
Minneapolis, Minnesota

Positive Attitude

> I know that there is nothing better than for people
> Than to be happy and do good while they live.
> (Ecclesiastes 3 vs 12)

It is interesting to think about what makes us happy, excited, and pleased with our lives. Each of us is different, but I suspect that he had certain things in mind in Paul's letters. I doubt they were what we consider life experiences.

Yesterday on the golf course, I was nervous on the first tee because my game has been suffering all summer. I was in England with my nephew Matt and wanted to do well. My drive went long straight, stopped perfectly, and my approach held the green less than 20 feet from the hole. That is happiness but not what Paul meant by "do good."

Paul was a teacher with a mission. We are tasked to carry on his mission in our faith. The Lord has not given many of us the ability to be preachers or to talk the talk every day. We are not all Evangelists. However, if we are Christians, we are all ministers of the gospel. We preach every day through our actions and the example we set in our daily lives. Knowing that, how do we preach the word?
We need to be "… happy and do good…" always.

Thought for Today: Today, we will be tested; things will not all go well. We need to find a way through our faith to be an example to those around us, an example of good living and happiness.

Prayer for Today: Heavenly Father, today we pray that we may help your cause. We pray for the opportunity to help. Amen

Lake Harriet
Minneapolis, Minnesota   **October 19**   **Page 305**

Operating Style

Walk in his ways, and keep his decrees
and commands, his laws and requirements,
as written in the Law of Moses,
(1 Kings 2 vs 3)

Recently I mentioned the following John Madison quote to a non-believing friend. "We have staked the whole of all our political institutions upon the capacity of mankind for Self-Government, the capacity of each and all of us to govern ourselves, to control ourselves, to sustain ourselves according to the Ten Commandments of God." This story is not a political statement; it is just a story.

His comment was you were doing all right until you got to that last part. So I asked him if he would accept the quote if we substituted "ethical behaviors" for the commandments. He was OK with that. I missed an evangelical opportunity here, but he was looking for an argument, and I was not in the mood.

My two points today are: Political rhetoric is un-godly, self-serving, and often malicious, and human nature's ten commandments and common courtesies are often left aside. We need to pray about that. Second, I find it interesting that my non-believing friend was happy when I removed God from the quote but still accepted the ethics specified in the commandments.

My conclusion is that we need to keep on keeping on. People like my friend are closer than they think. Accepting the ethics of the Commandments is just one step away from receiving the spirit.

Thought for Today: Let's lead by example through obedience to our Lord's commandments.

Prayer for Today: Dear Lord, we thank you for the opportunity to lead and demonstrate that your way is the correct way. We pray we will overcome the many temptations set before us and follow your laws ton the letter. Amen

October 20

West Waushacum Pond
Sterling, Massachusetts

Operating Results

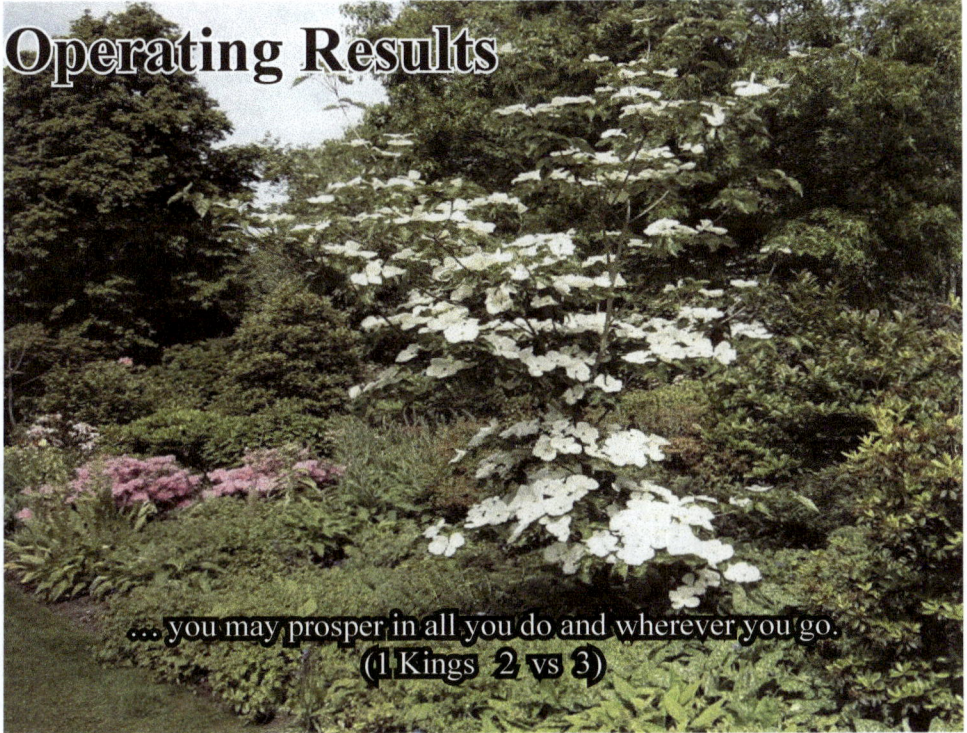

... you may prosper in all you do and wherever you go.
(1 Kings 2 vs 3)

Yesterday we talked about operating within God's laws and Christian ethics. They are essential to us, and we feel good when we function within those limits. Feeling good is important.

Beyond feeling good, I have observed that ethical business was good and led to long-term profits in my forty years of doing business. The bad guys seem to get all the publicity; Ponzi schemes, Enron, and fraud generate headlines. It appears that the new generations believe that profitable business is ripping off people. A low online price replaces the win-win of the 1980s.

My point is that yesterday the quote was about self-governance and the commandments. My point today is that successful businesses also follow and meet those same standards. When they do, we are all blessed.

Thought for Today: Let us follow those same standards and commandments in our business and personal activities.

Prayer for Today: Dear Lord, we thank you for the opportunity to lead and demonstrate that your way is the correct way. We pray we will overcome the many temptations set before us and follow your laws ton the letter. Amen

RHS Wisley Grarden
Wisley, Sussex, UK

Faith And Life

Photo by Stephanie Symmes

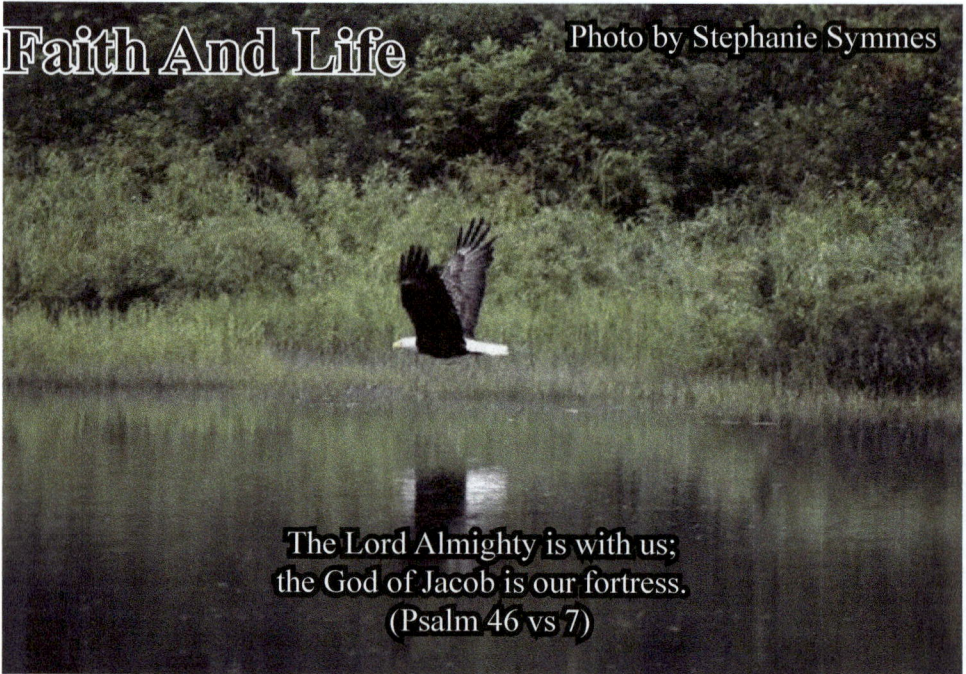

The Lord Almighty is with us;
the God of Jacob is our fortress.
(Psalm 46 vs 7)

Since September 11, 2001, the World has changed drastically. For the first time in history, Americans realize the fear of attack. In 2020, COVID and its variants changed our social structure and how we interact. Our society has become more violent, and Russia seems to have started a war that will affect the World.

June and I have developed a strong faith during our lives. We often quote the Psalmist who wrote the 23rd psalm- those familiar words, "Even though I walk through the valley of the shadow of death, I will fear no evil, for you are with me." The Psalmist does not say that we will not have to walk through the darkest valley or that evil does not exist. Instead, the Psalmist reminds us that we need not fear or be overwhelmed because God is present with us at all times and places. God will see us through. The ground and content of our hope is the promise that nothing in all creation can separate us from God's love.

Thought for the Today: Since those who walk with God are never alone, let us focus on our faith and live a normal life.

Prayer for the Today: Almighty God, when the foundations of our lives are shaken, hold us close to you and remind us that you will never leave or forsake us. You alone are our hope and security. Amen.

October 22 Eagle over the Ossipee River
Effingham Falls, New Hampshire

Courage

Be strong and very courageous.
Be careful to obey all the law my servant Moses gave you
(Joshua 1 vs 7)

Often we are tempted to take shortcuts to success. One technique is to leave someone out of the loop because we do not want to deal with their point of view. Sometimes take action on our own out of arrogance; we know it is the right thing to do. That is the operating style of some successful people. The word is control.

Another way to operate is to delegate that control. People who delegate often seem uninvolved, and some are. Successful delegators trust others to make decisions and manage with minimum supervision. In our homes and at work, this can be successful.

Now I have to ask if our style is what works? Or is it our beliefs? People with strong spirituality and a God-like manner tend to be successful players in life. They build trust with their peers, are liked, and generate a comfortable environment within their relationships. Successful people are "...strong and very courageous...do not turn from it to the right or the left...meditate on it day and night," When people follow those laws, they succeed no matter their operating style.

Thought for the Day: We have read, heard, and recited God's laws many times. We have slipped a few times and broken a few. Today let us focus on being "tough and courageous" in our efforts. Let us focus on keeping our spirituality and beliefs at the forefront of our activities.

Prayer for Today: Heavenly Father, we are approaching the great season of joy and Thanksgiving, a season when you are worshiped and thanked by many religions and languages. We pray that we may have the courage and strength to do your will during Thanksgiving. Amen

Harvest

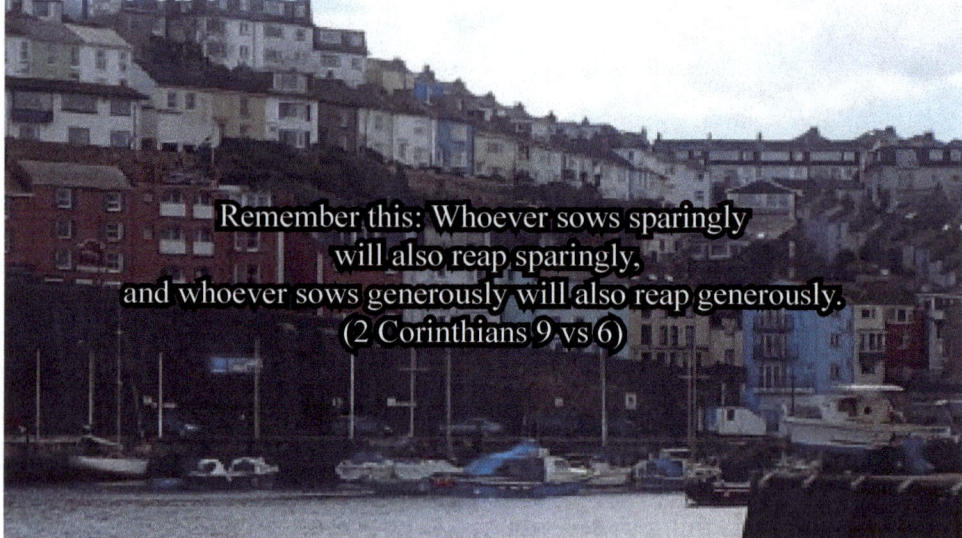

> Remember this: Whoever sows sparingly
> will also reap sparingly,
> and whoever sows generously will also reap generously.
> (2 Corinthians 9 vs 6)

Since retirement and downsizing in 2006, June and I have not had the benefit of gardens as we had at our home for twenty-seven years. Long hours were spent tending them, and we had a bountiful harvest. We do not miss all that work because we have other harvests.

As apartment dwellers, we have forty to fifty days a year to fill that used to be spent gardening. Those days are spent together sowing seeds in our relationship, spending time with others, and helping where we did not have time in the past. The crop is now a closer relationship with each other and friends.

This different harvest is a blessing. Paul's analogy of reaping crops in his message in Corinth is still valid. We all need to sow seeds daily in relationships, our minds, and each other to reap the harvest of love and friendship.

Thought for Today: Let's take a quick look at our calendar and see where we can sow seeds for our future, our worldly lot, and the Lord because He is our real future.

Prayer for Today: Dear Lord, we live in a world of hate and anger. This week we pray that we may sow seeds of love that will temper negativity and help spread love in our world. Amen.

October 24

Brixham Harbor
Devon, UK

Healing

> But for you who revere my name,
> the sun of righteousness will rise with healing in its wings.
> (Malachi 4 vs. 2)

Some diseases require medical treatment, and some by other means. Attitude helps with spiritual growth, especially with mental and chemical dependency issues. When I say "helped," please do not substitute the word "cured." Church workers, pastors, and lay ministers that do hospice-type visits seem to deal with serious illness better than people who ask, "why me."

I want to go with this to discuss depression, a disease that seems to be growing in today's fast-moving society. Experience shows that those diagnosed have mostly lost touch with their spiritual side. They feel alone, hopeless, incapable of dealing with life, and unable to recognize God is with them. They are most often impatient with God.

A case in point is a friend who is clinically depressed but deeply religious. That seems like a catch-22, but it is true. On Sunday, many people in the church are searching for something, seeking peace and coming away empty. They leave it behind by having a closed mind. That's the disease.

As Christians, we need to learn to recognize our friends, reach out to them, and help them grow to know the spirit of Christ. Spiritual growth is the answer, and we are the tool placed here to help.

Thought for Today: Let's call or talk to a friend in need; let's help.

Prayer for Today: Dear Lord, today we are thankful for our many blessings; of the spirit, the mind, and the body. We appreciate what we are. Amen

Brixham Harbor
Devon, UK

Sincerity

> Love must be sincere.
> Hate what is evil; cling to what is good.
> (Romans 12 v 9).

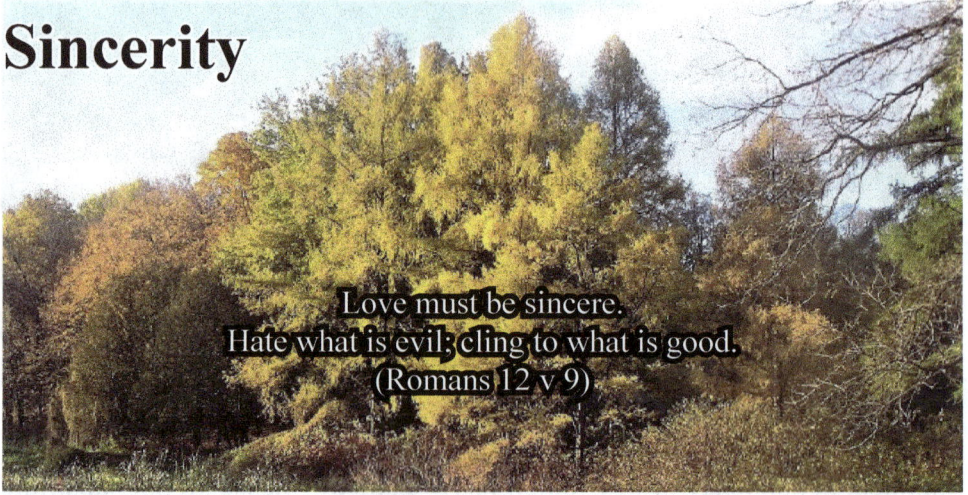

Love versus evil and hanging on to what is good sounds simple. In life and relationships, the definition of good and evil has a variety of meanings and are analog terms. Those meanings are often personal and evolve through relationships based on a person's point of view. They change from personal to business and become confused based on each individual's socialization.

In business, there are sociopathic managers (from Kurt Vonnegut); in our personal life, different lifestyles are considered "evil" or unaccepted by others. I am not talking about evil in murder, rape, and criminal activity- just simple things that are often unacceptable. For today let's take a few standards from my life observations.

Some issues are defined within a couple's relationship; considered "evil" by some acceptable to others. In divorce cases, issues of abusive behavior are often truly evil. I remember stopping at a friend's house at 9 am on a Saturday and sitting in his kitchen listening to him complain because his wife was still asleep and had not yet made the morning coffee. That standard was unbelievable to me. In his mind he was suffering abuse- in my mind, he needed to make some coffee. (Oh, and maybe bring her a cup in bed.)

Through the years we have all heard stressed couples express their spouse's evils: too much time at work; too much golf, hunting or fishing; shopping, spending, etc. These are all not evil but negotiable in a healthy relationship. These are communication issues rather than good versus bad.

In the business world, I agree with Mr. Vonnegut regarding sociopathic management; management that crosses the line between good management and abusive behavior. Recently there have been examples of management actions that have made headlines and hurt thousands if not millions. These are major league. My example is a simpler one.

For a short time in the 60's my engineering manager used to fire one engineer per quarter- Four a year just to make sure the rest were uncomfortable. Of course, I learned about this practice the day I started because I filled a cubicle that had housed the last victim the previous Friday. The style was to lay off someone on Friday morning and call in two or three in the afternoon and advise them to shape up of they would be next/ This was the most abusive person I ever worked for and he was very close to sociopathic in his management practices.

In summary, Paul's message works in all phases of life- Clinging to and living to acceptable standards generates happiness and long term success. Even in today's world.

Thought for the Day: Today let us be sincere in every activity.
Prayer for Today: Dear Lord and Father, today I pray to be at peace and see no evil. I pray that through my love and caring others will grow in your spirit. Amen

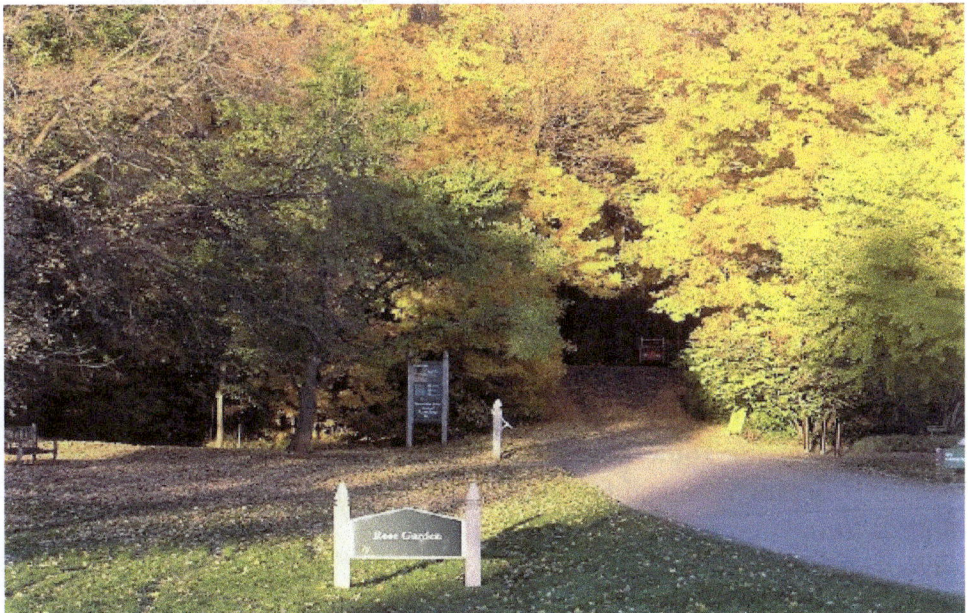

Fall Color
Minnesota Landscape Arboretum   **October 26**   **Page 313**

Our Rock

Photo by Stephanie Symmes

There is no one holy like the LORD;
there is no one besides you;
there is no Rock like our God.
(1 Samuel 2 vs 2)

Growing up in New England, we often fished in streams and frequently crossed them by stepping from rock to rock. We got cold and wet when we stepped on a loose one or slipped. The analogy to the passage is that we chose the wrong rock! That is not an option with God.

The Lord is the rock of our life, our foundation, and always with us. We forget that simple truth; we will not let Him in to help when we feel lonely. During those times, we can feel cold and lonely. (Hopefully not wet.)

Prayer and devotionals will help that situation. If you are reading this today, you are probably sitting squarely on the rock.

Thought for Today: Let's be aware of our foundation, our rock.
Prayer for Today: Heavenly Father, I recognize you and thank you for being my rock and foundation. I pray to identify someone who has slipped from your rock and help them.
Amen

Fear No Evil

But now, this is what the Lord says, "Don't be afraid,
for I have ransomed you;
I have called you by name; you are mine.
When you go through deep waters and great trouble, I will be with you.
When you go through rivers of difficulty, you will not drown.
When you walk through the fires of oppression, be burned up, the flames
will not consume you."
(Isaiah 43 vs 1,2)

Since 2001, with COVID, and other issues, our society has realized that we are at risk of harm at home. As Americans, fear seems to have become a resident in our neighborhoods, living rooms, and daily lives. Not the instantaneous fear felt when we have a close call in an accident or other one-time event, but a subtle hollow fear about our security.

After 911, our neighbor canceled a bicycle trip to the south of France. My doctor canceled a vacation trip to Italy. June and I went to the UK for a visit, and our children were concerned. Now, people generally feel different when going downtown.

Read Isaiah 43 carefully and understand the message. As Christians, we need not let fear change our lives. Yes, we have fear today but have a tool to alter that fear and convert it to concern: our faith through meditation and prayer. Spirituality is our ultimate protection plan.

Thought for the Day: Let us all focus on our fears. Recognize them as accurate; pray about them and ask God for guidance. Let us change our fears and move them down one level to concerns. Remember the 23rd Psalm, "Even though I walk through the valley of the shadow of death, I will fear no evil, for you are with me..."

Prayer for Today: Dear Lord, the last few years events are beyond our comprehension. We pray that through fear, terror, and war, there will emerge a global understanding, peace, and a world where love and respect are at the forefront. We ask for your guidance in all of this. Amen.

Ossipee River
Effingham Falls, New Hsmpshire   **October 28**   **Page 315**

Hide

Photo by Stephanie Symmes

:Can anyone hide from me?
Am I not everywhere in all of Heaven and Earth?
(Jeremiah 23 vs 24)

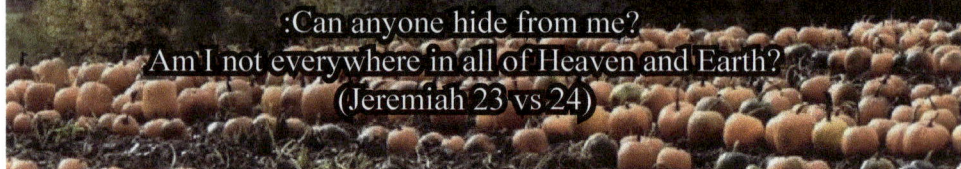

How do we do God's work here on earth? How do we make sure that what we are doing follows His plan? These are questions that are often in our minds. When we awake, we dive into our daily routines, off to the office, school, or whatever. We rarely set a goal to "follow the Spirit," but somehow, we experience the fruits mentioned by Paul in his letter to the Galatians.

In September, a friend asked me about a career opening that he needed to fill for his nonprofit company. As I thought about it, my contacts that fit were unavailable, and those available did not work. God was not ready yet.

That Friday, I called to console an application engineer laid off that day. She mentioned that her dream would be "to find a career where she would be working for more than just money. Perhaps a nonprofit." WOW, was God ready?

The parties are together now, and we are thankful God's will was done. The Spirit is present, and the fruits of "love, joy, peace, and patience" somehow came together because three people were willing to follow the Spirit.

Life is good when we do.

Thought for the Day: As we go through this week, let us think about the millions of people in transition. Let us each make a call to someone and console them. If they talk, let us listen. You never know where the discussion may lead.

Prayer: Heavenly Father, we live in a confusing and angry world. People are feeling economic pressure. There is terrorism, war, conflict, and deceit everywhere we turn. Somehow we pray that we can continue to follow the Spirit and experience its fruits. Amen

God Is Ready

But the fruit of the Spirit is love, joy, peace, patience,
kindness, goodness, gentleness, and self-control.
Against such a thing, there is no law.
...Since we live by the Spirit, let us keep in step with the Spirit.
(Galatians 5 vs 22-25)

How do we do God's work here on earth? How do we make sure that what we are doing follows His plan? These are questions that are often in our minds. When we awake, we dive into our daily routines, off to the office, school, or whatever. We rarely set a goal to "follow the Spirit," but somehow, we experience the fruits mentioned by Paul in his letter to the Galatians.

In September, a friend asked me about a career opening that he needed to fill for his nonprofit company. As I thought about it, my contacts that fit were unavailable, and those available did not work. God was not ready yet.

That Friday, I called to console an application engineer laid off that day. She mentioned that her dream would be "to find a career where she would be working for more than just money. Perhaps a nonprofit." WOW, was God ready? The parties are together now, and we are thankful God's will was done. The Spirit is present, and the fruits of "love, joy, peace, and patience" somehow came together because three people were willing to follow the Spirit.

Life is good when we do.

Thought for the Day: As we go through this week, let us think about the millions of people in transition. Let us each make a call to someone and console them. If they talk, let us listen. You never know where the discussion may lead.

Prayer for Today: Heavenly Father, we live in a confusing and angry world. There is terrorism, war, conflict, and deceit everywhere we turn. Somehow we pray that we can continue to follow the Spirit and experience its fruits. Amen

Pumpkin Harvest
Kingston, New Hampshire

October 30

Halloween

On October 31st, 1991, Halloween was a significant event in the northern part of the United States. We had two events to prepare for; children trick or treating and June's departure to the UK for a family visit on November 1st. Mother nature also had a plan that she had not consulted with me on; the great Halloween three-day blizzard in Minnesota was a piece of what is now known as "The Perfect Storm."

Paul told the Philippians, "Do not be anxious about anything..." but millions of Americans were anxious that weekend. People died on lost ships on the Grand Banks, and Minneapolis had 30 inches of snow. But it was not all bad on our end. Let me explain.

We had a temperature drop in the early afternoon, and a snowstorm started. There were six inches of snow on the ground, and we prayed for the children's safety. That is not unusual in Minnesota in the fall, and we did not expect it to be anything but a fun Halloween. We had already decorated the outside of the house with Christmas lights, so we turned them on. The lights drew a large group of Halloween revelers. We met them with a special greeting, "Ho Ho Ho, Happy Halloween."

There were 15 inches of snow in the morning, and the visibility was near zero. A trip to the airport seemed impossible. We decided to depart after lunch for a 6:30 flight, and the twenty-minute drive took over two hours and was very dangerous. June's flight departed 3 hours late, and I had a three-hour ride home. Happy Halloween.

Tonight is Halloween; enjoy it with your neighborhood goblins.

Thought for Today: Halloween is a special day, and we should enjoy it with the revelers. We should also think back to 1991 and be prayerful.

Prayer for the Day: Heavenly Father, we pray for children on a day they look forward to each year. We pray that they are safe and have a great evening. We give thanks for their presence in our lives. Amen

November

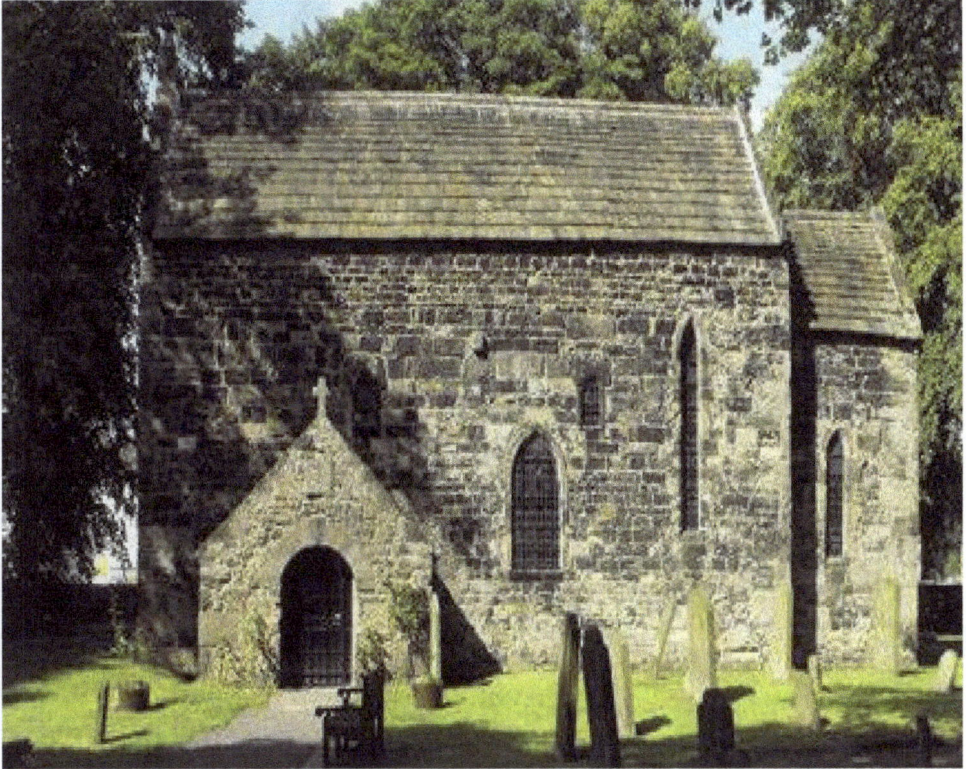

St. Johns Church

St Johns Church, Escomb ,was built in the 7th or 8th century AD when the area was part of the Anglican Kingdom of Northumberland, and has been called "England's earliest complete church."

Be Real

Love must be sincere.
Hate what is evil; cling to what is good.
Be devoted to one another in brotherly love.
(Romans 12 vs 9)

Open and honest is a great way to go through life. Where did Jesus end up when he tried it? There are two answers. One is "On the Cross." The Christian answer is "At the right hand of God." It is sometimes a good idea to keep our thoughts to ourselves in our world. Sometimes being open or honest will cost you, and in workplaces differing from the leadership's opinion can hurt your career. At church, differences are often divisive, and we need to pray about that.

In 2005, at my workplace, I chose to be open and honest with a new company vice president. My openness accelerated my retirement and ended my employment. It is something that is OK at age 65 but would have been a crushing blow at age 50. It is an issue for all faithful Christians.

As we travel through life, we must work to keep bread on the table. Sometimes we will be tempted to hold back for self-preservation. We need to *"Never be lacking in zeal, but keep your spiritual fervor, serving the Lord. Be joyful in hope, patient in affliction, and faithful in prayer."* (Romans 12 vs 11 & 12) In the long run, we work for the Lord, but there is a fine line that we need to walk in life.

Thought for Today: We often have to decide about "being real." Today let us focus on demonstrating sincerity, zeal, and joy through the patience we are blessed with through Jesus.

Prayer for Today: Dear Lord, we are surrounded by the love of Jesus as we approach the holiday season. It is a time of social pressures as well as great joy. Today we pray for those who have a problem experiencing this joy. We pray they find the belief and experience the circumstance to give them everlasting peace. Amen

Bill's Big Book

> He replied, "Blessed rather are those
> who hear the word of God and obey it."
> (Luke 11 vs 28)

Twelve-step programs are based on Dr. Bill's Big book written for Alcoholics Anonymous. It guides spiritual growth through twelve steps and is a way to let go of negativity. It is used for weight loss, drugs, and numerous other complex personal challenges the human race faces.

A vital piece of it is an admission of past wrongs and recognizing we will be forgiven. That is an essential piece of life that we need to acknowledge. (Or at least I do). We were not and will not live perfect lives, and our humanness gets in the way. For example, a senior pastor in our bible study keeps talking about his thoughts regarding Sophia Loren. Another younger man mentions Madonna, and there are lawyers in the group who need to represent clients who need protection from an unknown truth. These issues can lead to guilt.

Growing up, my church did not have confession at any level. Massachusetts was a Catholic-dominated state, so I had many Catholic friends who were required to go to confession weekly. I did not even understand why. I do now. Accumulating wrongs or guilt at any level is dangerous, creates a negative personality, and inhibits spiritual growth. Our faith is sure, we have a guarantee, but in our weakness, we sometimes fail. Recognizing our mistakes and learning to accept Christian forgiveness keeps us on a path to spiritual growth. That is the real reason for confession.

Thought for Today: Let's tell it like it is, or at least as we understand it.

Prayer for Today: Heavenly Father, today, tomorrow, we pray that truth will win out. With your help and our honesty, life will prevail. Amen

Deal With Worry

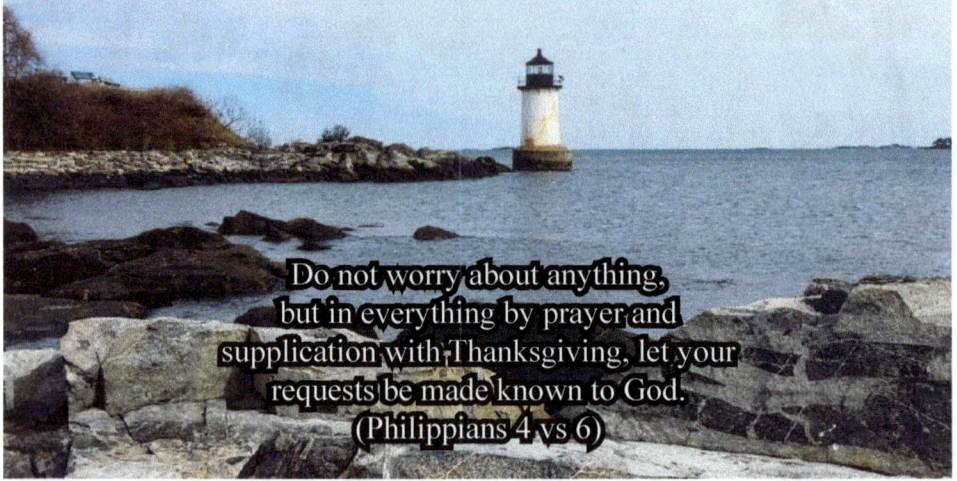

> Do not worry about anything, but in everything by prayer and supplication with Thanksgiving, let your requests be made known to God.
> (Philippians 4 vs 6)

We are in the holiday season, a time of great joy, Thanksgiving, and love. We share with others, we give more freely than we do at other times of the year, and often it is a time when we miss loved ones that are not with us. We need to pray about that.

Yes, the term "blue Christmas" applies to everyone to some degree. It is easy to mask sadness during this period of celebration. Each year in our family, we follow a tradition started by my mom. The children and grandchildren come help trim our tree. It is chaotic with the excited grandchildren. It is a blessing and a joy that my mom started years ago. She is gone now and missed every year.

It is essential to acknowledge the blue piece of Christmas rather than bury it in celebration.

Thought for Today: Let us focus on the spiritual piece of the holiday season. Take an honest look at our whole selves. Acknowledge the many blessings we are experiencing and the sadness of things and people we will miss. Let us pray to God, giving thanks for the blessings while asking for relief from our sorrow. Let us use prayer to help fade the color "blue" in our celebrations.

Prayer for Today: Heavenly Father, we are in a joyous season of celebration. Many of us have lost loved ones. We pray for personal peace, knowing our lost loved ones are with you. Amen

November 3 Fort Pickering Light
Salem, Massachusetts

He Comes Through

**With my whole heart,
I will praise his holy name.
(Psalm 103 vs2)**

Every day the Lord gives us blessings. It is easy to forget the role He plays in our lives in our busyness. Here are three events that made me think of the Lord this week.

Early in the week, a friend and I discussed what we prayed about. They were guidance, support, internal peace, and several others. It was apparent that neither of us prayed for favors or help. We realized that through prayer, good things would happen.

Later in the week, a young athlete competing for a chance to compete in the Olympics collapsed and died. Why? That is a big question and certainly something that makes people doubt. When the final reports are in on this, somehow good will come from his young life. It is too soon for mortals to understand.

The third event that brought the Lord to the forefront was a Good News buddy from San Diego correspondence about his return home after a firestorm that ravaged his neighborhood. There were 15 of 47 houses destroyed on his street, plus the sanctuary of his church. Here are the words he used in closing his correspondence:

"Truly, God is good. Many lessons are to be learned, and many prayers are answered. To God be the Glory."

Thought for Today: Today will be just like many others. Our calendars are crowded, we will have unreasonable demands on our time, and we will need to focus on making it all happen. Let's take a few minutes and think about the Lord's role in our lives with that in mind. Let's let Him into our day.

Prayer for Today: Dear Lord and Father, today we pray to see the results of your participation in our lives and the ability to accept what we do not understand. We trust that good things will happen. Amen

Hampton Beach State Park
Hampton Beach, New Hampshire   **November 4**   Page 323

Personal Care

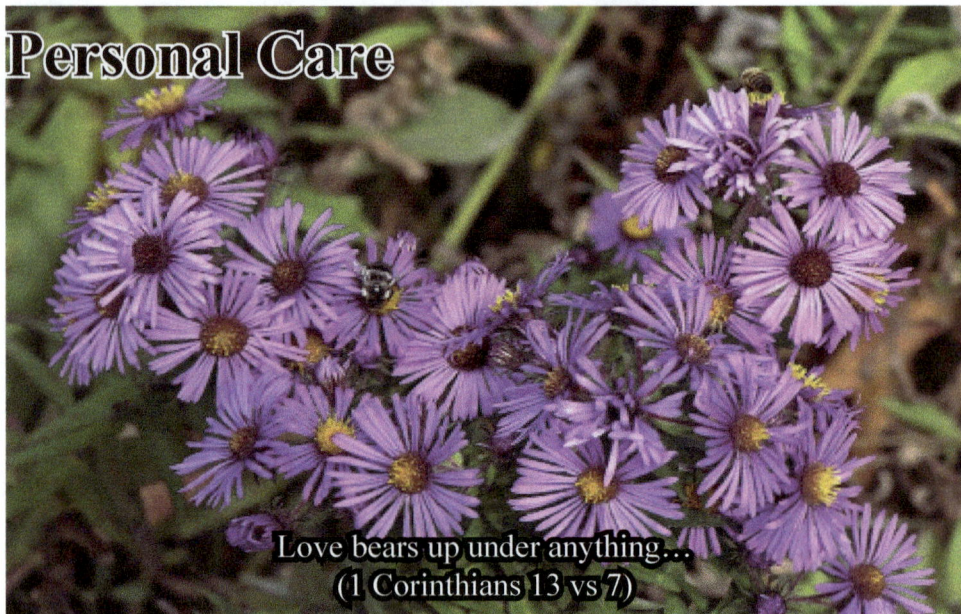

Love bears up under anything...
(1 Corinthians 13 vs 7)

The Pandemic has created a new normal. In 2001, the attacks of September did the same. There is deep-seated resentment regarding the changes. There are concerns regarding our safety; travel is more complex, and we are changing our style of operation and the way we live our lives.

Those are some of the reasons these devotionals exist. Meditation works and helps bring us back to reality. A good example is a friend with chronic degenerative back problems for over 15 years, tired of pain killers and muscle relaxants and meditated to the point of self-hypnosis. She reduced her drugs to one-quarter of her previous dosage.

Taking time to pray and to love will improve our lives.

Thought for Today: Let us take time with our families and God. Let us contribute to peace and tranquility rather than helping increase stress.

Prayer for Today: Heavenly Father, please guide us to contribute to peace and friendship. Please help us do your will through our presence here on Earth. Give me the good judgment to stop and pray rather than react. Amen.

Home Care

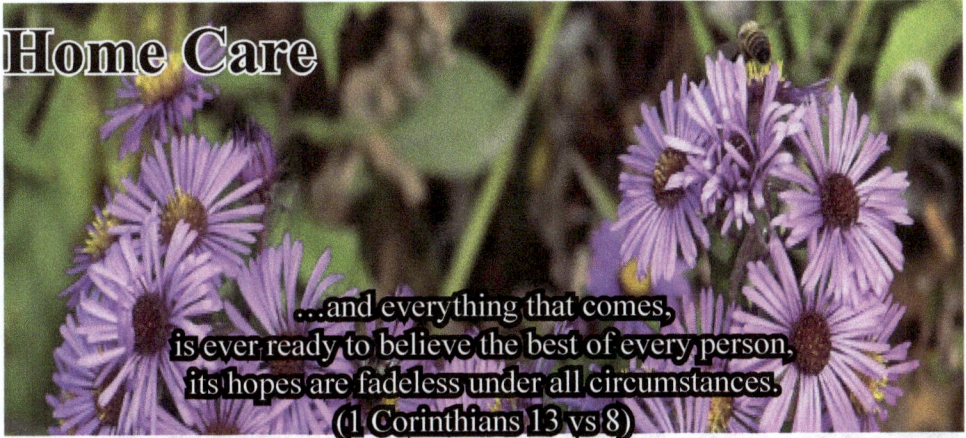

…and everything that comes, is ever ready to believe the best of every person, its hopes are fadeless under all circumstances.
(1 Corinthians 13 vs 8)

Following from yesterday:

One of the things they teach in sales training is always to be ready for the "sales call" or meeting. Sit in the car before entering the building and review in your mind why you are there and what you hope to accomplish; focus. It works in sales and life. We always need to be ready for the events of the day.

We tend to carry our work problems into the home at night and let our frustrations affect our family. The children bring home their frustrations from school, mom and dad from their jobs (or from a bad round of golf), or the evening traffic. Tonight, when you go home, try sitting in the driveway and read this week's passage and leave the stress behind. Why? Pray that you can go into the house in a loving and caring mood and contribute to a peaceful and loving environment called home.

Thought for Today: Someone once said that we are all salesmen at times. My example of preparing for a meeting is a serious part of business life and success. This week, let us focus on "preparing for the meeting" with our families and God. Let us contribute to peace and tranquility rather than helping increase stress.

Prayer: Heavenly Father, in our world today, there is war, fear of attack, theft, and many hostile forces. Please help us do your will through our presence here on Earth. Somehow, please guide us to contribute to peace and friendship, show me how to act when stressed, and give me the good judgment to stop and pray rather than react. Amen.

Protect Our Hearts

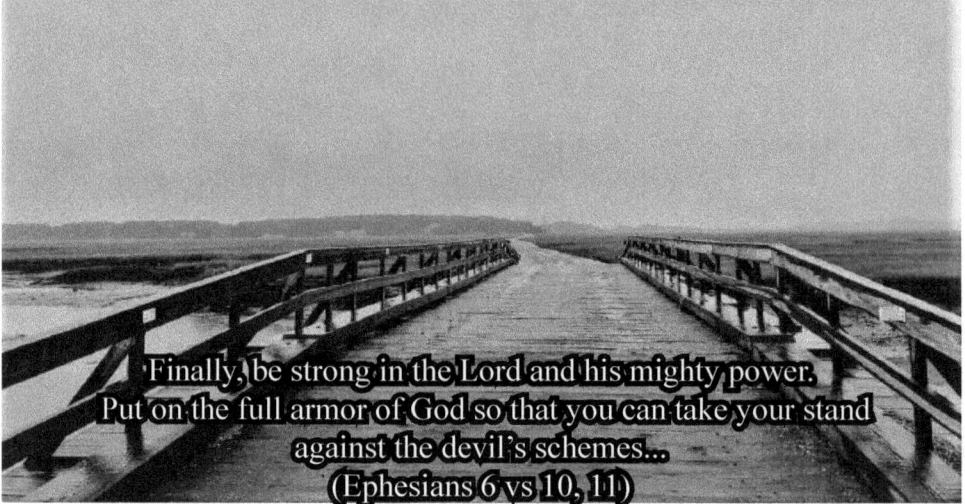

Finally, be strong in the Lord and his mighty power. Put on the full armor of God so that you can take your stand against the devil's schemes...
(Ephesians 6 vs 10, 11)

Today we need to protect ourselves from our self-induced stress and the negativity in the World that we cannot control. The question is, how? Mac Hammond from the Living Word Christian Center says, "We need to protect our hearts."

Over the years, I have often heard the expression, "When the going gets tough, the tough get going." In business and sports, this meant that when the pain sets in, run harder; when it is a breakpoint, put the ball away; when the order is being lost, dig deeper. In each instance, "I" assumed full responsibility for correcting "my" problem. My male ego would come into the issue and apply pressure to the situation. I changed my thoughts on that in the 1980s.

I needed help from someone with more power, God. Think about that for yourself.

Thought for Today: Today is the first day of the rest of our lives. Let us move forward through daily prayer and let the Lord help..

Prayer for Today: Heavenly Father, life is good. The kids have food and shoes, there are two cars in the garage, and TV sets in every home- we are genuinely "fat cats" living under your domain. Today we all want to thank you for the physical needs that we have met and ask for help daily, meeting our spiritual needs. Amen

Bridge to Lieutenant Island
Wellfleet, Massachusetts

November 7

Protect Our Hearts 2

Stand firm then, with the belt of truth buckled around your waist,
with the breastplate of righteousness in place,
and with your feet fitted with the readiness that
comes from the gospel of peace...
And pray in the Spirit on all occasions
with all kinds of prayers and requests.
With this in mind, be alert and always keep on praying ...
(Ephesians 6 vs 13, 18)

Continuing from yesterday:

When my two youngest were in private colleges, my ego-driven logic failed like many parents. The financial pressure combined with the desire to serve the educational needs was too much to get through. This independent guy needed help, and it came through the simple saying, "Let go and let God." Funny how that works. Everything turned out OK.

When deeply involved with our loved ones, we must protect our hearts, keep our feet on the ground, and make caring decisions through love. Keep on asking for support through prayer. If we allow the Lord to help protect our hearts and listen to Him and accept His part in our lives, our lives will be better and more straightforward.

Thought for Today: We have a chance to renew ourselves, forgive others, and move forward with positive thoughts.

Prayer for Today: Heavenly Father, life is good. Today we all want to thank you for the physical needs that we have met and ask for help daily, meeting our spiritual needs. Amen

Lieutenant Island
Wellfleet, Massachusetts

November 8

Global Peace

> Whatever you have learned or
> received or heard from me,
> or seen in me—put it into practice.
> And the God of peace will be with you.
> (Philippians 4 vs 8,9)

There are over 300 million people in America and billions worldwide. As individuals, we are not statistically significant. But we all know that statistics can be manipulated and misrepresented. Indeed, each of us is significant to God within our Christian faith. In many of Paul's letters, he advised that "God will be with you." I will add, personally, upfront and close.

As statistically insignificant as the mathematicians make us, God gives us meaning, power, and faith. We are the power of one. As Christians, we can impact the world one individual at a time through our faith. When we demonstrate that we are at peace, we infect those around us. When we demonstrate good Christian ethics, we lead others to follow us. When we are at peace, others want to join us.

Our challenge as people of faith is to work our peace so others will join us. We all know of pyramid schemes and chain letters. Through our faith, we have an opportunity to be at the top of a living chain. Each day we are at peace through our faith, and we will positively affect our environment.

Thought for Today: It is challenging but exciting to think that we can affect others with our positive actions. This week let us consider others and, by example, share our hope regarding our future.

Prayer for Today: Heavenly Father, we see and hear ugliness in the world. There are wars, revolutions, and a worldwide refugee crisis. Our streets are unsafe, and our institutions have too many negative financial issues. It is hard to understand where you are when we are bombarded daily with these issues. We pray for an understanding of your role and that we may participate in an overall solution. Amen

November 9 Rye Harbour Nature Preserve
Rye Harbour, East Sussex, UK

Spiritual Gifts

Now about spiritual gifts, brothers,
...There are different kinds of gifts, but the same Spirit
There are different kinds of service, but the same Lord.
There are different kinds of working,
but the same God works all of them in all men.
(1 Corinthians 12 vs 1-6)

Often the bible mentions the gifts given to us by the Lord. However, in every case, the same Spirit is mentioned. Think about what that means to all of us. Think about us as a team, a Christian body, placed on earth to do God's work. Not alone but as a team.

I have always preferred working with a partner. I believe that two people working as a team is four times better than the best of the two working alone. If that is true, how powerful is a small congregation working together doing God's work?

In the 2004 super bowl, the New England Patriots came out to play without the TV Network's usual fanfare of individual introductions. They came and won as a team. Last week the newspaper's sports page was dedicated to the state girls' soccer championship. It listed the rosters of the two finalists and the state's all-star team. No all-stars were listed on the two teams' rosters playing in the finals. The championship teams won as a team without any all-stars.

We need each other; our Christian family needs to get the job done. So we all "have different gifts but the same spirit." We can all participate and use these gifts to do God's work, but we do not have the gifts to do it alone.

Thought for Today: Let us focus on our talents and God's gifts to us. Let us recognize our gifts and use them to do God's work.

Prayer For Today: Heavenly Father, we ask, "what is it all about?" We pray to you for the ability to better understand it all. We pray for the ability to recognize our gifts and the knowledge on how to utilize them to help. Amen

Always Friends

> Therefore, as God's chosen people, holy and dearly loved,
> clothe yourselves with compassion, kindness,
> humility, gentleness, and patience.
> Bear with each other and forgive whatever
> grievances you may have against one another.
> Forgive as the Lord forgave you.
> (Colossians 3 vs 12-14)

Most of us have a problem feeling like one of "God's chosen people." The control freak in us wants to believe that we chose to follow Him, which is ego-centric and introspective. We all know that we chase Him until he catches us. In our lives, who are "God's Chosen," and what do they do?

This month is Thanksgiving, and one of my traditions is to do Christmas greetings. Each card and letter that gets addressed is to someone special. The addressees have all played a role in my life, including friends, advisors, mentors, coaches, etc. It is a wonderful feeling to sit there and think about each of them (you). Are they God's chosen people?

The holiday season is an excellent opportunity to celebrate Christ's birth and life. It is also a chance to think of the many people God has placed into our lives that have demonstrated "… compassion, kindness, humility, gentleness, and patience..." A priest in the UK included me in his daily prayers during my cancer period, another is a running buddy of over thirty-five years duration, and several former pastors who were spiritual advisors… the list goes on.

Thought for Today: This week, let us think about our friends. Let us remember why they are, who they are, and what they mean to us.

Prayer for Today: Dear Lord and Father, we have many blessings you have given us. Among them are our friends and contacts, and each of them is a blessing. This week we offer our prayers for their health and happiness and thank you for presenting them to us and that we may all get through this 2020 holiday season healthy and thankful. Amen.

Sculpture Garden

November 11   Minnesota Landscape Arboretum

Love

Many waters cannot quench love;
rivers cannot wash it away. If one were to give
all the wealth of his house for love,
it would be utterly scorned.
(Song of Songs 8 vs 7).

In our over fifty years of marriage, one of the discoveries that June and I made is:

As we developed our spirituality, we became spiritually intimate. We had a deeper understanding of each other than I thought was possible. It minimizes walking on eggshells and the fear of raising questions and allows us to live confidently.

Worshiping together and sharing ourselves with others has created a special bond. This bond, in my mind, is a gift from God that we were somehow open to receiving and did not recognize when it arrived. Somehow we learned to share our hurts, concerns, frustrations, and joys.

We are glad and thank God that we received it.

Thought for Today: As we take our personal and corporate walk through life, let us keep the Lord a priority and a commitment.

Prayer for Today: Dear Lord, we pray that we can let Your love and spirit into our hearts; we renew our commitment to Christ so that we will be his sister or brother. Amen.

Red Barn
November 12 Minnesota Landscape Arboretum

Unseen

Therefore, we do not lose heart. Though outwardly, we are wasting away, yet inwardly we are being renewed daily. For our light and momentary troubles are achieving for us an eternal glory that far outweighs them all. So we fix our eyes not on what is seen, but on what is unseen. For what is seen is temporary, but what is unseen is eternal.
(2 Corinthians 4 vs 16-18)

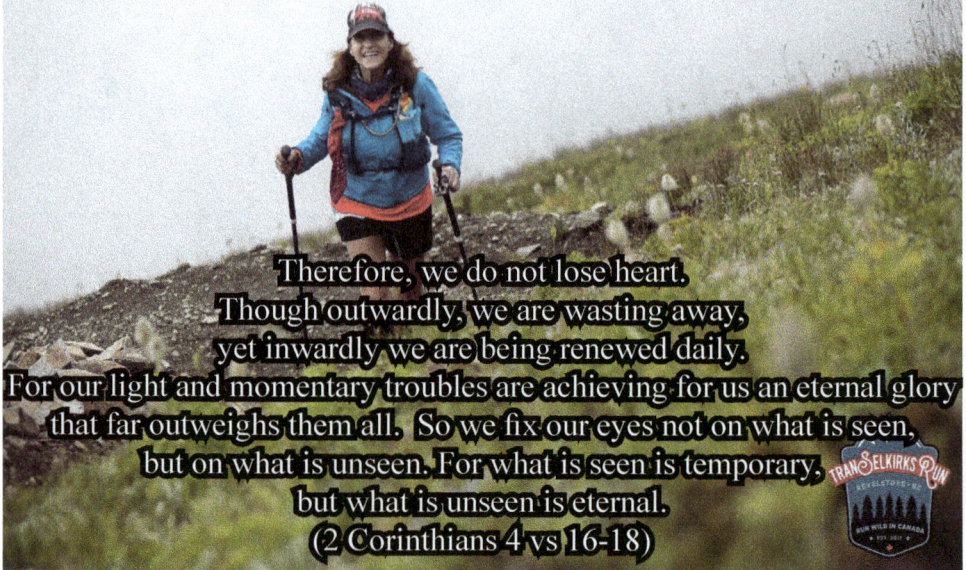

Life is not a sprint; it is an endurance event. Endurance athletes pride themselves on doing events from two hours to multiple days long, which is indeed commendable. I do not mean to sell them short, but we all need endurance and focus on getting through a 168-hour week, a four week month, and a fifty-two-week year.

Marathon runners do not get to the end of the race by being discouraged by the next hill; they focus on the finish they cannot see. An interesting piece of that is the pain suffered when nearing the end almost always subsides when the finish line comes into view, and that was always true for me in my Triathlons.

When we travel through our years, there will be peaks and valleys. Sometimes the hill out of the valley seems too steep to climb. One step at a time, we will get to the next peak when we keep our focus on the unseen prize.

Thought for Today: Let's think about what prize we want in life and focus on it.

Prayer for Today: Dear Lord, today we pray for a vision; your vision for us. We pray for the understanding of what your will is so that we may focus on it. Amen

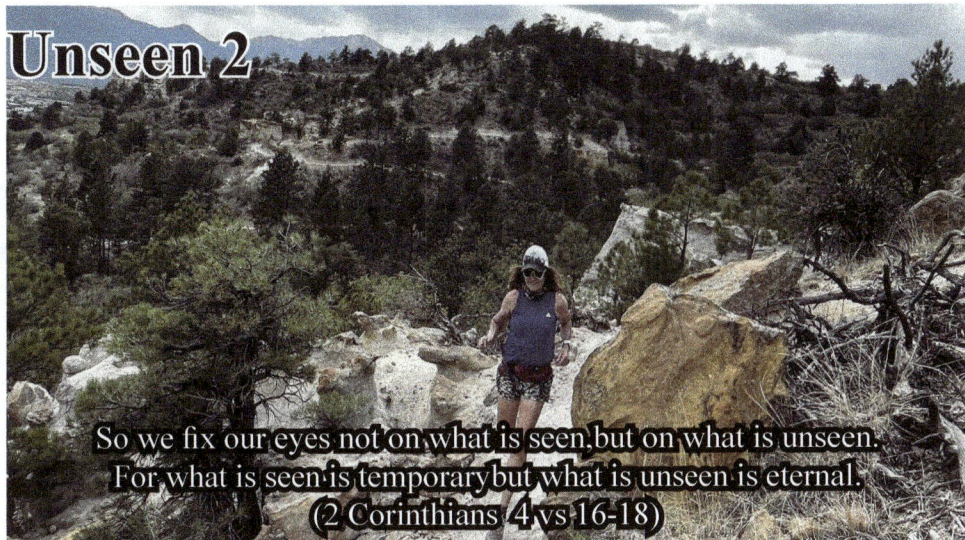

Unseen 2

So we fix our eyes not on what is seen,but on what is unseen. For what is seen is temporary but what is unseen is eternal.
(2 Corinthians 4 vs 16-18)

Following on from yesterday:

My friend and colleague will celebrate a significant birthday this summer. She is going to Colorado to celebrate and run the Pikes Peak marathon. Not only is that a challenge, but she is also one that can keep her focus on the prize "…that far outweighs them all." She has shown me tenacity and an example of excellence in lifestyle, in her athletics that carries over to her personal and business life; some people are secretly jealous, and some think she is nuts! Each of us needs focus and endurance to get through our lives.

We cannot see around the corners of our lives and must live one day at a time. Each day's challenges and problems dealt with appropriately is a step toward peace. Living each day in a Godly manner with our eyes on the eternal prize will bring us peace.

Thought for Today: Let us look ahead (in some cases think back about) in our families to our elders. In some ways, that gives us a preview of our future. However, there are no guarantees, positive or negative. Let us think about our dreams, fantasies, and goals. Let us remember what we see every day is"…temporary, but what is unseen is eternal."

Prayer for Today: Heavenly Father, we thank you for our blessings and can see them today. We pray that we have the endurance to reach the unseen, the ultimate prize. Amen

Having fun keeping fit
Colorado Springs, Colorado

November 14

Page 333

The Dalai Lama

June and I have the ability to enjoy our lives, both the pitfalls and the pleasures. We strongly believe that somehow the Lord has been involved in our lives and led us to enjoy simple pleasures. We both believe that the ability to put the events into perspective is our greatest blessing through our faith.

A Christian friend forwarded this to me. It does not describe a person of faith but is accurate for those who have not developed a spiritual lifestyle.

The Dalai Lama, when asked about what surprised him most about humanity, answered,

"Man. Because he sacrifices his health to make money.
Then he sacrifices his money to recuperate his health.
And then he is so anxious about the future
that he does not enjoy the present;
the result being that he does not live in the present or the future;
he lives like he is never going to die, and he dies having never really lived."

Maybe we can help the friends being referred to by the Dalai Lama.

Thought for Today: Who in our circle of friends resembles the Dalai Lama's description? It could be a family member, neighbor, friend, or someone in our church. Let's think about that and find a way to share our faith with them.

Prayer for Today: Dear Lord, today, let us pray for those who have not included Christ in their lives, those who are spiritually weak, worried about physical rather than Godly issues. We pray for them and ask you for a way to help, a way to share, and a way to contribute to their spiritual growth. Amen

November 15

RHS Wisley Arboretum
Wisley, Surrey, UK

Standing

"Standing on the promise of Christ my King,
Through eternal ages, let his praises ring;
Glory in the highest, I will shout and sing,
Standing on the promises of God."
(Promises, verse 1)
(written by R. Kelso Carter 1849-1926)

"Promises" is one of June's favorite Hymns that covers many issues in our lives. What do we stand for? What is "the promise"? They are simple questions that I will oversimplify today.

First, we stand for ethical Christian behavior that will benefit ourselves and everyone around us. We stand for living by following the Ten Commandments. Examples of being good in our world, and we are designated to show our Christian ethic.

Second, the promise is Grace, given to us by Christ when he died on the cross. We want to think there are more promises than that; when we need more money, self-control, time, more… etc. We want what we want when we want it. We already have what we need, Grace! Somehow we feel deserving.

We need to show off and stand for our faith.

Thought for Today: Let us stand out in the crowd; stand for our Christian beliefs.

Prayer for Today: Dear Lord, we find it easy to sit and watch. Today we pray for the opportunity and courage to stand up for you. Amen

Doubt

"Standing on the promises that cannot fail,
When the howling storms of doubt and fear assail,
By the living word of God I shall prevail,
Standing on the promises of God."
(Promises verse 2)
(written by R. Kelso Carter 1849-1926)

It is not a reality to get through this life without having crises. Every day has potential pitfalls. Our job is to focus on the ultimate promise and work through challenges to our faith. Doubt will be with us and how we deal with it is our challenge. It is OK to doubt and recognize the challenge. If I were a retailer, I would call my store "Temptations R Us." That's a business idea without a market; people would not have to come in and buy what they find daily for free.

In a recent bible study that includes several retired ministers (Ministers never really retire!), the concept of Grace was the subject. If you have accepted our savior, you have it; it is yours; accept it. It is our blessing.

Thought for Today: Let's walk around with a smile, realizing we have recognized our Grace.

Prayer for Today: Heavenly Father, we thank you for our peace and Grace. We pray that we may go through the day, standing on our beliefs and doing your work. Amen

Success

"Standing on the promises, I cannot fall,
Listening every moment to the spirits call,
Resting in my Savior as my all in all,
Standing on the promises of God."
(Promises verse 4)
(Written by R. Kelso Carter 1849-1926)

Faith and mystery are two words that weave their way throughout discussions regarding Christianity. People who do not believe use modern-day logic to negate Christian beliefs. That is their choice, their way, and certainly not my way.

The collection of stories called the bible is too many and too often repeated and confirmed to be ignored. When the bible was configured, they were listed as profits. Truly the profits advised people 2500 and 3000 years ago of future events.

Yes, people can challenge any one story. Did David go up against Goliath with a sling? Did Noah build an ark and save two of each species? There is the burning bush, the tablets with the commandments, etc. Logisticians can challenge each story, but why?

My choice is different. There is a totality in the good news stories repeated around campfires for thousands of years. A common thread certainly would have died if it were not true. They are lovely promises, an optimism, a kindred spirit, and Grace. Stand on these promises, and you will have success.

Thought for Today: Let us appreciate the mysteries of our faith. Let us stand on the promise and have success.

Prayer for Today: Dear Lord, we give thanks for the promise of your Grace. We appreciate the mystery of it all and stand by the promise. Amen

Prosperity

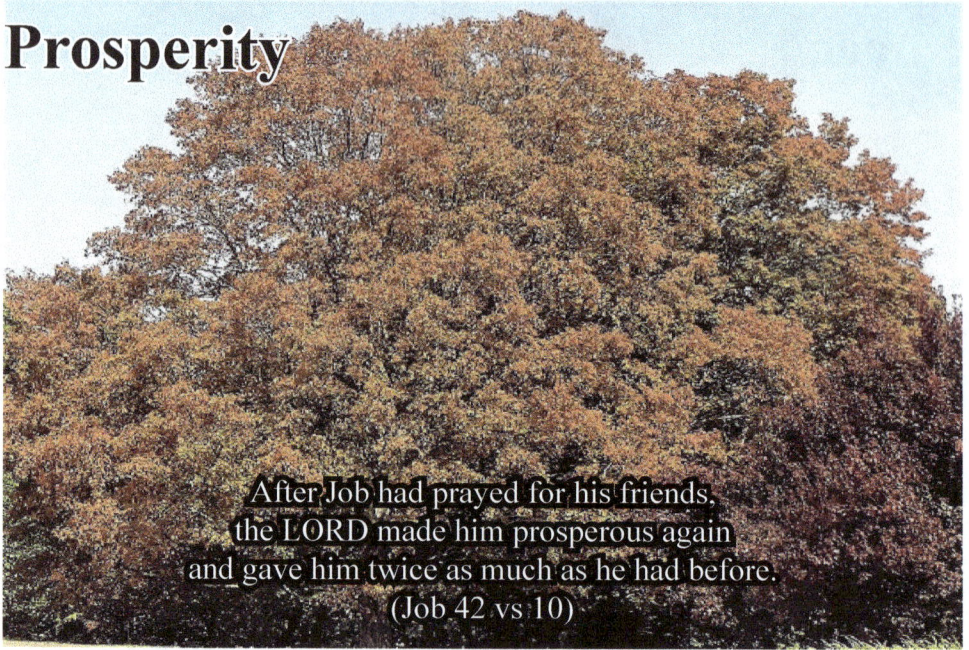

After Job had prayed for his friends,
the LORD made him prosperous again
and gave him twice as much as he had before.
(Job 42 vs 10)

In life, some people are prosperous, and some are not. Prosperity is generally the result of good work. The world economy works that way. It is competitive, and some people end up with more than others.

Today ask yourself where you are in this regard and become a guaranteed winner. You see, winning is not a financial thing at all. In our competitive business world, growth has been difficult. Regarding our physical selves, growth in fitness, weight loss, and staying healthy are challenges that change yearly. That is why New Year's resolutions go by the board.

One area where we can always grow healthier and have plenty of help is spiritual growth. Spiritual growth is always available, unlimited, and beneficial. If you are reading this devotional, you are on the right track. There is no limit to God's love and the benefits of being a spiritual being.

Thought for Today: Let's ask if we have had spiritual growth this year? …and why?

Prayer for Today: Lord and Father, help me grow in you and grow in my faith to be a better servant. Amen

Open Hearts

What does it take to be positive and happy? What is the best way to fix ourselves when we are sad, blue, or hurt? That's correct, "fix ourselves." We chose our moods and often cling to hurts and remorse. We are responsible for our attitudes and can work to adjust them.

Several years ago, while volunteering in treatment facilities, it was common to see a patient carrying a plastic garbage bag. It was called a "pity bag" and symbolized the emotional garbage that the patient had. I hope those bags did well for the patient because they did me a lot of good. Knowing that we can choose to throw away our troubles is a valuable concept. The tricky part is learning how.

We need to remember two messages to keep on the positive side of life. The first is to remember that God is with us, and the second is to be accepting his presence. With His help, we can throw away most garbage and stay positive.

Thought for Today: Our lives and weeks are full of routine and challenging choices that we need to make. Let us allow God to help us with the tough decisions and pray about them.

Prayer: Heavenly Father, this is a time of Thanksgiving and prayer, the start of the holiday season. We pray for the peace and hope promised through our faith. We give prayers of joy for your gifts and the many blessings in our lives. We pray that we may influence those around us through our example of love and joy. Amen

Universal Hope

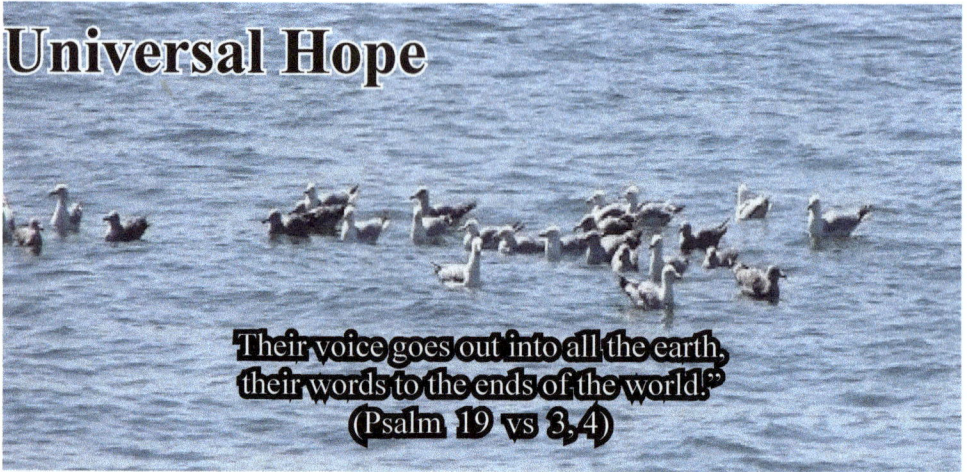

Their voice goes out into all the earth, their words to the ends of the world."
(Psalm 19 vs 3,4)

The holiday season is a time of hope. The Psalmist notes one clear message from the heavens, one God with one message in all tongues to all peoples. His word encourages us to believe there is hope for universal understanding and world peace.

We live in a troubled world. This year there have been natural disasters, pandemics, school attacks, war, and too many ungodly events. They capture the headlines—many question God's role in this.

We need to remember that "The heavens declare the glory of God; the skies proclaim the work of his hands," The press and media report on other issues, It is up to us to focus on the message, and with our example, we can infect the world with faith, peace, and hope.

The parable of the seeds points out the greatness of a well-planted thought. John F. Kennedy said it this way, "One person can make a difference, and every person must try."

Thought for Today: There will be bad news. We will hear it, see it, and sometimes feel it. We need to overcome it with the faith and hope of the Lord. Let us show others our hope for future generations.

Prayer For Today: Dear Lord, this is the time of year when all faiths celebrate you. We honor your presence in different ways with the common thread of thanks, love, and peace. This season we pray for the guidance to share our faith so that we may sow a seed in your name/ Amen

Spiritual Strength

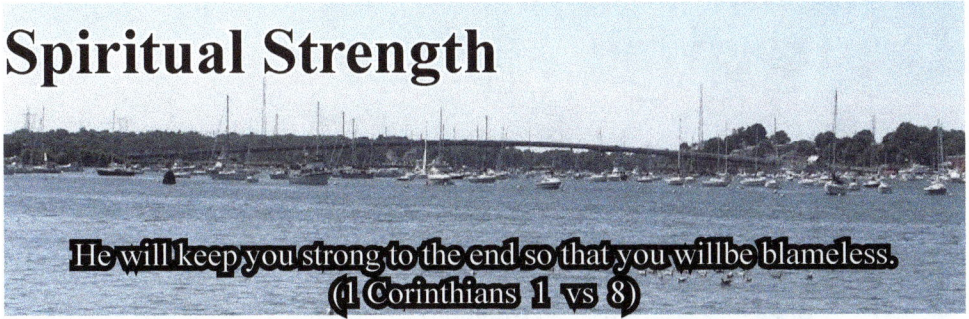

He will keep you strong to the end so that you will be blameless.
(1 Corinthians 1 vs 8)

If you have read this devotional since January, you will recognize that I have said this before; it is important, but the final time. We need to keep up our strength; spirit, mind, and body. June and I just returned from an after-the-early service walk at the zoo. We observed several things.

First, we observed the physical fitness of the people in line. It looked like a group of people waiting to get into their first Weight Watchers meeting; obesity was visible. People enjoyed themselves, a coffee in one hand (Probably a 750-calorie mocha.) and breakfast in the other. The people were not physically fit and were half of our age.

Secondly, many excited children were bursting with energy, running around the lawn. They were having a great time anticipating their trip to the zoo. June and I enjoyed watching these children as they visited the animals throughout the morning. Nothing makes June and I happier than observing families as they have fun spending time together. That is always a beautiful scene on a warm sunny morning.

I asked June, "Do you suppose that even one of these families considered taking these kids to Sunday school today?" You see, we arrived there at 10:15, and there were hundreds of children. Many faiths were represented in the crowd and were not charging their spiritual batteries. Also, many religions worship on Friday and Saturday, and I apologize to them and pray for the others.

As you know, I preach about physical fitness a lot; June says too much. I am hard to live with because of it. Above Paul is preaching about Spiritual strength and fitness. We need to exercise to keep our bodies feeling good and moving. We also need to exercise our minds to keep up the spirit.

Thought for Today: Let's allow time for our spirit to recharge and grow.

Prayer for Today: Dear Lord, we pray that we may keep our spirit, minds, and bodies strong and serve you well. Amen

Thanksgiving

As therefore you received Christ Jesus the Lord,
so live in him, rooted and built up in
him and established in the faith,
just as you were taught,
abounding in thanksgiving.
(Colossians 2 vs 6, 7)

June and I are incredibly thankful for a family running event we started in 1990 called the Turkey Day 5K. Each year we are tearfully proud when 10,000 plus runners, walkers, pets, and wheelchair participants enjoy their Thanksgiving morning in downtown Minneapolis. There will be contributions of food and cash to the Second Harvest food shelf will receive. We both feel blessed that the Lord inspired us to start this event and placed people in our path who have made it special.

Thanksgiving is the traditional start of what we call the holiday season. While giving thanks, we must be aware and focus on the good rewarding parts of our lives.

In his book, With All My Strength, H. Norman Wright puts it this way, "Thanksgiving is not to be limited to only the times when we are aware of blessings. We thank God for unconditional love and goodness, unlimited wisdom, and abundance at these times. Let us give thanks even when we have a problem to solve when there are difficulties to be met. We are rejuvenated when we give thanks continually- spirit, mind, and body."

Let us hold those thoughts and be thankful for all of our blessings.

Thought for Today: Let us focus on giving thanks to God for our love for each other and the support we both give and receive.

Prayer for Today: Dear Lord and Father, we give you thanks for our friends, families, and our troubles. We thank you for our financial crises, family stress, and the waves in our seas of tranquility. Through our problems, we learn to pray and appreciate the many blessings that seem greater than life's ripples. We thank you for our lives, love, and Grace. Amen

November 23 Looking North on the Ridge Trail
Minnesota Landscape Arboretum

Thank You

The best part of my writing these devotions is many of you who contact me whom I have never met. Our Good News email list of friends includes CEOs, many salespeople (because that is my world), several pastors, and people in 172 countries. Thanks to you all because you each enhance my life at some level.

In addition, readers of the Christian Blog, God Is My Spinach, and Facebook Group, Christian Friends, regularly share their thoughts and troubles. We have become a mutual support team helping each other with prayers and love.

Several years ago, my pastor spoke of "returning thanks" to God this week rather than "Giving Thanks." It was something his grandfather used to do three times a day. His basis was that God gave us the things we are thankful for, and he wanted to hear from us but that we were giving back or returning thanks.

This week, I return thanks to you and God and share my love of people and life with you.

Prayer for Thanksgiving: Dear Lord and Heavenly Father, we return blessings and thanks to you today for the many beautiful experiences, the love we feel from our friends and acquaintances, and the guidance you give us in our daily lives. We pray that people learn to appreciate your blessings worldwide and live the life you desire for us, one of peace and goodwill for all. Amen

Foot Bridge In the Fall
Minnesota kandscape Arboretum

Thanksgiving

Enter into his gates with Thanksgiving
and his courts with praise.
Give thanks to him and praise his name.
(Psalm 100 vs 4)

This week we celebrate Thanksgiving Day. But wait a minute, every day is a thanksgiving day. Thanksgiving is more than a day of football games, reunions, and eating. Every day of our life is a day of gratitude.

Have you ever made a list of all you have received that you are thankful for? An extensive list compiled over time and added to as you feel appreciative. If we were to start today, we could not finish the list before Thursday. Our lives are full of blessings. A great family activity for the holiday is to share this list of our blessings and recognize God's contribution's to the list.

The pilgrims knew what gratitude was, at least those still alive. Many had died on board ship and wintering in a harsh new country. They were grateful because they were now free and not oppressed for their beliefs. They faced hardships, but being thankful doesn't happen without difficulties; it happens amid problems.

God gave us a grateful heart, and he does want to hear about our gratefulness to him.

Thought for Today: This is the week of Thanksgiving. We are blessed, and you are all on my list. Let us give thanks for our blessings and pay close attention to what we mean to others.

Prayer for Today: Heavenly Father, this week, let me be more aware and thankful for your presence in my life. Let me share my gratitude with others and contribute positively to the world we live in. Amen

November 25 Quiet Place, On Green Heron Pond
Minnesota Landscape Arboretum

Love

Love the Lord your God
with all your heart, with all your soul,
with all your mind and strength.
Love your neighbor as yourself.
There is no commandment greater than these.
(Mark 12 vs 30.31)

Love is a choice. Yes, there are many feelings of love, but they come and go. It is a choice, especially agape love. This word is used over 200 times in scripture. It is the type of love that will make your marriage come alive. It isn't easy, and you can not do it independently. You need God infusing you with this love and the strength to be consistent with it. There are three words describing love in the Bible: Eros, Philos, and Agape. Agape is a love that serves, regardless of changing circumstances, Jesus's way.

We are loved unconditionally. He loves us whether we are flawed and no matter how bad we are. That's unconditional love. To be like Jesus, we must also love others in this way. We are loved willfully. Do you understand what this means? He wants to love you. Jesus was not forced to go to the cross for you. He chose to. How do we love others? By choosing to. We are loved sacrificially. Sacrificial love gives all, expecting nothing in return.

Thought for Today: Let's focus on two or three individuals who cause us angst. How can we find forgiveness and love for them?

Prayer for Today: Let us pray that there will be loving peace in our lives and around the world through some miracle. Amen

Fall Birches
Minnesota Landscape Arboretum   **November 26**   **Page 345**

Thanksgiving Prayers

Photo By Simon Halsey

Come to me, all you who are weary and burdened,
and I will give you rest.
Take my yoke upon you and learn from me,
for I am gentle and humble in heart
and you will find rest for your souls.
For my yoke is easy and my burden is light.
(Mathew 11 vs 28-30)

The Holiday season has arrived. Thanksgiving just passed, and surely we all spent four days meditating and offering prayers of thanks for our blessings. WHAT?? That's not what we did at my house. What we did was have a wonderful gathering with both friends and family. Yes, prayers and thanks combined with some outdoor games, football, Christmas shopping, and a 5K race. Put the weekend's activities on a list, and most of us would realize why we were tired the following week.

As Christians, we are coming to a very special day, a day to celebrate the birth of Jesus Christ. Our calendars are full of special events: holiday parties, Winter sports, Christmas pageants and services, shopping, and yearend business meetings. However, our focus is often on gifts, parties, and getting our acts together for the New Year. Is all this activity a bad thing? I think not, especially if somehow we can get through it all by keeping Christ at our side and on our minds. Sometimes it just gets out of control.

Christianity and spirituality are beautiful allies during busy times.

Thought for Today: Let us focus on finding more time for ourselves during this busy period. Let's take a few minutes each day to let Christ help us enjoy the season. Let us be selfish once a day and take time out from our obligations to society.

Prayer for Today: Heavenly Father, we are overburdened with problems. People are dying at war and on the streets of our cities. We are busy with final year business activities and planning for Christmas. Many of us will be traveling over the holidays. Please give me the power to be aware of Christ's presence through all of this. Help me find a way to walk through this activity with God as my co-pilot. Amen.

River Nene

Express Yourself

Photo By Simon Halsey

The only thing that counts is faith expressing itself through love.
(Galatians 5 vs 6)

As Christians, we need to demonstrate our best every day in every event. That does not mean walking around handing out roses and hugging everyone we see, which would scare many people off.
Therefore there must be another way.

Greeting people in biblical times included a hug, a cheek kiss, and sometimes water to wash off dusty feet and cool their heads. If we did that, people would be uncomfortable. Times have changed over 2000 years; however, expressing our faith through love still works.

You may do simple things that will help, and you can see the effect immediately. When you open a door for someone, make eye contact and smile; they will almost always smile back and seem more relaxed. We often see a crying child with a frustrated mom in public places. Don't look away or walk away. Try to make eye contact, smile, and wave to the child; say something nice. Inevitably if you do, both the mom and child will relax. You would have expressed love.

In photos and movies, Jesus is portrayed with piercing, loving eyes, often a stare. No one knows if that is a truism, but it works. If we are to be the light of the world it can be through simple acts of consideration and love.

Thought for Today: Today, let's smile at people and see their difference; they will be more comfortable with us.

Prayer for Today: Heavenly Father, I pray that I demonstrate your love and faith through my behavior toward others. I pray that I shine your light brightly. Amen.

River Nene
March, Cambridgeshire, Uk   **November 28**   Page 347

Invisible Qualities

For since the creation of the world, God's invisible qualities, his eternal power and divine nature have been seen, being understood from what has been made, so that men are without excuse.
(Romans 1 vs 20)

The holiday season is a hectic time of the year. Next year's budgets at home and work, the snow needs to be shoveled (for us northerners), and increased activity at church, holiday parties, and all the holiday sports tournaments added to our schedule. Getting caught up in human activities and leaving our spirituality behind is easy. Merry Christmas.

Interestingly, activity surrounding Christ's birthday celebration may often deprive us of the time to meditate and appreciate the wonders of his gifts. It is a glorious time of the year, full of memories of our youth and the excitement of growing closer to our families. Where is God in all of this?

First and foremost, God is with us, even when we are too busy to be conscious of His presence. His "…invisible qualities, his eternal power, and divine nature" are available to us daily. All days are not created equal. We all have our ups and downs. When we are out of touch, where is the Lord? He is precisely where we left Him, waiting to support us.

Thought for Today: We face holiday activities added to the norm. It is a blessed time of the year. Let us focus on ensuring that we bring the Lord with us daily. Yes, He can go shopping, to a youth Holiday tournament, to a business meeting, or any place we will take Him. This week let us silently recognize His presence through meditation and prayer.

Prayer for Today: Dear Lord and Father, today we thank you for the gift of grace received through your son Jesus. We are blessed this time of year through the memories of his life and the celebration of his birth. We thank you for your presence in our lives and the ability to reach out to you when stressed. Amen

River Wey Navigation
West Byfleet, Surrey, UK

A Day of Joy

> For in six days, the Lord made the heavens and the earth,
> the sea and all that is in them, but he rested on the seventh day.
> Therefore the Lord blessed the Sabbath day and made it holy.
> (Exodus 20 vs 11)

During the holiday season, obligations increase. You can feel the stress building; at work, at home, and elsewhere if you are paying attention. Often, I talk about being the best you can be and refer to the YMCA logo, Spirit, Mind, and Body.

We need to rest physically and mentally. There is a rhythm to the seventh day of rest. It gives some balance to our life. God says that we need to take a break once a week. He is saying there is more to life than work. He is also urging us to follow his pattern.

Spiritually we need this time to refocus our lives. God wants us to spend one day looking to him and thanking him for being liberated. Listen to what the Lord said to Isaiah 58 vs 13.

> *If you keep your feet from breaking the Sabbath*
> *and from doing as you please on my holy day,*
> *... then you will find your joy in the Lord.*

Our friend and former neighbor showed more respect for the Sabbath than any other modern family I know. Mom does not even have to cook on Sunday. They are a family that has a lot of love and joy. That is our lifelong goal.

Thought for Today: Take some time to meditate and pray for rest and peace in our lives. Take some time to recharge your spiritual batteries. Take some time to find Joy.

Prayer for Today: Dear Lord, today we pray for people who can't take time for you.. May they somehow grow to find joy in the Lord. Amen

December

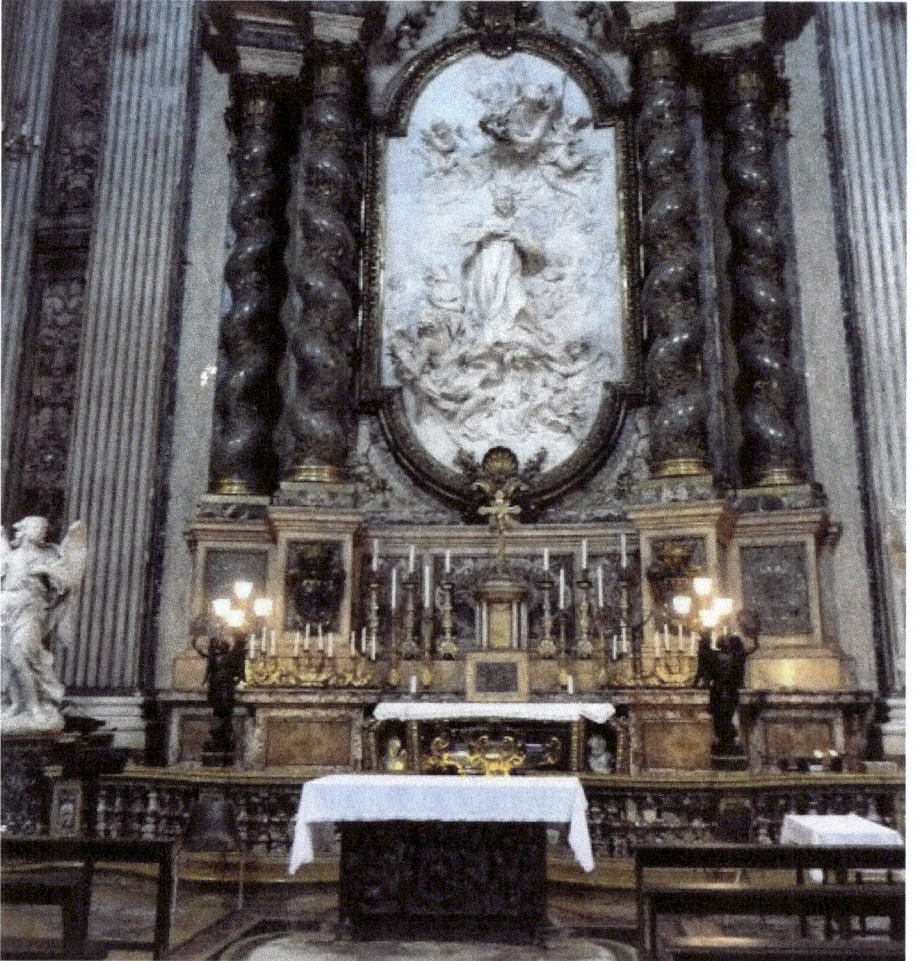

Church of Saint Ignatius in Rome
The history is linked to the origins of the Collegio Romano
founded by Ignatius of Loyola in 1551. When the number of students
increased, Pope Gregory XV entrusted the project of building a church
dedicated to Saint Ignatius of Loyola to Orazio Grassi. The new church
was consecrated in 1722.

Glory of St Aloysius Gonzaga
Church of St. Ignatius, Rome Italy

Happiest Season

"But what about you?" he asked. "Who do you say I am?"
Peter answered, "You are the Messiah."
(Mark 8 vs. 29)

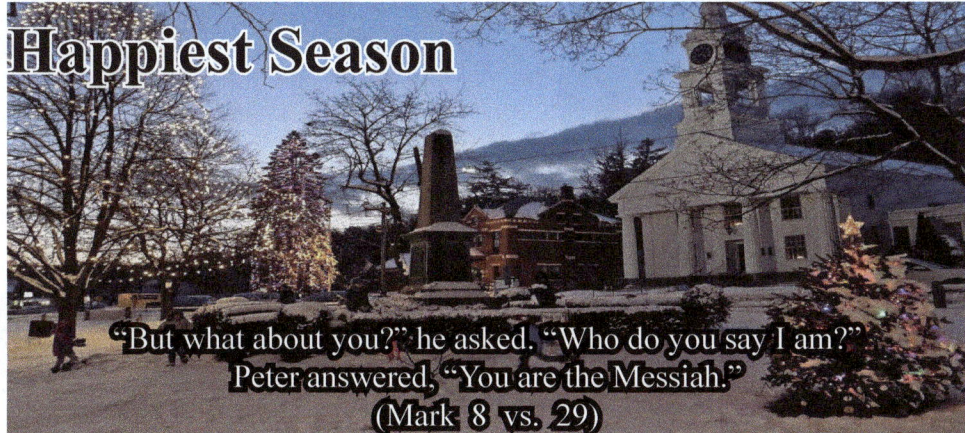

It is a wonderful time of the year when we look forward to celebrating Christ's birth. We are blessed because of His presence in our everyday lives. We have a God-given relief from the daily stresses our society places on us.

Interestingly, 30-plus years after his birth, Jesus was asking who they believed he was. My thoughts are that the Christmas story would be enough. But then, nothing in this world is ever easy; not then and certainly not now.

So what is Christmas really about? Gifts, material giving, and recharging of our spiritual batteries. It is a great time of the year, the happiest time. We must enjoy the season while recharging our batteries, reinforcing our beliefs, and preparing for the New Year.

Katharine McPhee said in her song:
"Have yourself a merry little Christmas
Let your heart be light
From now on, our troubles
Will be out of sight."

Blessings to you all for a great season of Joy!

Thought for Today: The Christmas season is not all joys. We will encounter stress, financial hardships, bad weather, and all the events of winter life. They are all blessings that are part of our lives. We need to keep Christ as our focus.

Prayer for Today: Heavenly Father, we give thanks for Christmas and festivities. Through prayer, we give thanks that "our troubles will be out of sight." Amen

Sterling, Massachusetts   **December 1**   **Page 351**

Relaxing

Come to me, all you who are weary and burdened,
and I will give you rest.
Take my yoke upon you and learn from me.
(Mathew 11 vs 28)

If this passage sounds familiar, you read November 27th. Often a strong message is worth repeating during such a busy time. It suggests that we have tools through our faith to help us enjoy the season. However, just like the tools in the garden shed, they will not help us if we don't reach out and pick them up.

The many tools of Christianity are available to us all, and "picking them up" means taking the time to allow them to work. Here are some suggestions.

Try changing your daily routine for the season. In the morning, shut off the news, put down the paper, sit alone with your beverage and think about the season in quiet. That may change your outlook for the day.

When you feel out of control or stressed, keep today's message in your presence, take a break, and read it. Give your faith a chance. There are many options, and God is available to us, but we must let Him into our lives.

Thought for Today: The Christmas story is one of wonder and genius, the genius of the wise men to read and follow the signs shown to them. They took the time to go and answer a call. They took a leadership role. As we go through this busy time, let us understand our role as Christians and be leaders in spirituality.

Prayer for Today: Heavenly Father, we are experiencing unusual times. The weather is confusing, and there is unrest in our society. We are approaching a New Year with hesitance and, in many cases, fear. We need you beside us in times like this. We pray for the presence of mind to stop and let you come with us. Amen

Medicine Lake
Plymouth, Minnesota

Endurance and Encouragement

> May the God who gives endurance and encouragement
> give you a spirit of unity among yourselves...
> (Romans 15 vs 5)

Instant gratification is something that we always seem to want and often expect. We have national lotteries around the world, and people become instant winners. (They may have played for twenty years!) The desire is clear; we want what we want when we want it.

If that is where you are at in your life, you need not read any further today. That is not my message! Paul's message to the Romans is about endurance and encouragement, two things given to us through our faith and prayers that will make us successful. There will be no lightning bolt that makes us winners.

In the years that June and I were associated with my son's music business, we dealt with hundreds of starry-eyed musicians waiting for their big break. Some made it, but all that succeeded earned it. The ones that worked at it 24/7; the ones with an undying passion for writing and performing; those who were too serious about it to enjoy the party atmosphere succeeded.

In our own lives, we need to endure. Life is not a sprint, it is more like a marathon, and there are no days off. We will feel weary and need encouragement. We need a place where we can find encouragement; we have it because God is with us. We do need to reach out and grab it through prayer.

Thought for Today: Let's think about who we could reach out to for encouragement; our pastor, significant other, child, or bartender. There is always someone.

Prayer for Today: Dear Lord, we thank you for your support and pray that we can let you in when we are tired. Amen

Lake of The Isles
Minneapolis, Minnesota

Recovery

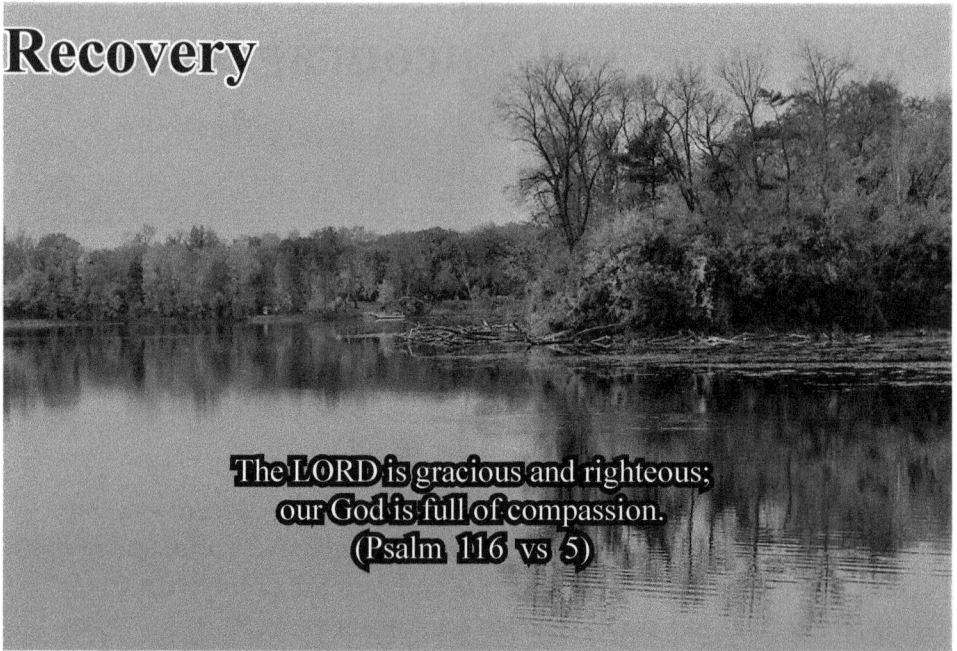

The LORD is gracious and righteous;
our God is full of compassion.
(Psalm 116 vs 5)

The following is a story about a close associate with over fifty years of hardship. He was a star college hockey player and married a beautiful lady, which did not work. Tried marriage again two more times and failed. He worked his way out of a career over ten years ago and nearly lived on the street. He tried everything but living a faithful lifestyle and was addicted to alcohol and gambling. At his bottom, he "Recognized that a power greater than himself could restore him to sanity. That person is God."

Stories of recovery are common, and many of you recognize that quote as the second step of a twelve-step program. At age 60, my friend went to AA rather than a sports bar that facilitated both of his destructive habits. He took a step I took in March of 1978 and never looked back. Read tomorrow for more on him. It is a blessed story.

Thought for Today: Let's think about who we know that needs to allow the Lord into their life. Let us reach out to someone and see if they are ready.

Prayer for Today: Dear Lord and Father, we are blessed to have you. We pray that we honor your presence and help others let you into their lives. Amen

Hockey Players

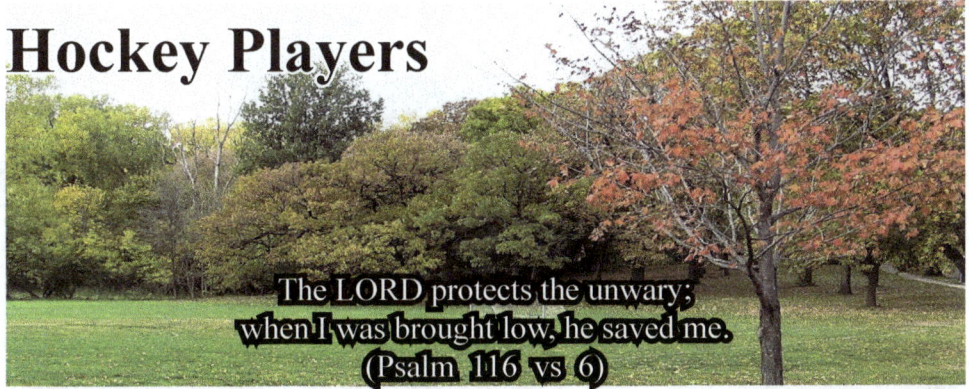

> The LORD protects the unwary;
> when I was brought low, he saved me.
> (Psalm 116 vs 6)

More from yesterday:

That story was over ten years ago, and we do not have enough time to tell the whole story of spiritual growth, so you get the short version. After four years without a job and one year after finding a higher power, a former business associate sought him for a six-month contract, his first job using his degree and experience in five years. It became a full-time management career with full benefits and a retirement package.

Well, now comes one of those coincidences that, in my mind, are God moments. He needed to be interviewed by the VP of operations. He was a bit nervous, but he knew how to pray by now. He walked into the office, and the fifteen years younger VP had a photo of Bobby Orr, the great Boston Bruin defenseman, on his wall. The conversation started with him asking the VP, "Did you ever see him play?" They both grew up on the north shore of Boston and played college hockey. There were mutual friends and a lot of hockey chitchat. Hey, this was in California, where hockey players are scarce. I do not believe in coincidences. He got the job.

Accepting a higher power ten years ago has changed his life. The Lord was always with him and available and is to us. It is important to let him in.

Today's thoughts and prayers are repeats of yesterday. They are important.

Thought for Today: Let's think about who we know that needs to allow the Lord into their life. Let us reach out to someone and see if they are ready.

Prayer for Today: Dear Lord and Father, we are blessed to have you. We pray that we honor your presence and help others let you into their lives. Amen

Why Fear

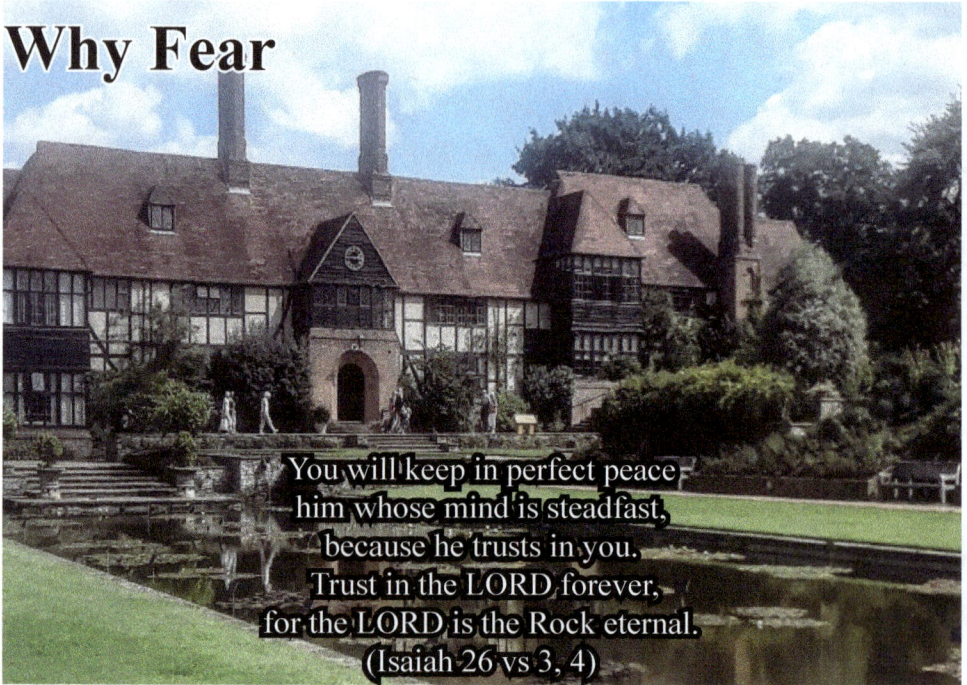

You will keep in perfect peace
him whose mind is steadfast,
because he trusts in you.
Trust in the LORD forever,
for the LORD is the Rock eternal.
(Isaiah 26 vs 3, 4)

The terms "shaky ground" and "solid ground" generate strong visual images that are easy to understand. Growing up in Massachusetts, we played in the grassy marshlands alongside the tidal rivers north of Boston. The land was around six inches above "mean high tide." We often ran into shaky ground, ground that was virtually floating. That was always scary because several times, one of us broke through the sod and had to be helped out. Breaking through could be fatal.

Solid ground is also very definable; a rock or piece of ledge. When fishing in these tidal streams, we would fish from the rocky corners where we would be safer. The tidal flows had eroded the mud bank back to the ledge, and the water was often deeper. That's where we felt safest.

In life, we are safest when we are firm in our faith, have time for God, and remember our rock. Our rock protects us emotionally and physically. Our rock is eternal.

Thought for Today: Let us remember to stand on our rock.
Prayer for Today: Heavenly Father, today we pray that we can stay grounded in our faith when we have issues. We pray that we remember our rock when we are stressed.
Amen

RHS Wisley Garden
Wieley, Surrey, UK

Infamy

Surely, as I have planned, so it will be,
and as I have purposed so that it will happen.
(Isaiah 14 vs 24)

Today is a famous day described as a Day of Infamy. It is one of the most celebrated days in the history of war. There are many famous battles in our history books, David and Goliath, Troy, Gettysburg, and the list goes on. I need to wonder and ask why. Most wars since WWII have been un-Godly nobody wins situations that do not seem to resolve anything. It does not make much sense to me.

So, where is God in all of this? What would Jesus do? How come both sides can think God is with them? These are great questions, and I will not answer them but refer them to Abraham Lincoln as he analyzed God's presence in war.

In Abraham Lincoln: A History by Nicolay and Hay, Lincoln is quoted: "The will of God prevails. In great contests, each party claims to act following the will of God. Both may be, and one must be, wrong. God cannot be for and against the same thing simultaneously. In the present civil war, God's purpose may be something different from the purposes of either party—and yet the human instrumentalities working just as they do, are of the best adaption to effect His purpose. God wills this contest and wills that it shall not end yet. He could give the final victory to either side any day. Yet the contest proceeds."

Today we need to remember Pearl Harbor, a day in infamy. We need to contemplate world peace. We also need to pray for an end to all conflicts.

Thought for Today: Contemplate world peace.

Prayer for the Day: Dear Lord and Savior, today we wonder where it will end. Throughout history, the world's people have found ways to battle. Today we pray for some understanding of your role in all of this. We pray for wisdom to represent your will in search of peace. Amen

Slow Down and Enjoy

...give thanks in all circumstances,
for this is God's will for you in Christ Jesus.
(1 Thessalonians 5 vs 16)

This Saturday morning, it is evident that the Christmas season has taken over my life. Yesterday I was booked from 7 am to 3 with no breaks and tasks I would not get done. Thursday evening, I was so tired that I only skimmed through my bible study. On Friday, I had a meeting set up with a friend to tour his robotics lab at his school. It would be fun, and I had two business appointments following that.

The day did not go as I had planned. At 6:45 am, a tire blew out in ten-degree temperatures as I entered the freeway. Fortunately, an immediate exit led to a strip mall that included a coffee shop. Oops, there goes the men's breakfast and bible study and the lab tour.

After a trip to the tire store, I made a quick stop at the office to check email and do a few things on the list. There was a message canceling my tour. So, I did not miss anything and had time to prepare for a meeting over lunch. Everything worked out.

I do not like to think that God works at the daily line item level because that would make Him very busy. But I carried some guilt while waiting for AAA to change my tire. Just maybe I was being punished for skimming over the bible study material. When I got home, there were messages that arrived after I left, canceling both my appointments. Maybe God was trying to keep me from making an unnecessary trip. Thus, no more guilt.

My summary is: God is with us, and God is good.

Thought for Today: Today and throughout the holiday season, let us shed the stress, pray for the moment and find the joy.

Prayer for Today: Heavenly Father, today we ask that we find the joy of the holiday season. We ask to share it with others and be leaders in our faith. Amen

December 8

Birch Tree, RHS Wisley Garden
Wisley, Surrey, UK

Yule Fire

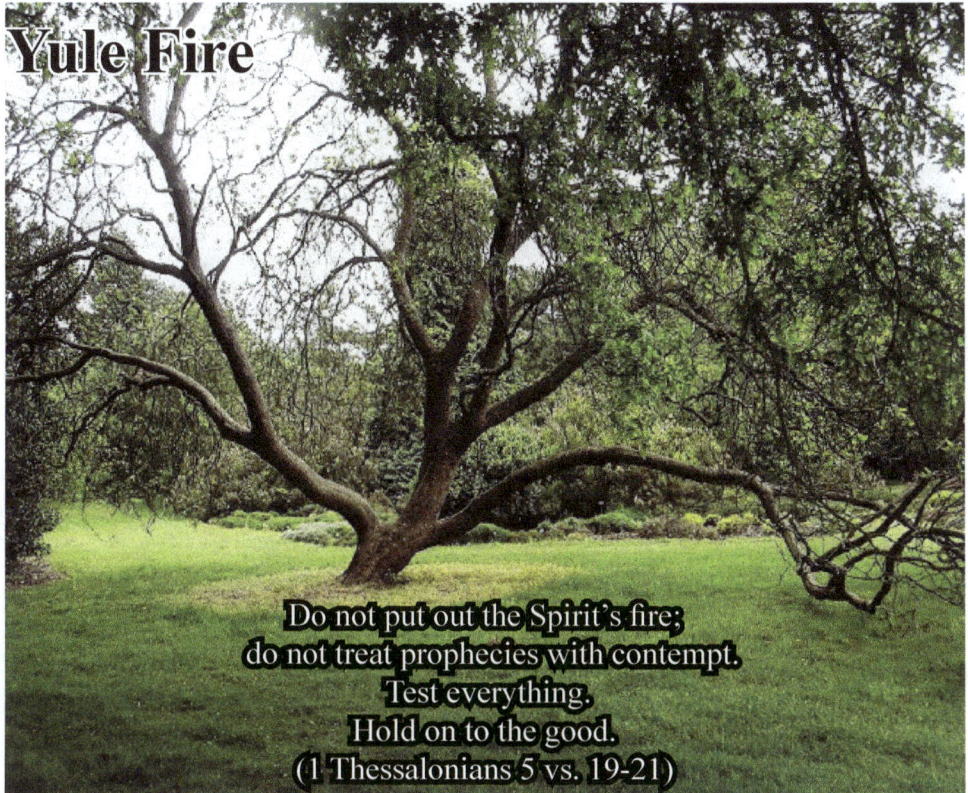

Do not put out the Spirit's fire;
do not treat prophecies with contempt.
Test everything.
Hold on to the good.
(1 Thessalonians 5 vs. 19-21)

The Christmas season in Minnesota is cold. A cable TV station stops programming, runs a video of a Yule log burning as a symbol, and backs it up with Christmas music. It is very peaceful and meaningful.

The symbol of the Spirit's fire warms our hearts during this season, and here in the northland, it is very welcome. Christmas is a blessed season, and we all need to focus on the spiritual blessings as we work toward the year-end.

Thought for Today: Let us think about our spiritual goals and carry the joy of Christ's birth with us, and the materialistic pieces of the season will fall into place.

Prayer for Today: Dear Lord and Father, we thank you for the love that we feel when you are in our hearts. Today we pray for a chance to help serve you after the season and find opportunities to do your will here on earth and contribute to a loving, peaceful world. Amen

Joy

Be joyful always,
pray continually,
give thanks in all circumstances,
for this is God's will for you in Christ Jesus.
(1 Thessalonians 5 vs 16-18)

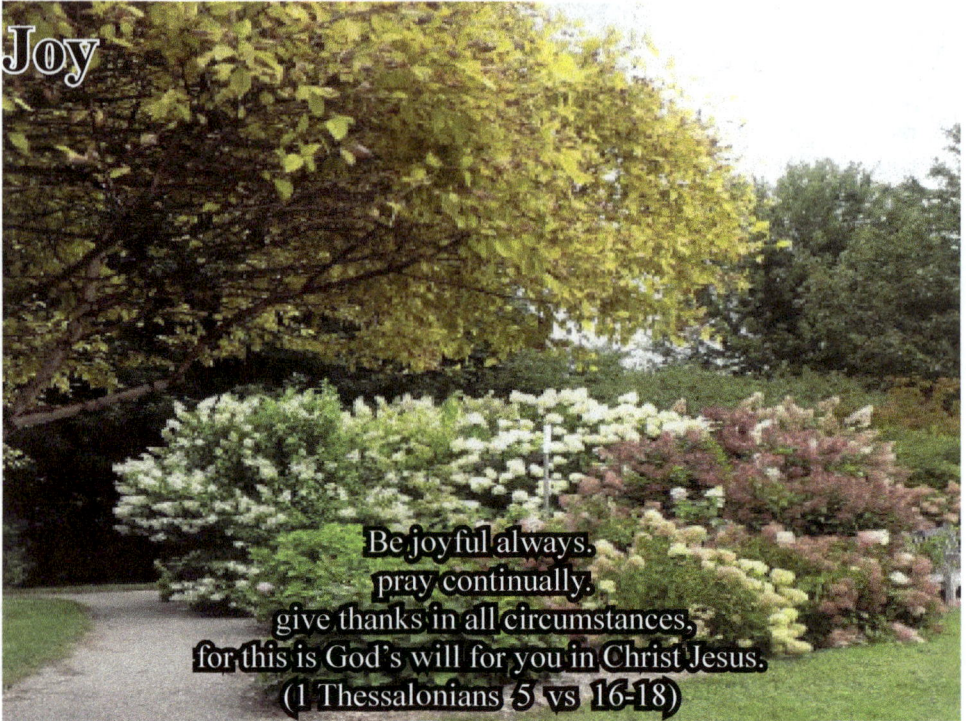

Christmas is a joyful time. The joy of the celebration generally pushes the stress and negativity into the background. A friend recently commented that he wanted to bottle up the holiday spirit. He needs to learn that the bottle is the bible on his bookcase. The bible is more than a bottle; it is a large jug of joy. A drink a day will keep miseries away, and you can take as many drinks as you want from it.

Ok, so that's enough analogy for today. If you are reading this devotion, you know where to go when in need, seek out a spiritual mentor, a sponsor, or even grab your favorite prayer guide and pray. That is what spirituality is about; having faith and snatching joy from the heat of the moment rather than getting bogged down in negativity.

Thought for Today: Today and throughout the holiday season, let us shed the stress, pray for the moment, and find joy.
Prayer for Today: Heavenly Father, today we ask that we find the holiday season's joy and spirit. We ask so that we may share it with others. Amen

The Shrub Walk

Problems

From them will come songs of thanksgiving
and the sound of rejoicing.
I will add to their numbers,
and they will not be decreased;
I will bring them honor,
and they will not be disdained.
(Jeremiah 30 vs.19)

Every day is a day to rejoice. We are between our formal day of Thanksgiving and Christ's birthday celebration. Most of us are enjoying what we call the holiday season. The message above tells us that God wants us to rejoice, to be happy. We need to pay attention to that.

Thought for Today: We will be happy as we will work through the busy schedule, deal with holiday stress, and in the end, let us rejoice.

Prayer for Today: Dear Lord and Father, today we rejoice in your name and thank you for giving the Grace and spirit of your son, Jesus. Amen

My Body

Do you not know that your bodies are temples of the Holy Spirit, who is in you, whom you have received from God ?
(1 Corinthians 6 vs 19,20)

Yes, we own our temple, and it needs constant maintenance. Those who know me are expecting a dialog regarding diet and exercise. As an octogenarian, those are important. But being a happy elder is all about the Spirit.

Many octogenarians are angry, and I do not mean unhappy. Life is not perfect, and how we deal with negativity makes the difference. Yes, in aging, we lose capabilities and hopefully taper into our "end of life experience." As Christians, I plead with you to be elderly and happy. Let your family remember your smile and your laugh.

Thought for Today: Let's do what we need to be happy.
Prayer For Today: We Pray that as we approach our end on earth, people will remember us as grateful and happy stewards of our Christian faith. Amen

Purification

All men are like grass,
and all their glory is like the flowers of the field;
the grass withers, and the flowers fall,
but the word of the Lord stands forever.
(1 Peter 1 vs 22, 23)

Somehow Love seems needed in our world today. There are wars and hate; doing business has become cutthroat. Unemployment remains leftover from the pandemic, but there are for-hire signs everywhere. We are competing for what seems to be limited resources. There is a scramble for the top. Why?

We need that second SUV, the lake home, and the 60-inch TV for Sunday's game. Yes, we have undoubtedly become very materialistic. But is it all necessary?

We all know the answer to that is no, but somehow we all participate at some level. Many people have "things" but are not at peace. The need in our society for spiritual growth is as essential as the need for economic growth. We need a strong faith community to support an economic and political system that seems in need. We need to demonstrate through our behaviors that we are at peace.

Christmas time is a season when we focus on Christ's birth. While concentrating on spiritual messages, the materialism of it all is ever-present. This time of year is our opportunity to refresh our spirituality and a great chance to grow in faith.

Thought for Today: Let us demonstrate that we are at peace through our behaviors. Let's deal with the demands placed on us in the way that Jesus would advise us; through forgiveness and prayer.

Prayer for Today: Heavenly Father, the world still seems to be suffering many ills. The lack of love, trust, and the violence of terrorism seem to dominate the news. We pray for some understanding of the situation. We pray for a way to bring your love into the international and interracial differences equation. Amen

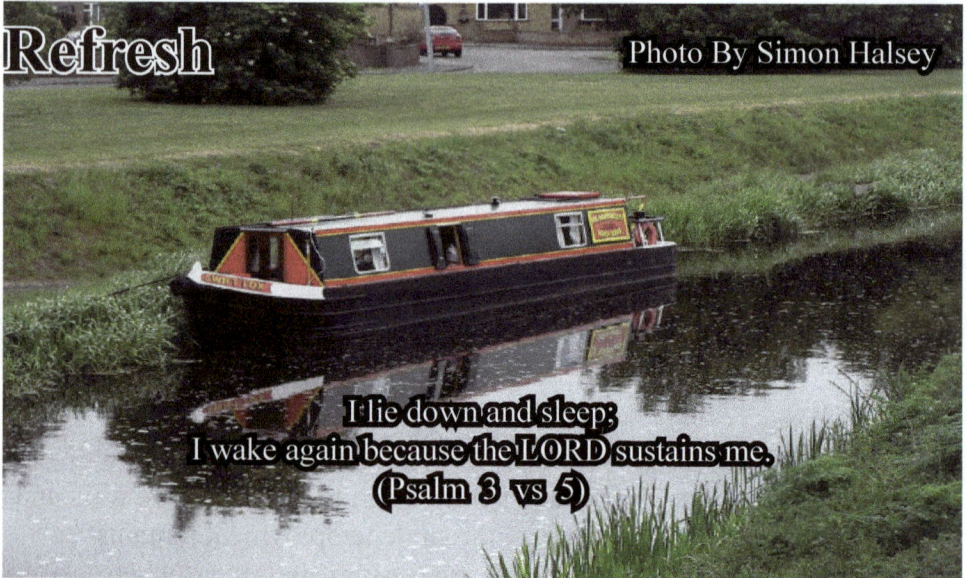

Photo By Simon Halsey

I lie down and sleep;
I wake again because the LORD sustains me.
(Psalm 3 vs 5)

Almost every night, we go to sleep without fear, knowing that we will awaken refreshed and ready to make it through another day. We walk one step at a time, live one day at a time, and sometimes the days break down into minutes and hours. But we get through them.

As an endurance athlete, I assure you that you try to avoid thinking about the distance and keep up that one-step concept. That is hard because endurance athletes must focus on the balloon arch covering the finish line. That's a conundrum because you need to visualize the finish without thinking about the distance. The expression "one day at a time" in AA programs refers to another day without using alcohol or drugs.

Making it through a day without addiction, running miles, and just getting through to the end is always easier when you have faith. You need to believe you can make it, and the best way to believe that is through the spirit of the Lord. With his help, we will be sustained and succeed.

Thought for Today: Today, we awoke refreshed. Tonight we will be tired. Let's go to bed proud of what we did today.
Prayer for Today: Dear Lord and Father, today was a day of progress. Tomorrow we pray that we may believe that you are with us as we walk through the pitfalls of life. Amen

December 14 Swift Fox, Narrowboat, River Nene
Cambridgeshire, UK

Encouragement

*Be strong and let us fight bravely
for our people and the cities of our God.
The LORD will do what is good in his sight.
(2 Samuel 10 vs 12)*

We experience great memories and thoughts surrounding Christmas during the holiday season. Some temptations arise during the many celebrations. Life is never a sprint; it often takes courage to stay the course and do what is right.

My biggest temptation is at what my friend calls grazing parties; overeating. Before 1978 the attraction was to drink too much alcohol; it was almost a tradition in my family. It seemed that the women cooked and the men drank too much. They were not the greatest of days.

There is a trend to overspend. The credit card society we live in is difficult to control, and peer pressure to ensure that kids have what they want can be extreme. We must be careful in all cases to meet our needs and separate them from our wants. Sometimes that takes bravery.

During the month between Thanksgiving and Christmas, we tend to burn the candle at both ends. Often it takes strength and sometimes feels like a battle. We need to keep the Lord's insight as he keeps us in his.

Thought for Today: Let's fight bravely as we deal with the issues of life.

Prayer for Today: Dear Lord, we pray for the strength to do your will here during this busy season. Amen

River Nene
Cambridgeshire, UK

December 15

Faith and Illness

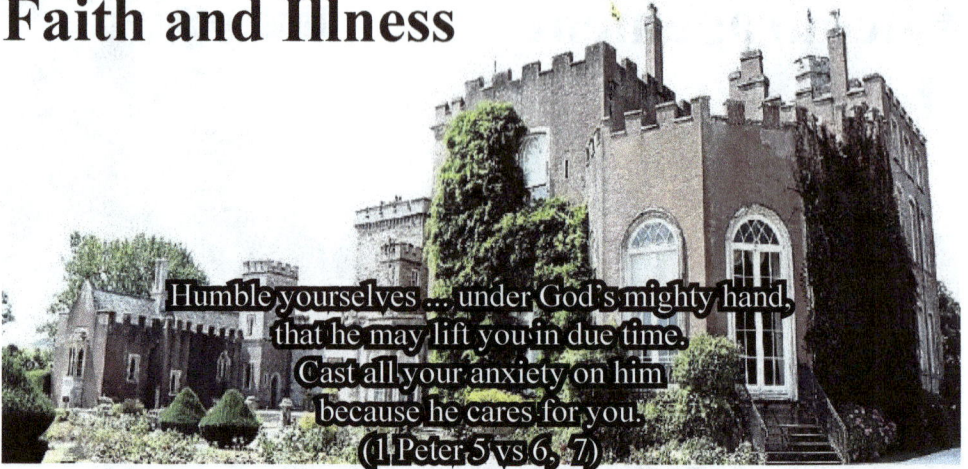

Humble yourselves ... under God's mighty hand,
that he may lift you in due time.
Cast all your anxiety on him
because he cares for you!
(1 Peter 5 vs 6, 7)

Holiday cheer is a great and wonderful thing. It is a time when it is easy to be happy in our society there are bright lights, merry music, and more smiles and eye contact as we walk along the streets. Yes, the holiday season brings us great joy.

There are, however, those that are experiencing tough times. We cannot ignore those critically ill loved ones who fear this is their last holiday together; some are experiencing their first holiday alone after losing a loved one, and others are ill and frightened. These are friends of ours that are experiencing a "Blue Christmas."

Many of us do not know how to deal with people with this emotional need. We would love to help but do not want to interfere. I pray that all of us think about that. We need to take time to share, listen, pick up the phone, and say hello to ask someone if they would like to share a prayer. We can reach out to someone out of love and share God's faith.

Thought for Today: Let us focus on those around us experiencing a blue Christmas, identify and reach out to them with love.

Prayer for Today: Heavenly Father, we pray for ourselves, our friends, and our loved ones. Many are ill and experiencing fear, uncertainty, loneliness, or hurt. Many need you in their lives and have not found You. This week we pray that we may help be the conduit that strengthens their faith and eases their anxieties. Today we pray for a way to do your will in this way. Amen

December 16   Powderham Castle
Exeter, Kenton, Devon, UK

Christmas Love

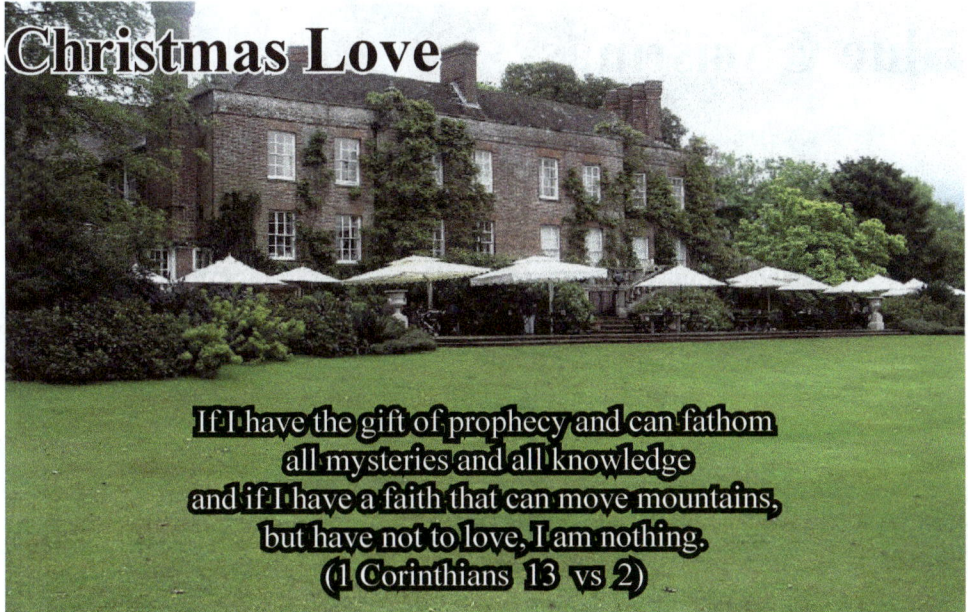

> If I have the gift of prophecy and can fathom
> all mysteries and all knowledge
> and if I have a faith that can move mountains,
> but have not to love, I am nothing.
> (1 Corinthians 13 vs 2)

The holiday season is a time of great joy and symbolism. There are bright lights in almost every neighborhood, stores are full of shoppers buying gifts for loved ones, and Christmas trees light up our homes. We sing special carols only once each year, a sound pleasing to our ears. Yes, the celebration of Christ's birthday is a beautiful experience.

As Christians, we proceed through this season, and love abounds within our society. When we donate to the food shelf, Toys for Tots, serve at a shelter, or say Merry Christmas, we feel good because we demonstrate our love for each other; through Christ. Love is a beautiful gift we have through our faith.

Thought for Today: As we go through this week before Christmas, stress tends to build. Year-end activities pile up on top of holiday parties, annual budgets, and all the "to do" about Christmas. As we go through the day, let us focus on why we do all this.

Prayer for Today: Heavenly Father, we are all wrapped up in the season's activities. We are concerned about all of the "hate" in the world. Everywhere there seems to be unrest and fear of terror and violence. We pray that somehow love can shine through all of this and that we as people may see through the negative forces and learn that love is possible. Amen

Pashley Manor
Wadhurst, East Sussex, UK

Blue Christmas

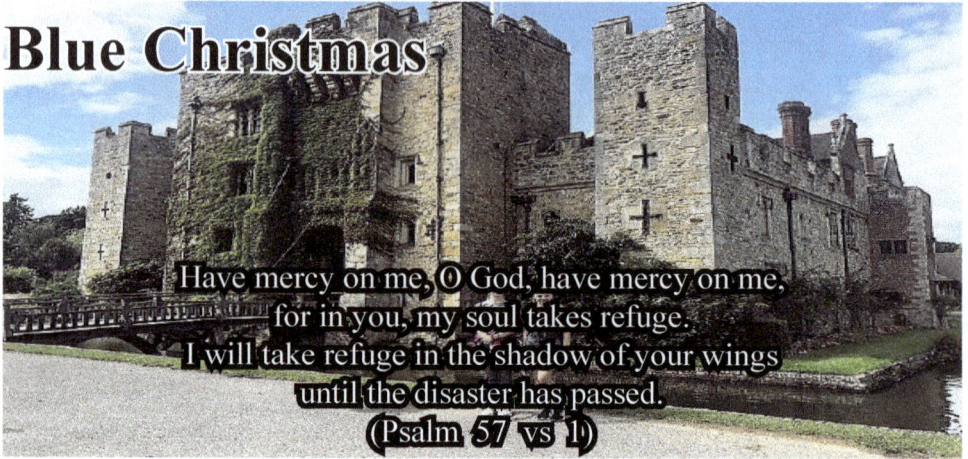

> Have mercy on me, O God, have mercy on me,
> for in you, my soul takes refuge.
> I will take refuge in the shadow of your wings
> until the disaster has passed.
> (Psalm 57 vs 1)

This week Christian Churches have a particular service for people having a sad time over the Holidays. Often called a Blue Christmas Service after the Elvis Presley song, but also exists as a Service of Light and Hope. We can always find reasons to be blue over the holidays, and it is good to take a look at those feelings, put them in perspective and pray to God for the support available to us.

Many miss spouses who passed this year. There are too many to list with severe ailments and others with challenging career and financial situations. Also, we need to pray for what seems to be our new COVID lifestyle.

Christmas is a time of celebration. Through it, we remember those who are experiencing loss. June and I pray about aging, living in a new society with COVID, and our growing family's future. We must accept the season's joy as we move toward the holiday. Take refuge in the shadow of God's wings.

Thought for Today: Let us take note of our sad feelings over the holidays. Let us recognize that they exist. Rather than mask them with joy, let us pray about them and turn them over to God so we can enjoy the celebration of Christ's birth.

Prayer for Today: Heavenly Father, we have special holiday prayers. We pray that your presence brings trust and love to the world. We pray for people who have lost loved ones and are spending their first Christmas with an empty place at the table. We give thanks for your role in our lives and the help you have given us. Thank you for being available for us each day. Amen

December 18

Hever Castle
Hever, Kent, UK

Bottle ?

There is a time for everything, and a season for every activity under the heavens.
(Ecclesiastes 3 vs 1)

Today we awaken a week before the Christmas celebration. We are tired, weary, and excited. Our hearts are full of the joy and spirit that this beautiful season creates. It would be great if we could bottle it all up so we could drink it year-round.

Several years ago, my good friend Paige said it well on her Facebook site, "I wish it could be Christmas every day..... I'm getting the best present of all this year." She was moving into a new home near her daughters and grandchildren, and they will celebrate Christmas together.

Each year one of my best gifts is you, what I like to call my Good News buddies (Those of you that put up with my weekly emails.), and all in my Christian Friends group worldwide. You drive me to read, write, and consider what Christ means to me and the world. Wow, that is a fantastic gift-Thanks.

> "Down in a lowly manger
> The humble Christ was born,
> And God sent us salvation
> That blessed Christmas morn."
> (Verse 3, Go Tell It on the Mountain)
> (John W. Work Jr. 1907)

Thought for Today: Let us all enjoy the celebration. The birth of Christ is fast approaching. Today let's focus on the excitement, blessings, and spiritual meaning of it all. Also, remember that this spirit can be with us all year long- we do not need a bottle; it is in our hearts.

Prayer for Today: We pray for the many families that are experiencing holiday loss. It is sad when there is an empty place at the Christmas table. Amen

Mallards, River Nene
Peterborough, Cambridgeshire,UK **December 19** Page 369

Midnight Clear

"It came upon a midnight clear,
That glorious song of old,
From angels bending near the earth,
To touch their harps of gold;
"Peace on the earth, goodwill to all,
from heaven's gracious King"
The world in solemn stillness lay,
To hear the angels sing."
(Methodist Hymnal 218)
Words by Edmund H. Sears, 1849

In Minnesota, the idea of clear air at midnight on a sub-zero evening is a great setup to think peaceful thoughts. Outside in that setting, the fantastic feeling of quiet, beauty, freshness, and the wonders of the evening seem endless.

Yes, God has created a fantastic place for us.

The following is a comment from a relatively new Minnesotian, "I'm officially embracing winter (though it took a while). Snowshoeing at Murphy in the early morning and breaking paths was great fun, and cross-country skiing this afternoon was awesome…." Winter is a beautiful time of year, and the beauty, stillness, and invigorating atmosphere are a gift for us all. It is easy to sense how the three Wiseman must have felt while following that star many years ago.

Luke put it this way:
"Suddenly a great company of the heavenly host appeared with the angel,
Praising God and saying, "Glory to God in the highest heaven,
and on earth peace to those on whom his favor rests."
(Luke 2 vs. 13, 14)

Thought for Today: We live in a wondrous world; enjoy, appreciate, and protect it.

Prayer for Today: Heavenly Father, we thank you for our worldly blessings, and the bountiful lives have through you. Amen

Grays Bay, Lake Minnetonka
Wayzata, Minnesota

December 20

Universal Hope

"The heavens declare the glory of God;
the skies proclaim the work of his hands.
Day after day, they pour forth speech;
night after night, they display knowledge.
There is no speech or language
where their voice is not heard.
Their voice goes out into all the earth,
their words to the ends of the world."
(Psalm 19 vs 1-4)

The holiday season is a time of hope. We are encouraged to believe there is hope for universal understanding and world peace. The Psalmist notes that there is one clear message from the heavens, one God with one statement in all tongues to all peoples.

We live in a troubled world with natural disasters, civil unrest, war, and COVID persists again this year. They capture the headlines. Indeed, people question God's role in all of this.

We need to remember that "The heavens declare the glory of God; the skies proclaim the work of his hands." The press and news media report on other issues. It is up to each of us to focus on the message. We can infect the world with faith, peace, and hope with our example.

John F. Kennedy said, "One person can make a difference, and every person must try."

Thought for Today: OK, there will be bad news this week. We will hear it, see it, and sometimes feel it. We need to overcome it with the faith and hope of the Lord.

Prayer for the Season: Dear Lord, this is the time of year when all faiths celebrate you. We honor your presence in different ways with the common thread of love and peace. We pray for the guidance to share our faith so we may sow a seed in your name. Amen

Grays Bay, Lake Minnetonka
Wayzata, Minnesota   **December 21**   **Page 371**

In The Bleak Mid-Winter

"In the bleak midwinter,
Frosty wind made moan,
Earth stood hard as iron,
Water like a stone;
The snow had fallen, snow on snow,
In the bleak-midwinter long ago."
(Christina Rossetti, 1872)

Merry Christmas, HoHoHo! Often here in the northland, the weather and the holiday season can make one weary; ice scraping the windshield, brushing off the car after a long day at the office, stuck in traffic on the way home, and then trying to be smiling for the family at dinner. It can be trying, even depressing.

It is a season to be jolly, spiritual, and be with family and friends, and we certainly compound the issue. There are extra events in all areas of our lives; sports tournaments, holiday parties, shopping, gift wrapping, and cooking! Through it all, we recognize the fun and spirit of the season.

There is an entity within our Christian faith that all this activity cannot conquer. That is the Love that is in our hearts. It seems to swell up in magnitude during Christmas. Our energy levels increase, and through all the activity, we can say Merry Christmas and mean it- we have an embedded passion and Love.

And the child grew and became strong;
he was filled with wisdom,
and the grace of God was on him.
(Luke 2 vs. 40)

Thought for Today: Let us feel the wonders of the season- The Love in our hearts for Jesus and those around us. Let us share it with others.

Prayer for Today: Dear Lord and father, today we pray for people who are overstressed by holiday activity. We pray that they may find peace through it all. Amen

December 22

Grays Bay, Lake Minnetonka
Wayzata, Minnesota

There's A Song In The Air

*"There's a song in the air!
There's a star in the sky!
There's a mother's deep prayer
And a baby's low cry!
And the star rains its fire
While the beautiful sing,
For the manger of Bethlehem
cradles a king."*
(1989 Methodist Hymnal #249)
(Josiah G. Holland 1874)

There is a lot of joy around the Christmas season. There are pop songs that create fun played with the spiritual Christmas Carols. Songs of Rudolph, Jingle Bells, White Christmas, Grandma Got Run Over by a Reindeer, and many more usually do not help increase the spirituality but do add to the happiness of the season.

Several years ago, at lunch with a pastor, the restaurant was playing pop Christmas music. He was having a bad day and grabbed onto the music to symbolize his angst. He did not want to hear about Rudolph, Santa, or Grandma. I failed to manipulate the mood to be positive and in the season's spirit. .

Christmas pop music adds to the joy and maybe even brings someone to Church. It allows people to think about what it is about and adds to the season.

*Glory to God in the highest heaven,
and on earth peace to those on whom his favor rests.*
(Luke 2 vs. 14)

Thought for Today: As we wrap up our last-minute preparations for Christmas, let us take a few moments, forget the stresses and enjoy the moment.

Prayer for Today: Heavenly Father, today we approach the celebration of Jesus' birth. It is a wonderful season, and we are blessed. We thank you for the Grace guaranteed us through him. Amen

Hoar Frost
Amesbury, Massachusetts

Joy To The World

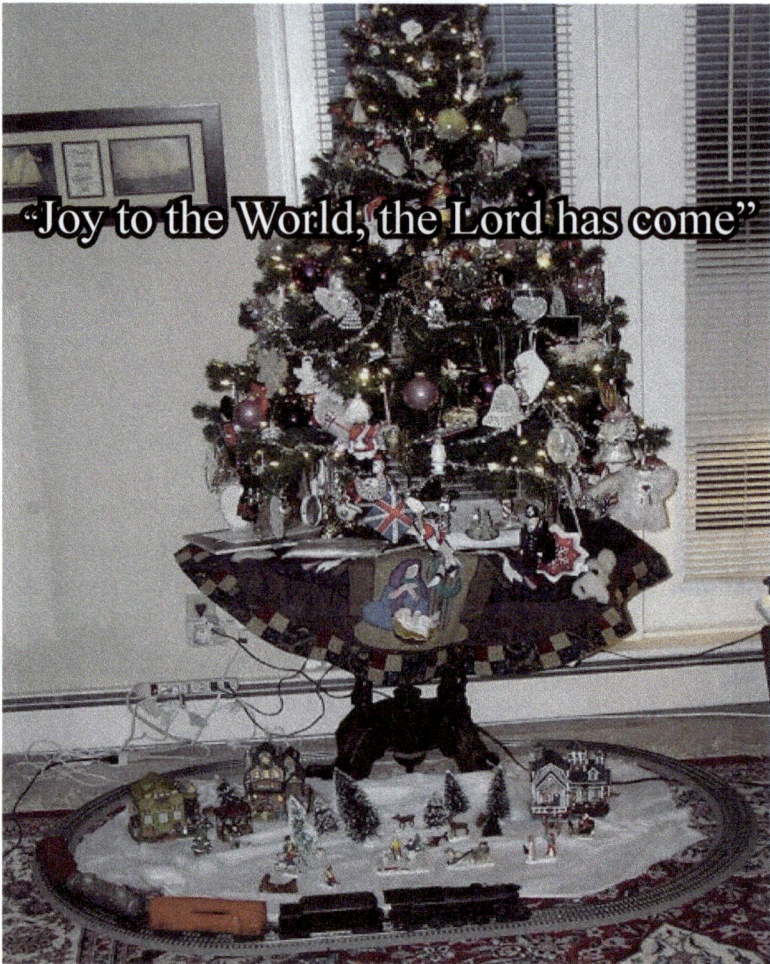

"Joy to the World, the Lord has come"

There are many one-liners in Christmas carols. The opening of "Joy to the World" says it all. It summarizes our Christian lives, lives of joy through the forgiveness of our faith and our Christian peers. Let us all feel the joy of the season, the love for each other, and keep our faith strong throughout the season.

With blessings, have a great Christmas.

December 24   Tree Train
                                              Pickering Family Tree

Rejoice

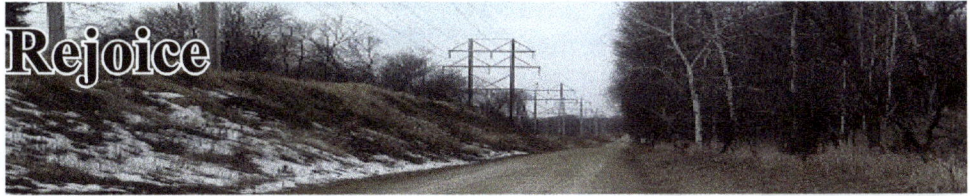

This is the day the Lord has made. Let us rejoice and be glad in it. Christmas is a special day in our faith and our society. The public displays representing our faith, the music, the crowded stores, and special events impact the world, as has Jesus.

June and I lived in a complex over half occupied by Jewish families for several years. In the lobby, there was a Christmas tree alongside a menorah. Several of the Jewish families put up lights and had Christmas trees. One of June's friends, Cheryl, recently invited her to see her first Christmas tree. Religion was not the issue. It was about happiness, sharing joy, and a beautiful tree.

My Jewish friend Bobby has a daughter in college. Every year since she was very young, they set up a tree for Christmas, and Bobby and his wife shared gifts to celebrate Christ's birthday. Bobby also attends bible study and often contributes using his Old Testament knowledge. He and his wife wanted to acknowledge the spirit of the Christian celebration, allowing them to openly discuss the differences that exist in the world.

My family is Unitarian, and view Christ as a great teacher or philosopher. They do not recognize the holy trinity. However, Christmas is undoubtedly the most important day on their Church calendar. They share in our Joy of Christmas.

So they hurried off and found Mary and Joseph,
and the baby, who was lying in the manger."
(Luke 2 vs 16)

Thought for Today: This is the day the Lord has made:
Jesus Christ is born today!
Jesus Christ was born for this!
Jesus Christ was born to save!

Prayer for Today: Dear Lord and Father, we pray that we may follow Jesus' teachings and do your will here on earth on this joyous day. We pray for a world of peace and love. Amen

Let Go

> But he who unites himself with the Lord
> is one with him in spirit.
> (1 Corinthians 6 vs 17)

I have watched hundreds of people take a step to believe a power greater than themselves would restore them to sanity, people that were so down and out that the concept of God was beyond them. That is how someone who is chemically dependent starts their journey to sanity. It is a process of spiritual growth.

Several people I worked with could not grasp the concept, even when God was referred to as a higher power. Those were too afraid to let go of the control. Most of us try to control too much and do not like letting go.

We will experience New Year's Eve in a few nights, and many of us are making resolutions and setting goals. Today, please think about something other than exercise and weight. Think about adopting the slogan "Let go and let God." Make that your New Year's resolution, and you will have a great year.

Thought for Today: Let us think about what we can turn over to God so that we may have a less stressful New Year!

Prayer for Today: Dear Lord, we pray that we may trust in you and allow your control and spirit into our daily lives. Amen

Gifts

> For by the grace given me, I say to every one of you:
> Do not think of yourself more highly than you ought,
> but rather think of yourself with sober judgment,
> In accordance with the measure of faith God has given you.
> Just as each of us has one body with many members,
> And these members do not all have the same function,
> so in Christ, we who are many form one body,
> and each member belongs to all the others.
> We have different gifts,
> according to the grace given us.
> (Romans 12 vs 3-6)

Christmas has passed, and we were all involved in its materialism at some level. The advertising, the gift-giving, and the holiday cards all lead us away from its meaning. It is not about the gifts that were given and received by people.

Earlier this year, we read about the gifts that God gave us. Paul's letter to the Romans has a special meaning. Verse nine of Romaans twelve lists seven of God's gifts. It is essential to understand God's blessings and recognize our gifts. We need to know where we fit in God's world and how to apply His gifts in our lives. These gifts matter- They are not advertised on TV or in the newspaper. They are given to us by Him to use.

Thought for Today: As we approach the New Year, let us think about who we are and what gifts God has given us. Let us learn to use these gifts to make our lives and the lives of others better.

Prayer for Today: Dear Lord, self-improvement always seems to be an objective at this time of the year. Each year I focus on "my improvement" and sometimes do not recognize the tasks you may have set forth for me. I pray that this will be the year that "my improvement" is accomplished by identifying your gifts to me and finding a way to do your work with them. Amen

Lake Bde Maka Ska
Minneapolis, Minnesota

December 27   Page 377

Renewal

but those who hope in the LORD
will renew their strength.
They will soar on wings like eagles;
they will run and not grow weary,
they will walk and not be faint.
(Isaiah 40 vs 31)

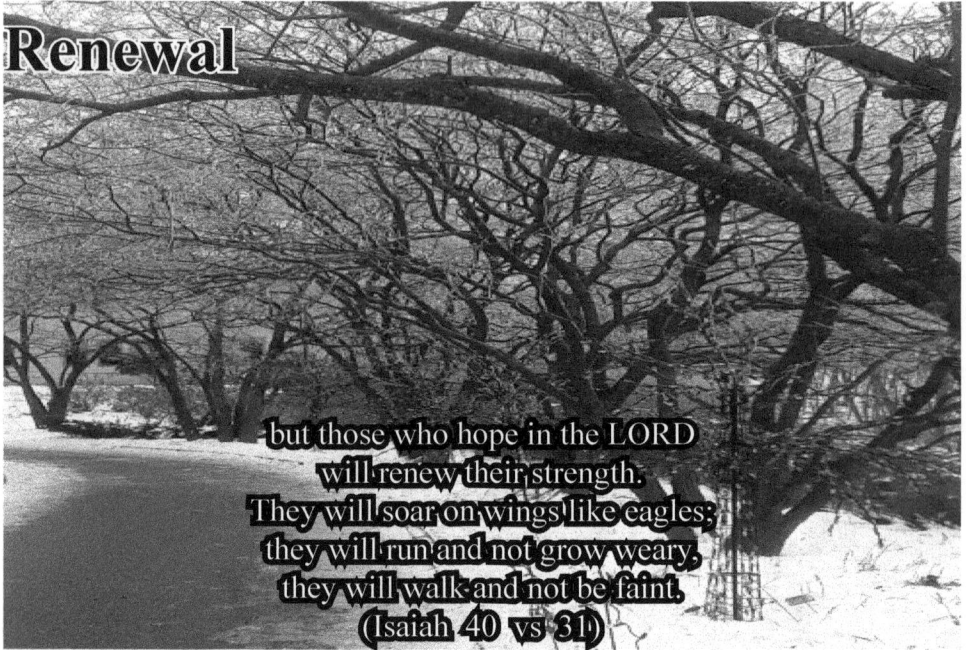

We are in the Holiday recovery mode and are weary. From time to time, it is necessary to take a break. It is vital to prevent burnout and refresh ourselves. We need rest to be the best we can be and do our jobs as parents, employees, and citizens.

Along with resting, we need meditation. Ok, if you are reading this, I am preaching to the choir again. However, many rest and renew their minds and bodies without thinking of renewing their spirit. They forget to pray or recognize the Lord's role in their lives.

Others neglect their bodies. It is easy to overeat during the holidays and skip a workout. That's a double-edged sword that I have been guilty of for years. That's what New Year's resolutions are all about. We will do fine next year. The message from Isaiah above is to keep hope in the Lord, keep him in your life, and he will help you soar like an eagle.

Thought for Today: Let us think about keeping God in the forefront of our minds.
Prayer for Today: Father, we ask that you fill us with your spirit and strength and guidance. Amen

, Lake of the Isles
Minneapolis, Minnesota

Show Off

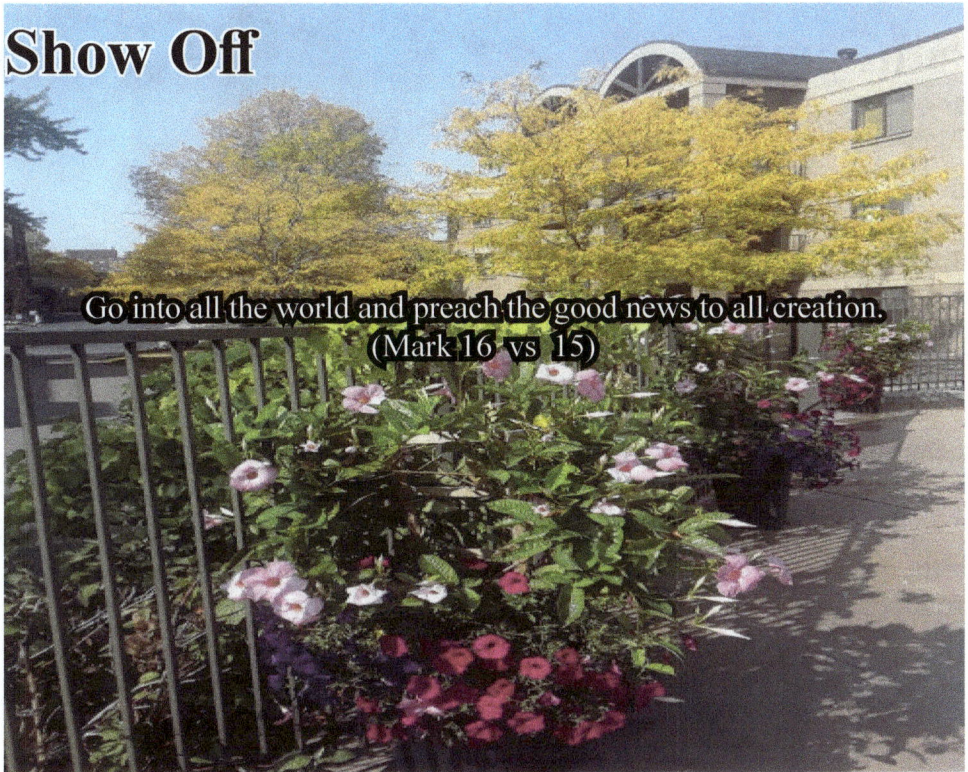

Go into all the world and preach the good news to all creation.
(Mark 16 vs 15)

We are staring New Year's Eve in the face at the end of the year. Resolutions and promises abound, and we have thoughts on improving our lives. I ask, "What will you do next year to improve other people's lives?"

We suggest that you try living a Godly life. Make your choices by asking, "What would Jesus do?" That would be something significant; people would notice. It would be a very loud but subliminal testimony of your faith.

Go out and show it off.

Thought for Today: Let's consider our behavior a subliminal testimony of our goodness and faith. Next year let us demonstrate we are the children of God.

Prayer for Today: Dear Lord, today we pray for our pending New Year. We pray that our Christian behaviors and ethics impress others so they may want to join us. Amen

Pool Side Garden
Avana Minnetonka, Minnesota December 29   Page 379

Sincerity

> Love must be sincere.
> Hate what is evil; cling to what is good.
> Be devoted to one another in brotherly love.
> (Romans 12 vs 9)

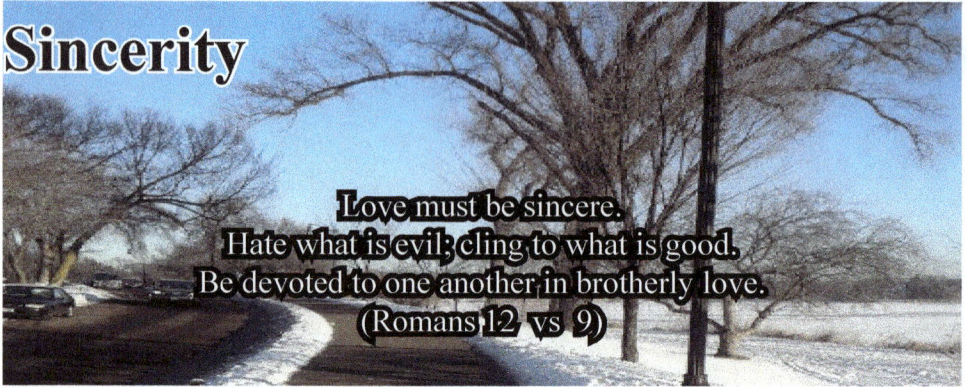

During the Christmas season, we all share material gifts. It is a beautiful time of year. It is a time of love and caring with lots of hugs, kisses, and tears of joy. The love and spirit of Christ are a blessing.

Now we are faced with a New Year and the resolutions that come with it. We tend to go back to the grind of daily life and settle into our routine with very few changes. However, we need to continue to share this love, this zeal, and this joy. When we do, we all benefit and live better lives. Here are two of my favorite quotes worth thinking about for the New Year.

John F. Kennedy: "One person can make a difference, and every person must try."

John Wesley:
> "Do al the good you can,
> by all the means you can,
> in all the ways you can,
> in all the places you can
> at all the times you can,
> to all the people you can,
> as long as ever you can."

Thought for Today: As we proceed toward the New Year, let us focus on ourselves and our talents. Let us recognize that we have unique gifts from the Lord to use for Him.

Prayer for Today: Heavenly Father, we are entering the New Year, and we wonder where it will have in store for us. We pray we can apply our talents and gifts in the New Year to pursue your will. Amen

New Year's Eve

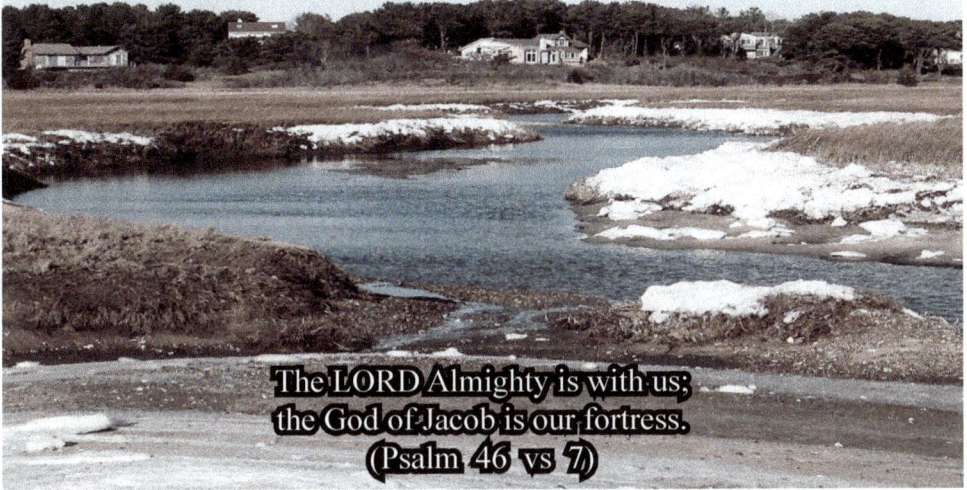

The LORD Almighty is with us;
the God of Jacob is our fortress.
(Psalm 46 vs 7)

Today rather than focusing on a new beginning, let's give thanks for the blessed year that has passed. There are both positive and negative memories, and we may ask why we did some dumb things? Or why something great happened? Whatever the case, the Lord was with us, and we need to be thankful.

Thought for Today: Let us be thankful for last year and prayerful about our future. As we move forward, let's remember two of my favorite themes. Keep healthy in spirit, mind, and body. Also, when in doubt, "Just do it!"

Prayer for Today: Father, we thank you for all our blessings lest year and pray for peace and prosperity throughout the world.

Thank you.
It has been my pleasure to stay in touch
with Christian friends through these
devotions. I invite you to stay in touch
online through these sites.

Facebook: Christian Friends Page
https://www.facebook.com/
groups/1537792806542165

Blog: God Is My Spinach
https://godismyspinach.blogspot.com/

Web Page
https://www.bobpickeringauthor.com/

With Christian love,
Bob

God is *Still* My Spinach

God is *Still* My Spinach

God is *Still* My Spinach

Index Page 3

God is *Still* My Spinach

God is *Still* My Spinach

God is *Still* My Spinach

www.ingramcontent.com/pod-product-compliance
Lightning Source LLC
Chambersburg PA
CBHW060305030426
42336CB00011B/947